BASIC
MEDICAL
LABORATORY
TECHNOLOGY

Basic Medical Laboratory Technology

Editor
CLIVE J C KIRK, *TD, FIMLS*
Senior Chief Medical Laboratory Scientific Officer
Department of Surgery
Charing Cross Hospital Medical School, London

Authors
R NIGEL PEEL, *MB, BS, MRCPath*
Consultant Microbiologist
York District Hospital

KEITH R JAMES, *FIMLS*
Senior Chief Medical Laboratory Scientific Officer
Department of Histopathology
Charing Cross Hospital and Medical School, London

KEITH S LEWIS, *FIMLS, MIBiol, MSc*
Senior Chief Medical Laboratory Scientific Officer
Department of Chemical Pathology
Charing Cross Hospital and Medical School, London

A DOUGLAS WAFT, *FIMLS*
Senior Chief Medical Laboratory Scientific Officer
Department of Haematology
York District Hospital

Second Edition

Pitman

PITMAN BOOKS LIMITED
39 Parker Street, London WC2B 5PB

PITMAN PUBLISHING INC.
1020 Plain Street, Marshfield, Massachusetts

Associated Companies
Pitman Publishing Pty Ltd, Melbourne
Pitman Publishing New Zealand Ltd, Wellington
Copp Clark Pitman, Toronto

First Published 1975
Second Edition 1982

British Library Cataloguing in Publication Data
Basic medical laboratory technology. – 2nd ed.
  1. Medicine – Laboratory manuals
  I. Kirk, Clive J. C.
  610′.2   R852

  ISBN 0-272-79630-1

Text set in 9/11 pt Linotron Times, printed and bound
in Great Britain at The Pitman Press, Bath

Contents

Preface to second edition   ix

Preface to first edition   xi

Acknowledgements   xi

PART 1—GENERAL TECHNIQUES

1   Professional Conduct, Health and Safety   3
Code of behaviour – Staff health and immunisation – Safety – Reception of specimens – Posting of specimens – Disposal of specimens and cultures – First Aid

2   Glass and Plastic Laboratory Ware   10
Glass – Apparatus – Cleaning glassware – Plastics

3   Pure Water, Solutions and Storage of Chemicals   18
Distilled and deionised water – Solutions – Storage of chemicals

4   General Equipment   25
Balances – Centrifuges – pH Meters – Gas cylinders – Water-baths

5   Spectrophotometry   32
The Beer-Lambert Laws – Instrumentation – Sources of error in colorimetry

6   The Microscope   38
Illumination – Lenses – Specimen stage – Focusing – Setting up the microscope

PART 2—MICROBIOLOGY

7   Introduction to Microbiology   43
Bacterial cultivation – Inoculation – Anaerobic culture

8   Examination of Specimens   49
Apparatus – Blood – Cerebrospinal fluid – Urine – Other specimens

9   Preparations for Microscopy   61
Preparations – Staining

10   Identification of Common Bacteria of Medical Importance   66
Introduction – Gram-positive cocci – Gram-negative cocci – Aerobic gram-positive bacilli – Anaerobic gram-positive bacilli – Mycobacteria – Pseudomonas and Alcaligenes – Enterobacteria – Small gram-negative bacilli – Gram-negative anaerobic bacteria – Spirochaetes – Vibrios – Spirilla

11   Fungi   108
Yeasts – Yeast-like fungi – Filamentous fungi

12   Parasitology   114

13   Culture Media and Biochemical Tests   118
Constituents – Liquid media – Blood culture media – Solid media – Biochemical tests – Diluents – Control of culture media

14   Serology   139

15   Counting bacteria   142
Total counts – Viable counts

16   Laboratory Tests of Therapeutic Antimicrobial Agents   146
Sensitivity – Sensitivity tests – Assay techniques

17   Laboratory Aspects of Sterilisation and Disinfection   155
Physical methods – Chemical methods

18   Introduction to Experimental Animals   165
Introduction – Techniques – Guinea-pigs – Mice

PART 3—HISTOLOGY AND CYTOLOGY

19   General Outline of Procedures in a Routine Histopathology Department   173
Reception – Trimming and block selection – Processing – Embedding – Cutting and staining – Reporting and filing

20   Fixation   175
General routine fixing mixtures – Special fixing mixtures

21   Decalcification   179
Acids – Chelating agents – Proprietary fluids – Ion-exchange resins – Electrolytic decalcification – Testing for decalcification – Surface decalcification

22 Processing 181
Paraffin wax method – Celloidin or Low-viscosity Nitrocellulose method

23 Microtomes and Microtome Knives 187
Microtomes – Microtome knives – Knife sharpening

24 Microtomy 191
Paraffin wax-embedded material – Celloidin or LVN-embedded material

25 Section Staining and Mounting 194
Paraffin wax sections – Celloidin and LVN sections

26 Frozen Sections 205
Section cutting – Section staining – Staining methods

27 Cytology 209
Specimen collection and preparation – Fixation – Mounting – Staining methods

PART 4—HAEMATOLOGY

28 Introduction to Haematology 217
The nature of blood – Haemopoiesis – Anticoagulants – Collection of blood – Quality control – Documentation

29 The Blood Count 223
Haemoglobin – Estimation of haemoglobin – Visual methods of counting cells

30 The Blood Film 228
Preparation of blood films – Staining – Erythrocytes – Leucocytes – Platelets – Observation of the film – Reticulocyte counts – Bone-marrow biopsy – Supplementary staining methods

31 Packed-Cell Volume and Absolute Values 238
Packed-cell volume – Absolute values

32 Haemostasis 240
Platelet function – The vessel wall – The coagulation factors – The coagulation process – Fibrinolytic system – Investigation of disordered haemostasis

33 Automation in Haematology 246
The electrical resistance method – The electro-optical method – Automatic differential counters – Coagulometers – Aggregometers

34 Further Considerations of Haemoglobin 251
Haemoglobins A, A_2 and F – Haemoglobins S and C – Methaemoglobin, sulphaemoglobin and carboxyhaemoglobin

35 Miscellaneous Investigations 255
Haemolytic disorders – Systemic lupus erythematosus – Erythrocyte sedimentation rate – Infectious mononucleosis

PART 5—BLOOD GROUP SEROLOGY

36 Introduction to Blood Group Serology 263
Antigens and antibodies – Demonstration of antigen–antibody reactions – The inheritance of blood groups – The ABO blood group system – ABO grouping methods – Selection and preparation of ABO grouping sera – The Rh blood group system – Selection and preparation of Rh grouping sera – Other blood group systems

37 Blood Transfusion Techniques 275
Compatibility tests – Preparation of anti-human globulin reagent – Low-ionic-strength saline (LISS) – Investigation of a transfusion reaction – Haemolytic disease of the newborn (HDNB) – Automation in blood group serology – Quality control in blood serology

38 Blood Bank Procedures 283
The blood donor – Storage of blood – Blood products – Blood bank organisation

PART 6—CLINICAL CHEMISTRY

39 Quality Control in Clinical Chemistry 295
Pre-analytical quality control – Analytical quality control – Post-analytical quality control

40 Tests of Carbohydrate Metabolism 302
Glucose – Reducing substances in urine – Chromatography – Ketone bodies

41 Electrolytes 309
Sodium and Potassium – Calcium – Chloride – Bicarbonate

42 Kidney Function Tests 315
Urea – Urine examination – Detection and measurement of protein in urine – Urinary acidification tests – Specific gravity of urine

43 Tests of Liver Function 320
Excretion of bile – Tests of bile pigment metabolism – The plasma proteins

44 Chemical Tests for Diseases of the Alimentary Tract 327
Measurement of gastric acidity – Blood in faeces – Malabsorption

45 Miscellaneous Tests 331
Commercial urine tests – Cerebrospinal fluid

46 Enzymes 334
Factors affecting enzyme analysis – Methods of measurement – Units of enzyme activity – Serum alkaline phosphatase – Estimation of trypsin in duodenal contents – Amylase – Ultraviolet spectrophotometric methods of enzyme analysis – Lactate dehydrogenase – Isoenzymes – Enzymes as reagents

47 Automation in Clinical Chemistry 343
Continuous-flow systems – Small dedicated analysers – Centrifugal analysers – Reaction rate analysers – Multiple discrete analysers

Index 355

Preface to the Second Edition

Since the publication of the first edition changes have been made in the educational schemes for medical laboratory scientists in the United Kingdom. From the point of view of this book the most important of these changes has been the replacement of the Ordinary National Certificate by the Technician Education Council's Certificate in Science. However the body of technical knowledge required of medical laboratory scientists at this stage in their careers remains essentially the same, with due regard of course to the advances made since the publication of the first edition.

Another aspect of laboratory work that has seen considerable changes in recent years is safety. The introduction of the Health and Safety at Work Act, and the publication of the Howie Report, along with numerous other reports and items of legislation, have brought about a far greater awareness of factors affecting safety. This edition has attempted to highlight the more important safety precautions necessary in the somewhat hazardous environment of the medical laboratory. However it is not possible to cover all such precautions and the reader is reminded that no procedure should be attempted without due regard to its possible health and safety implications.

With these changes in mind, what was written in the Preface to the first edition concerning the aims of this book remains true for this edition.

In the first edition we thanked a number of people for their assistance. This assistance has proved to be of value either directly or indirectly in this edition and we would like to reiterate our gratefulness. In addition our gratitude is due to the following for their helpful advice and criticism of the sections indicated: Mr. D. Freer (Microbiology), Mrs. J. Gauntlet (Cytology), Mr. R. Hall (Haematology), Mr. N. Harling (Experimental Animals) and Mr. M. Pepper (Blood Group Serology); also to Mrs. C. Hiscoke, Miss A. Matcham and Miss E. Simpson for their able secretarial help.

C.J.C.K.

Preface to the First Edition

This book has been written primarily for the technician studying for the Ordinary National Certificate in Medical Laboratory Sciences but it is hoped that it will prove of value to all newcomers to Pathology Laboratories. It is intended to provide a working knowledge of the basic range of techniques in each of the major branches of Pathology.

The authors felt the need for a book that would provide instruction in those practical aspects of laboratory work that form part of the student's inservice training and that would augment the instruction in theory which is available at Technical Colleges. It is therefore essentially a practical book, although some theory has been included where required for the intelligent use of the methods described.

The methods recommended have all been proven in routine use as also have any commercial products mentioned. No claim is made that others may not be just as useful.

The authors wish to thank the following people: Miss M. Kenwright, Mr. L. C. Wilson and Mr. K. S. Lewis for their helpful criticisms of the Haematology, Microbiology and Clinical Chemistry sections respectively, Miss J. Willoughby for the effort and ability necessary to produce the line drawings, and Mrs. L. Thomas and Mrs. S. Paxton for their painstaking secretarial assistance. Professor A. J. Harding Rains has given us much help, encouragement, and the benefit of his considerable experience as an author and editor. Mr. Stephen Neal of Pitman Medical has brought us through the long gestation period to the birth of this book as painlessly as is possible. Our families also deserve our grateful thanks for tolerating the upheaval that seems inseparable from authorship. Naturally any mistakes remaining are our own.

C.J.C.K.; R.N.P.; K.R.J.; Y.K.

Acknowledgements

The authors acknowledge with thanks the following for permission to reproduce the illustrations referred to:

Mr. R. Barnett *Fig. 22.1*
Corning Ltd. *Figs. 41.3* and *47.11*
Coulter Electronics Ltd. *Fig. 33.1*
Griener Electronics Ltd. *Fig. 47.15*
Miss M. Hudson *Fig. 40.4*
Jencons (Scientific) Ltd. *Fig. 2.2*
E. Leitz (Instruments) Ltd. *Figs. 6.1, 23.1* and *23.2*
Medical Illustration, York District Hospital *Fig. 38.1*

Pye Unicam Ltd. *Figs. 5.1* and *5.2*
SLEE Medical Equipment Ltd. *Figs. 26.1* and *26.2*
Sartorius Instruments Ltd. *Figs. 4.1, 4.2* and *4.3*
Technicon Instruments Ltd. *Figs. 33.2, 33.3* and *47.2* to *47.9*
Union Carbide (UK) Ltd. *Fig. 47.14*

For permission to quote the Code of Conduct we are grateful to the Registrar, Council for Professions Supplementary to Medicine.

PART ONE

General techniques

1. Professional conduct, health and safety

CODE OF BEHAVIOUR

Medical laboratory science is a profession supplementary to medicine and a high standard of ethics is required of those who practise this profession. In the United Kingdom the Professions Supplementary to Medicine Act of 1960 requires the Disciplinary Committee of the Medical Laboratory Technicians Board, in consultation with its Board and with the Council for Professions Supplementary to Medicine, to prepare a statement as to the kind of conduct which the Committee considers to be infamous conduct in a professional respect, and to send it to every registered practitioner of the profession. This statement is as follows:

No registered medical laboratory scientific officer should:

1. Hold himself out as a person who, by training and experience, is professionally qualified to diagnose or treat disease in man or animal.

2. Knowingly accept, obtain, assist in obtaining or report on any specimen for the purpose of the diagnosis and/or treatment of disease, or make any investigation for those purposes unless the diagnosis and/or treatment are to be performed by a registered medical, dental, or veterinary practitioner.

Unless there is specific evidence to the contrary, it is considered that a medical laboratory scientific officer who has carefully followed procedures which have been approved by local health managements for requesting laboratory tests will not be considered to be in breach of this requirement. Even in those cases where there is specific evidence, the Disciplinary Committee of the Board may take into account special circumstances, such as emergencies, which may enable them to consider that a breach of this rule should not make the registrant guilty of infamous conduct in a professional respect.

3. Knowingly disclose to any patient or to any other unauthorised person the result of any investigations or any other information of a personal or confidential nature gained in the course of practice of his profession. Unless there is specific evidence to the contrary it is considered that a medical laboratory scientific officer who has carefully followed procedures which excep-

tionally have been approved by local health managements for reporting results to patients (or in the case of children, their parents or guardians) will not be considered to be in breach of this requirement.

4. Advertise, whether directly or indirectly, or associate himself in any way with advertisement for the purpose of obtaining specimens for laboratory investigations.

5. Knowingly falsify or suppress a report of any laboratory investigation with which he may be concerned.

STAFF HEALTH AND IMMUNISATION

Before persons are employed in a pathology laboratory in the United Kingdom the employing authority will insist on a medical examination to see if they are fit. This will include a chest X-ray examination and this will be repeated every 3 years, except for staff who handle known or suspected tuberculous material, where it will be carried out annually. Prospective employees will also be given a skin test for tuberculosis, e.g. Mantoux or Heaf test, which if negative will be followed by inoculation with BCG (Bacille Calmette Guérin) since they must not handle tuberculous material until they have a positive reaction. All staff will also be tested for presence of hepatitis B surface antigen for their record, and females of child-bearing age for the presence of rubella (German measles) virus antibodies. If a high enough titre of rubella antibodies to suggest immunity is not found she will be offered the rubella vaccine. Pregnant women will not usually work with the rubella virus, cytomegalovirus or *Toxoplasma gondii* because of the risks of intrauterine infection.

It is clear that staff in pathology laboratories are at risk from a number of infective agents by the nature of their work. In addition to good working practices and proper conditions, protection from some infectious diseases can be achieved by artificial active immunisation. It is recommended that each member of the laboratory staff should be offered such protective inoculations (see Table 1.1) as are considered to be necessary by the medical staff of the laboratory or the local occupational health service unless there are individual contraindications. This will necessitate liaison with the general medical practitioner of each person and a knowledge of previous immunisations and other medical history. Employing authorities should make some immunisation procedures a condition of employment, such as BCG in those who are tuberculin-negative. Until recently it was advised that smallpox vaccination should be repeated every 3 years but now that Africa has been declared free of smallpox by WHO the advice is likely to be changed for laboratories not known to keep or handle this dangerous virus. Sometimes passive immunisation with gamma-globulins may be used, such as following an accident where a member

Table 1.1. Examples of diseases for which protective immunisation is available

Anthrax	Plagus	Tetanus	Paratyphoid fevers
Cholera	Poliomyelitis	Tuberculosis	Typhus
Diphtheria	Rubella	Typhoid	

of staff has been accidentally inoculated with material containing a pathogen-like hepatitis virus. In this case, if it is virus B, a hyperimmune serum containing anti-virus B antibodies or gamma-globulin will be given.

SAFETY

Medical laboratories are potentially hazardous working environments and this has been increasingly recognised in recent years. Consequently several relevant Acts of Parliament and Codes of Practice have been promulgated in the United Kingdom. Foremost among these are the 'Health and Safety at Work [etc.] Act 1974' and the 'Code of Practice for Prevention of Infection in Clinical Laboratories and Post Mortem Rooms 1978', commonly known as the Howie Report after the Chairman of the committee which produced the code. In addition several books, papers and circulars have been published and a short safety bibliography is appended to this chapter.

In general terms safety can be viewed in the light of common sense, specialist knowledge and statutory requirements. Most of the dangers encountered in clinical laboratories stem from infectious material, chemicals, ionising radiations, fire, faulty apparatus and careless behaviour. The safety information given in this chapter is by no means complete; that would be impossible. However this chapter includes some general safety considerations and elsewhere in this book mention is made of hazards associated with particular techniques.

Two points should always be borne in mind. Firstly it is the duty of all members of the laboratory staff to co-operate in the prevention of accidents. Secondly some hazards seem more applicable to one laboratory discipline than another; this can lead to complacency.

All laboratory personnel automatically have a responsibility for their own safety as well as that of other workers. Ultimate responsibility for safety is shared between employer and employee.

Safety officers

In the United Kingdom the Health and Safety at Work Act requires the appointment of Safety Officers and the formation of Safety Committees. The Safety Officer will be a senior member of staff and will have specific responsibilities aimed at ensuring a safe environment and safe techniques. The advice of the Safety Officer should be sought before any new technique is introduced into the laboratory, after any accident or if any potential danger is identified.

The duties of the Safety Officer will also include keeping written records of all accidents, ensuring that new staff are adequately instructed on safety matters, periodic safety 'auditing' of methods and equipment and advice on the safe handling and disposal of hazardous materials and spillage.

Infection

The hazards of working with live germs in a microbiology laboratory are well recognised. There is an obvious danger from direct contact with cultures of pathogenic organisms, but the greatest danger is from breathing aerosols produced by careless handling of infected material. All materials sent to pathology laboratories are potentially infectious with the possible exception of tissues in histological fixative. Specimens sent for chemical or haematological examinations are just as likely to contain pathogens as specimens sent to the microbiology laboratory.

In the United Kingdom the 'Code of Practice for the Prevention of Infection in Clinical Laboratories and Post Mortem Rooms 1978' describes the way in which infective materials should be handled. The code divides micro-organisms, viruses and materials into four groups denoting their relative hazard levels and the minimum standard for handling them. A brief resumé of some aspects of the code of practice follows. However the code will be available in all UK laboratories and should be studied by all members of staff. For those readers outside the UK the code can still be used as a guide to good laboratory practice in conjunction with any relevant local codes or legislation.

Classification of micro-organisms, viruses, and materials

The most hazardous organisms are viruses in Category A which includes rabies, smallpox and haemorrhagic fever viruses. Fortunately these viruses are not normally encountered in routine clinical laboratories and as only a limited number of specially approved centres are allowed to work on them further discussion of them would be out of place in this book.

Category B1 contains organisms, viruses and materials that present special hazards to laboratory workers and therefore require special containment precautions. Included in B1 are *Mycobacterium tuberculosis* and *Salmonella typhi*, which are not infrequently isolated in clinical microbiology laboratories in the UK. In addition materials and reagents containing hepatitis B viruses that are deliberately introduced into the laboratory as test materials and controls are included in this category.

Category B2 is mainly concerned with specimens known to be hepatitis B surface antigen (HB_sAg)-positive or those specimens coming from 'at-risk' patients who have not been screened and shown to be HB_sAg-negative. The at-risk groups include patients suffering from infective or suspected infective diseases of the liver, those in renal units and drug addicts.

Category C covers those organisms, viruses and materials not covered in the above groups which, provided that high standards of microbiological technique are maintained, do not present any special hazard to laboratory workers.

Laboratory accommodation for Category B1

Special accommodation, as described in the code, must be provided for work on Category B1 material. Naturally the organisms in this group may be isolated unexpectedly during normal laboratory work. When this occurs all the materials, cultures, etc., must be transferred to the special accommodation before any further work is carried out.

Work on materials that are tuberculous or might contain mycobacteria, the testing of sera for the presence of HB_sAg and on other organisms on the B1 list must be performed in a separate room which should not be used simultaneously for handling Category C items.

In addition to facilities normally associated with a microbiology laboratory the room must have at least a Class 1 exhaust protective cabinet and sufficient deep-freeze, and storage space so that all Category B1 specimens, materials and reagents are kept exclusively in the room.

Adequate security must be maintained by restricting admission to authorised personnel and locking the door when the room is not in use.

The door must have a glass panel so that the occupants of the room can be seen from the outside. The door, refrigerators, incubators and all equipment containing B1 items must be labelled 'Danger of Infection' with the international 'Biohazard' symbol (*see* Fig. 1.1).

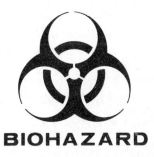

Fig. 1.1. The International biohazard sign (red on yellow ground).

Aerosols

As is stated above infective droplets are probably the major source of laboratory infection and some droplets are formed whenever a fluid surface is broken. The smaller droplets evaporate at once to form nuclei of dried airborne material which can travel some distance in the area and which, if inhaled, may reach the alveoli of the lung. Aerosols may persist in the air for some time. Careful technique can reduce the droplet formation but they are formed in many procedures, some of which are detailed in Table 1.2 together with specific ways to reduce the aerosol risk. As many of these procedures as possible should be done in an exhaust protective cabinet and always if there is a likelihood of material being infected with particularly dangerous organisms such as tubercle bacillus. After accidents in which there has been an aerosol produced, it is recommended that the windows should be opened and that the room be evacuated for 10 minutes before clearing up and disinfection.

If the skin becomes contaminated it should be washed immediately and contaminated clothing should be removed and autoclaved or disinfected. If the accident involves the breakage of a glass vessel containing infective material the area must at once be covered by cloths soaked in a phenolic disinfectant. After at least 10 minutes the broken glass is picked up, using a pan and brush, and discarded into an infected waste container along with the cloths. The pan and brush should then be autoclaved or disinfected for 24 hours. All such accidents must be reported to the safety officer or a senior member of staff.

Personal hygiene

The individual laboratory worker can do a great deal to ensure his or her own safety and the safety of others by following a few simple rules of hygiene. These include:

1. Never eat, drink, smoke or apply cosmetics in a laboratory. Food and drink must not be taken into or stored in laboratories.

2. Always wear the appropriate protective clothing.

3. Hand-washing and the removal of protective clothing before leaving the laboratory will help to prevent the spread of laboratory hazards.

4. Remove immediately any chemical or biological contamination from clothes or skin.

5. Avoid such activities as nail-biting, pencil-chewing, sitting on benches and licking gummed labels.

6. Report all accidents however trivial they may seem.

Protective clothing

The simple white coat with buttons down the front has traditionally been the standard, and often only, form of protective clothing issued to laboratory workers. For many purposes it remains adequate so long as it fits properly and is buttoned up. However more advanced designs are now available and these are to be recommended especially in environments where infective material is handled. The new design of coat includes a wrap-over double-front, fastened at the side with press studs, a high neck, long sleeves and close-fitting waist bands. Coats should be changed at least twice a week, and immediately if contaminated or thought to be contaminated.

An impervious wrap-around plastic or rubber apron reaching from ankle to chest should be worn whenever HB_sAg-positive plasma is being handled. In addition plastic over-shoes or rubber boots should be worn under these conditions.

Disposable gloves must be used for handling Category B1 and B2 materials and are recommended at any time when the hands could become contaminated (e.g. with blood) or when there are cuts or abrasions on the hands. Heat-resistant gloves should be available in the laboratory for handling hot apparatus and standard household rubber gloves are useful for such tasks as washing up.

Goggles or face visors should always be used where there is a danger of splashing of chemicals or other potential eye hazards such as when cutting glass.

Table 1.2.   *Common causes of aerosol production and methods of prevention*

Cause	Prevention
Pipetting (Pasteur)	Discharge the pipette slowly; forceful ejection of contents is usually inaccurate and causes aerosol formation
Centrifuging	Use sealed centrifuge buckets (*see* Chapter 4)
Decanting supernatants	Pipette whenever possible; pouring produces aerosols and usually contaminates the outside of containers
Opening screw-top bottles	Open carefully; avoid if possible filling or tipping to prevent the contents getting into the thread or cap
Opening snap-off caps or plug stoppers	Use screw-tops whenever possible
Bacteriological loops	Short loops cause less spraying than long ones. Use micro-incinerators for flaming rather than open burners. Use disposable swabs for viscous material (e.g. sputum)
Use of discard jars	Place items into disinfectant carefully, submerge completely, change disinfectant daily
Accidents	Keep benches tidy, do not hoard infective material unnecessarily, work carefully and methodically. CONCENTRATE

Suitable protective clothing properly fastened must be worn at all times in the laboratory and removed before leaving.

Biological safety cabinets, laminar flow cabinets and fume cupboards

All laboratories must be provided with cabinets and fume cupboards, of an approved design and standard, appropriate to the nature of the investigations carried out. These installations should be regularly inspected to ensure that they are functioning to the required specification of their type. If there is any doubt as to the suitability of the cabinet for a particular function the safety officer or a senior member of staff should be consulted.

There should be a minimum of equipment and material in the cabinet when in use and gas burners should not be used in biological safety or laminar flow cabinets. If it is necessary to flame loops a micro-incinerator should be used, but disposable plastic loops are often suitable.

To disinfect the cabinet 25 ml of formalin should be boiled away on an electric heater with the front closed down. The cabinet is then left overnight before opening the front and turning on the fan to vent the remainder of the formaldehyde.

It should be noted that exhaust protective cabinets are not the same as fume cupboards found in chemistry laboratories. Fume cupboards are designed to remove toxic or unpleasant vapours and to provide a measure of protection in certain chemical procedures, and should only be used for these purposes.

Chemical hazards

Chemicals may be hazardous in one or more of many different ways. The potentially hazardous properties of chemicals are dealt with under storage in Chapter 3. The same considerations must be borne in mind when using these chemicals.

Mouth pipetting is always potentially dangerous and some form of safety pipette *must* be used instead (*see* Chapter 2). Procedures involving boiling solvents, toxic gases and vapours must be carried out in an efficient fume cupboard such as that described by the British Standards specification.

Equipment including rubber gloves, goggles, rubber boots, a respirator, dust pan and brush, mop and sand should be available for dealing with spillage of noxious chemicals. The procedure to be adopted will depend upon the nature of the spilt chemicals and should be directed by a senior member of the staff. To help prevent spillage bottles and other containers should be carried with both hands, with one hand underneath giving support. Larger bottles, particularly those containing dangerous chemicals, should be transported in carriers.

Carcinogens are chemicals capable of provoking uncontrolled neoplastic change in tissues—in simple terms, cancer production. These chemicals are avoided as far as possible in the laboratory. Like infection, exposure can occur from inhalation, through the skin, and by ingestion. The risk involved depends mainly upon the length and frequency of exposure and the concentration of the carcinogen, but it is possible for even quite small exposures to be potentially hazardous. Junior laboratory staff should not, in general, be expected to use these substances.

Organic solvents are toxic and can be absorbed through the skin as well as being inhaled or ingested. Recent evidence suggests that they may cross the placental barrier and harm the developing fetus. Care should be taken to minimise the exposure to these solvents by adequate ventilation and protective clothing.

Fire

Fire is one of the most serious and most likely hazards to occur in a laboratory. All laboratory staff should know where the fire extinguishers are and how to use them, the rules concerning the fire-alarm system, and action to be taken in the event of a fire and the location of the fire exits. The most generally useful fire extinguisher in the laboratory is the carbon-dioxide cylinder which can be safely used with most chemicals and electrical equipment, and is clean. Dry powder extinguishers are also useful and may be more effective with some types of fire but are messy in use. Carbon tetrachloride, and water-based extinguishers such as the foam extinguisher, can be dangerous in laboratories and should be avoided. Glass-fibre blankets are useful for smothering small fires and clothing which is burning. These should be placed near at hand in the laboratory for instant use. Only the absolute minimum of flammable solvents should be kept in the laboratory. Serious laboratory fires have been started by ignition of flammable liquids by sparking contacts in electrical apparatus, and for this reason such liquids if necessary should be stored in spark-proof refrigerators. Laboratories, corridors and fire exits should also be kept clean, tidy and free of rubbish. This will help prevent the outbreak or spread of fire. Rooms containing special hazards (e.g. gas cylinders, radioactive substances and large quantities of inflammable liquids) should be suitably labelled on the outside as a warning to the fire service.

Electrical hazards

It is possible to receive a fatal shock from as little as 60 V under adverse conditions. Mains-operated apparatus must be safely constructed with correctly connected earthing points and switches in the live wires. All electrical apparatus must be kept clean and dry, and must be regularly serviced by a competent electrician. Faulty apparatus must be labelled as such and withdrawn from service until properly repaired and checked.

RECEPTION OF SPECIMENS

There should be a separate room available for the reception of specimens to which access is restricted to authorised staff. Specimens should be delivered to the room through a hatch or across a fixed counter. Staff must be instructed in the way to deal with specimens and be aware of the risks involved such as contracting viral hepatitis from live viruses in blood on the outside of a leaking container.

Hypochlorite (e.g. 10% chloros) freshly prepared daily must be available to mop up any splashes or spillage, and pipettes must be completely submerged in hypochlorite (e.g. 2.5% chloros) overnight before being discarded.

Specimens known to be, or likely to come, within category B1 or B2 referred to above must be clearly labelled 'Danger of Infection' at all stages and special care must be taken. This will include the use of disposable gloves, visors and sealed centrifuge buckets.

Broken or leaking containers should be discarded in the normal way for infective materials and the sender should be informed of the loss and another specimen requested. The information on the soiled request form may be copied on to a fresh form (and the old one discarded) if the writing is still legible. If not, a copy from the sender is needed.

Specimens must be clearly labelled with the patient's name and the date as a minimum. Unlabelled and inadequately labelled specimens without proper request forms should not be accepted. Request forms must contain enough information for patient identification. The name alone is not enough since laboratory files contain records of thousands of patients, some of whom will have the same name. The patient's name; age or date of birth, if possible; hospital number and address, ward or department should be clearly written, as should the date, the name of the medical practitioner making the request, the nature of the specimen and the investigation required. In addition, it is always helpful to have some relevant clinical details to assist in deciding if further tests should be applied, and to help in assessing the result. The large variety of request forms in use suggests than an ideal form has not yet been devised, but they nearly all provide space for the above essential information.

POSTING OF SPECIMENS

Any of the smaller containers for pathological specimens selected for use from the large number on the market must be suitable for transmission through the post. The regulations which apply to the posting of specimens are to be found in the *Post Office Guide* under the heading 'Pathological specimens, Deleterious liquids or substances, Articles sent for medical examination or analysis'. The regulations are designed to protect the staff of the Post Office from infection. They may be summarised as follows. Specimens should be sent by first-class letter post and never by parcel post. The specimens must be enclosed in sealed containers which themselves must be placed in cases approved by the Post Office, and they must be padded with a quantity of some absorbent material such as cotton wool to prevent possible leakage from the package in the event of damage to the receptacle. The package must be marked 'Fragile with Care' and have the words 'Pathological Specimens' on it. Failure to comply with these regulations leaves the sender liable for prosecution. Receptacles supplied by laboratories should be submitted to the Postal Headquarters, Operations and Overseas Department, St. Martin's le Grand, London, EC1A 1HQ, in order to ascertain whether they are regarded as complying with the regulations. The Post Office totally prohibits Category A pathogens from carriage by the postal services.

Air mail

The Universal Postal Union has revised the regulations for the carriage of hazardous goods by air both on inland and overseas routes. In this respect hazardous goods are defined as 'any material which contains a viable microorganism or its toxin which causes or may cause human disease'.

In summary these regulations allow for the despatch of such material by authorised senders only. Packages of infectious goods must be specially labelled, packed in accordance with the recommendations of the World Health Organisation, and be accompanied by two copies of a special certificate provided by the sender for the Post Office to give the airline.

DISPOSAL OF SPECIMENS AND CULTURES

All infectious and potentially infectious materials must be rendered safe before disposal. Flasks, bottles, test tubes and other media-containing vessels must be autoclaved before being sent for wash-up. Cultures, slides, swabs and many specimens can be autoclaved; others can be incinerated. Plastic Petri dishes and tubes must be autoclaved separately before disposal or incinerated in a specially designed incinerator. Fluids and urines are treated with an equal volume of hypochlorite or phenolic disinfectant. Pasteur pipettes, microscope slides and other glass items thought to be infected should be discarded in discard jars containing hypochlorite or phenolic disinfectant which should be prepared fresh daily. Such items must also be autoclaved before disposal. Disposable syringe needles must be discarded into a rigid container immediately after use until they can be incinerated.

There must be an identification system, for example colour-coded containers, for different types of waste. If accidents are to be avoided, particularly to domestic staff, this system must be strictly adhered to.

FIRST AID

There are two prerequisites for effective first aid, suitable equipment and training.

The laboratory should be equipped with a first aid box and certain additional items necessary to counteract specific laboratory hazards. The tendency in some hospital laboratories is to rely on the close proximity and ready accessibility of the Accident and Emergency Department; this is by no means sufficient as immediate and effective first aid can often have a crucial bearing on the outcome of any accident. The first aid box should contain as a minimum the following items:

(a) sufficient numbers (say 12 of each) of small, medium and large unmedicated sterile dressings;

(b) an assortment of adhesive wound dressings;

(c) six triangular bandages;

(d) a supply of absorbent sterile cotton wool in $\frac{1}{2}$ oz. packets;

(e) safety pins;

(f) sterile eyepads;

(g) a roll of 1 in wide adhesive plaster.

In addition many laboratories keep an eye-irrigation bottle filled with water. There is a risk of infection from such bottles and it is usually preferable to use running water from a tap in the event of splashing a chemical into the eye. The first aid box should be well labelled, in an easily accessible place and the contents well maintained.

It is recommended that all members of the laboratory staff receive first aid training as not only will this be invaluable in case of a laboratory accident but the trained first aider can often be a considerable asset at home and elsewhere. The British Red Cross Society, St. Johns and St. Andrews Ambulance Associations and similar organisations in other countries organise suitable courses.

BIBLIOGRAPHY

1. *Code of Practice for the Prevention of Infection in Clinical Laboratories and Post-Mortem Rooms.* HMSO (1978).
2. Muir, G. D. (ed.) (1976). *Hazards in the Chemical Laboratory.* Royal Institute of Chemistry.
3. *Handbook of Laboratory Safety* (CRC Press Inc., 1971).
4. Collins, C. H. (compiler) (1976, 1977). *Safety in Pathology Laboratories* (bibliographies). Institute of Medical Laboratory Science.

2. Glass and plastic laboratory ware

GLASS

The modern laboratory worker is fortunate in two ways with respect to the glassware he uses. First, most laboratory glassware, especially that used in analytical work is much more resistant to thermal shock and chemical attack than was the case some years ago. Secondly, the graduations marked by the manufacturers are reliable within very close limits.

Borosilicate glass is now almost exclusively used for apparatus that will be heated, contain a chemical reaction or be used for measuring volumes. This glass consists of about 80% silica and 13% boric oxide with the oxides of sodium, aluminium and other metals. It is more resistant to thermal shock than ordinary soda glass but should not be abused to the extent of, for example, heating beakers containing liquid in a flame without the protection of a gauze, or of plunging hot glass into cold water. Glass is said to be as strong as its surface so that any surface flaws, such as scratches or cracks, will tend to weaken a piece of glassware and for this reason it is advisable to check for flaws before use. Such surface flaws also make adequate cleaning more difficult.

The reliability of graduation marks is ensured by Standards Institutes in various countries. In Great Britain, the British Standards Institution has published specifications for various types of glassware which very closely define the limits of tolerance and various other criteria to be followed in the manufacture of the items described. Some of these British Standards (BS) will be referred to below. Most British Standards for volumetric glassware correspond to the requirements of the International Organisation for Standardisation (ISO).

Generally, volumetric glassware is calibrated for use at 20°C.* Whilst most laboratories are kept at higher temperatures than this the error introduced is within the limits of tolerance for the item concerned. There are two classes, A and B, the first of which is the more accurate. There are also two basic ways in which volumetric glassware is calibrated: one is to *contain* a

* 27°C for use in tropical countries.

volume, these items are marked 'IN'; the other is to *deliver* and is denoted by 'EX'.

APPARATUS

Pipettes

Pipetting must not be done by mouth. There are various devices obtainable to fill and empty conventional pipettes. The pipette fillers include rubber bulbs, glass sleeves over the ends of specially designed pipettes that act in a similar way to a syringe, and various valve-operated designs. The valve-operated types are in general the most convenient to use, and since they allow the introduction of air the pipette can be emptied in the correct way.

Only the most commonly used pipettes are described below, there are, of course, many other designs of pipettes available for special purposes.

1. One-mark pipettes. Also referred to as volumetric or transfer pipettes (Fig. 2.1*a*). These pipettes are governed by BS 1583. The capacity is defined as the volume of water at 20°C delivered by the pipette when used in the prescribed manner, which is first to rinse it with the fluid to be used, then to fill it just beyond the graduation mark. The meniscus is then carefully adjusted to the mark (at eye level) and the outside of the pipette is wiped with a clean tissue. Holding the pipette vertically the contents are allowed to run out, then the tip of the pipette is touched against the inside of the receiver after the meniscus has come to rest. No attempt must be made to increase the speed of delivery or to expel the small amount of fluid remaining after draining. Class A pipettes, used for the most accurate work, are marked with both the delivery time and the drainage time. Since the tip plays a major part in the accurate delivery of the calibrated volume, any pipette with a chipped or broken tip should be discarded. Faults at the other end of the pipette that make control difficult can be cured by filing a notch with an ampoule file, carefully breaking off the end and polishing by heating in a flame. Care should be taken, however, to

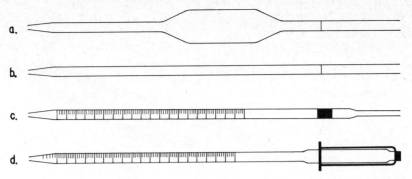

Fig. 2.1. Pipettes
(a) One-mark, bulb pipette (volumetric or transfer); (b) as (a) but without bulb (some smaller one-mark pipettes are made to this pattern); (c) graduated type 1 pipette; (d) graduated type 2 pipette with safety filler.

ensure that an adequate length of tube remains above the graduation mark.

2. Capillary pipettes. BS 1428 recognises four types of capillary pipette used for smaller volumes than those referred to above. Type 1 is graduated for delivery, and is therefore used in the same way as the one-mark pipettes. Types 2, 3 and 4 are calibrated for content, Type 2 being fully graduated, Type 3 having only one graduation mark and Type 4 having two. These types require washing out; the contents are blown out into the diluent, the diluent is drawn up to the graduation mark and blown out to wash out the remainder of the contents. This washing procedure should be repeated at least three times. A further type of graduated capillary pipette is the 'blow out' pipette which, as the name implies, does not require rinsing. This type has a number of useful applications particularly in serology.

3. Graduated pipettes (see Fig. 2.1). There are three types of graduated pipette recognised by BS 700. Type 1 consists of pipettes calibrated for delivery from zero down to any graduation line, Type 2 pipettes are graduated for delivery from any graduation line down to the jet. Type 3 is calibrated to contain a given capacity from the jet up to the graduation line corresponding to that capacity; it is used in the same way as a Type 2 capillary pipette. Type 2 graduated pipettes are used in the same way as the one-mark pipettes referred to above. For greatest accuracy the delivery should always be made down to the jet. Type 1 is filled in the same way, the contents are allowed to run down to the required graduation mark, the flow is then stopped and the tip lightly touched against the edge of the flask to remove the drop that will have collected on the outside

during delivery. For greatest accuracy each delivery should start at zero. 'Blow out' graduated pipettes are also available; they are not covered by BS 700 and are not recommended for the most accurate work, but are useful for some less exacting procedures.

4. Pasteur pipettes. These are uncalibrated pipettes that can easily be made in the laboratory or obtained commercially; they can also be made to deliver a set number of drops per ml. Full details of manufacture are given on page 50. Plastic pasteur pipettes manufactured with an integral teat can be obtained, and these are ideal for the transfer of biological fluids.

To prevent the formation of aerosols and to ensure complete delivery of the liquid being transferred by a Pasteur pipette the teat should be compressed slowly and carefully and released in the same way.

5. Disposable-tip pipettes. A number of pipetting systems have been designed using disposable plastic tips. They are controlled by a plunger, and the liquid being pipetted is separated from the plunger by an air gap. They are quicker to use than conventional pipettes. Fixed- or variable-volume patterns are available. The adjustable types can be quite easily and accurately set to the required value. The calibration can be checked by weighing the amount of water obtained by a convenient number of deliveries or, particularly for larger settings, by filling a volumetric flask and checking that the meniscus is on the graduation mark after the correct number of deliveries. Fig. 2.2 shows an adjustable pipette which also incorporates a tip ejection device which is advisable when biological specimens are being pipetted to prevent soiling of the operator's hand.

There is some variation in the mode of action of

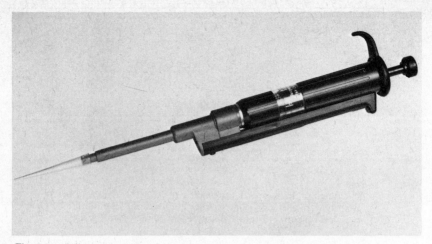

Fig. 2.2. Adjustable disposable-tip pipette with tip ejector (Finnpipette, Jencons).

disposable-tip pipettes, however many of them (including the type illustrated in Fig. 2.2) feature a plunger having a two-step depression sequence. This enables them to be used in one of two ways (*see* Fig. 2.3).

(a) Forward mode. This method is suitable for use with aqueous solutions.

(i) Put a clean tip onto the pipette.

(ii) Depress plunger to first step.

(iii) Immerse tip 2–3 mm below surface of solution and allow plunger to return, under control, to its starting position.

(iv) Remove tip from solution.

(v) Place end of tip against side of receiving vessel and depress plunger steadily through both steps.

(vi) Remove pipette from vessel and allow plunger to return to starting position under control.

(vii) Discard tip.

(b) Reverse mode. This method should be used for viscous samples, for example plasma.

(i) Put a clean tip onto the pipette.

(ii) Depress plunger through both steps.

(iii) Immerse tip 2–3 mm below surface of solution and allow plunger to return, under control, to its starting position.

(iv) Remove tip from solution.

(v) Place end of tip against side of receiving vessel and depress plunger to first step. Pause briefly.

(vi) Keeping the plunger in this position remove the pipette from the vessel.

(vii) Remove tip and allow plunger to return to starting position.

(viii) Discard tip.

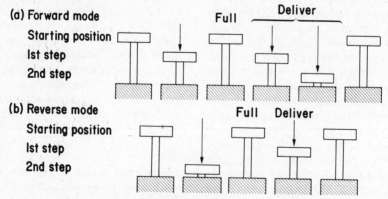

Fig. 2.3. Method of using disposable-tip pipettes in the forward and reverse modes.

Dispensers

For the repeated dispensing of a fixed volume of solution one of the forced-jet dispenser devices can be used. After setting, their accuracy and reproducibility is usually good. They normally depend on a syringe mechanism, although the plunger may or may not be in contact with the fluid. Some types have a fixed reservoir, others use a flexible side-arm that is dipped into the liquid to be used. Most refill automatically after each delivery but some require refilling after a few deliveries. Manual and electrically operated types are available.

The advantages of using these dispensers include speed of operation, reproducibility and safety. The disadvantages differ depending upon the design. Some types are not good at handling acids or alkalis. If the filling stroke is spring-operated the dispenser will usually be found to be useless for volatile solvents.

Graduated (measuring) cylinders

Graduated cylinders can have spouts or be stoppered. Since the surface area of the column of liquid is much greater than in a comparable-sized volumetric flask, cylinders are not accurate. They should not be used in making solutions where even a moderate degree of accuracy is required. It should also be noted that cylinders are graduated to *contain* a set volume and should not therefore be used to *deliver* that volume.

Volumetric flasks

Volumetric flasks are governed by BS 1792. The one illustrated in Fig. 2.4 is graduated to contain 500 cm^3 at 20°C and is of grade A. (The tolerance for this flask is therefore $\pm 0.25 \text{ cm}^3$ compared with $\pm 0.5 \text{ cm}^3$ for class B.) Details of the use of these flasks can be found on page 20.

Conical (Erlenmeyer) flasks

These are useful when making solutions, particularly when boiling is required. The sloping sides tend to decrease evaporation as the vapour condenses on them and runs back down to the solution.

Filter (Buchner) flasks

These are similar to conical flasks but have a side arm which can be attached to a vacuum pump (*see* Fig. 2.4). A Buchner funnel has a sintered glass platform; details of filtration through sintered glass can be found on page 160. Alternatively, the funnel can have a wide-mesh platform used for supporting a filter paper.

Filter funnels

The ordinary conical filter funnel can have plain or fluted sides. The fluted variety is recommended as the flow rates obtained tend to be higher.

Separating funnels

Separating funnels may be spherical, conical or cylindrical, of which the last are sometimes more useful as they can often be used with a roller mixer. Separating funnels are used in extraction procedures and to separate immiscible liquids. When mixing the contents during an extraction procedure, the pressure that builds up should be released occasionally by inverting the funnel and slowly opening the tap. When the pressure has been released close the tap and continue mixing. After extraction is complete clamp the funnel in a vertical position and allow the fluids to separate. Remove the stopper and drain off the lower liquid. Separating funnels may be obtained with PTFE stopcocks; these are recommended.

Care should be taken to avoid the formation of emulsions when using a separating funnel; gentle inversions will be found preferable to shaking. Fig. 2.4 shows a cylindrical model separating funnel.

Thermometers

There are a great number of types of thermometer designed for particular purposes over various temperature ranges. Mercury-filled thermometers calibrated in degrees Celsius (centigrade) will suffice for most laboratory purposes. Thermometers are calibrated to give the correct temperature either when totally immersed or alternatively when immersed over a given part of their length; this should be borne in mind for accurate temperature measurement. A useful type is the stirring thermometer which is thick-walled and, as its name implies, robust enough to be used as a stirring

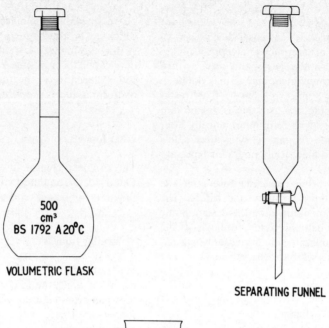

VOLUMETRIC FLASK

500
cm³
BS 1792 A 20°C

SEPARATING FUNNEL

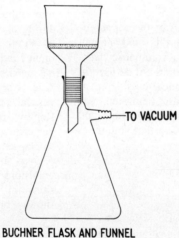

TO VACUUM

BUCHNER FLASK AND FUNNEL

Fig. 2.4.

rod. Occasionally the mercury column becomes divided. If this occurs, it can usually be cured by reducing the temperature until all the mercury is collected in the reservoir at the bottom of the thermometer. When the thermometer warms up it will be found that the mercury column has been rejoined. If mercury becomes trapped in the expansion chamber at the top of the thermometer the column can be rejoined by heating. This will force the gas past the trapped mercury until it is again in contact with the column.

Filter (Venturi) pumps

Fig. 2.5 shows a glass Venturi pump. The pump is connected to a tap, the water goes through the inlet and rushes through the constriction, drawing air in at the side-arm, before going to waste. The side-arm is attached to a trap bottle. If the water pressure falls there is a danger that water will be drawn back into the vessel being evacuated, unless a trap bottle has been fitted. Some pumps incorporate a non-return valve.

Venturi pumps are available in glass, metal and plastic. Depending of course upon the water pressure available, an ultimate vacuum of about 15 torr is possible with this type of pump.

Desiccators

Glass desiccators may be of vacuum or non-vacuum (Scheiber) type. The non-vacuum type can be used to maintain a dry atmosphere in which chemicals that have been previously dried can be stored. The vacuum type can be used to dry solids. Fig. 2.6 is a diagram of a vacuum desiccator. The desiccant (*see* Table 2.1) goes on the bottom of the desiccator and the chemicals to be dried are placed in beakers or evaporating dishes on the metal (usually zinc) gauze floor. The rims of the base and lid are greased and the lid is slid into place to form

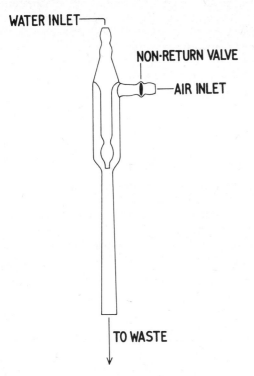

WATER INLET

NON-RETURN VALVE

AIR INLET

TO WASTE

Fig. 2.5. Filter pump.

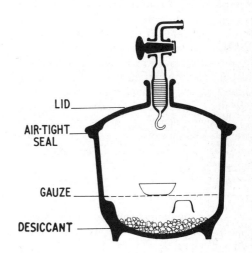

LID

AIR-TIGHT SEAL

GAUZE

DESICCANT

Fig. 2.6. Vacuum desiccator.

Table 2.1.   *Three commonly used desiccants in order of efficiency*

Desiccant	Advantages	Disadvantages	Other remarks
1. Phosphorus pentoxide	Very powerful.	Dangerous, reacts violently with water, causes burns.	Use only if strictly necessary. Discard when crust forms on surface.
2. Silica gel	Reusable, safe, incorporates an indicator.		Normally blue changing to pink when wet. Heat in oven to reuse.
3. Anhydrous calcium chloride	Cheap, safe.	Inefficient.	Satisfactory for storage of dried chemicals.

an air-tight seal. (Some desiccators have an inlaid rubber ring to form the seal and these do not require greasing.) When the lid is on, the desiccator is connected to a vacuum pump and evacuated. When sufficient vacuum has been obtained the tap is closed *before* disconnecting the pump. For most purposes the vacuum produced by a Venturi pump connected to the normal water supply is sufficient. In order to remove the lid the vacuum must be released. The tap should be opened slowly to prevent a sudden rush of air that might blow the chemicals from their containers.

CLEANING GLASSWARE

General laboratory glassware

The definition of 'clean' will depend upon the use to which the glassware is to be put. For general laboratory purposes glassware can be considered to be clean if an unbroken film remains after the item has been filled with distilled water and then emptied.

In recent years several detergents have become available. These have made the use of strong acid solutions (e.g. chrome-sulphuric) unnecessary since the detergents are at least as efficient as acid, safer and often cheaper. Ideally the detergent should be biodegradable and phosphate-free. Special low-foam detergents are available for use in automatic glassware washing machines.

For general laboratory cleaning the following routine will be found to be adequate.

(i) Gross contamination should be removed (after sterilisation if necessary) by vigorous rinsing with brushing if required.

(ii) The glassware should then be soaked in an aqueous solution of detergent. Overnight soaking, whilst not usually necessary, is often convenient.

(iii) After soaking the glassware is brushed if necessary, thoroughly rinsed in distilled water and dried, open end down, in a hot-air oven.

(iv) After inspection for damage the clean glassware should be stored in closed cupboards to prevent dust accumulating on it.

The following factors should also be considered when cleaning glassware. Do not allow dirty glassware to dry as this makes cleaning more difficult, and when soaking make sure that the item is completely submerged without trapping air bubbles, as a rim of dried-on detergent is often as difficult to remove as any other contamination. The manufacturer's recommended concentration

should be used; there is no advantage to be gained by exceeding the figure given. Although soaking in hot detergent is a rapid way of removing dirt a cold soak is sometimes preferable especially when dealing with biological deposits. A violent reaction can occur between strong oxidising agents (e.g. perchloric acid, strong nitric acid, etc.) and surfactants.

The quality of the results produced by a laboratory will be greatly influenced by the cleanliness of the apparatus used.

Finally, the majority of washing up in laboratories is done by unskilled staff. It is the responsibility of the trained laboratory staff to ensure that these unskilled people are protected from infection, the dangers of broken glass and dangerous chemicals and reactions, by adequately pretreating soiled glassware where necessary.

Cleaning pipettes

Pipettes may be cleaned as follows:

1. Soak overnight in cleaning solution.
2. Rinse in tap water.
3. Attach to water vacuum pump and wash through with distilled water.
4. Dry by drawing up acetone and air, alternately, ending with air, until completely dry.

Alternatively, large numbers of pipettes can be washed in a specially designed washer, several types of which are available. The pipettes are placed (with their tips uppermost to avoid damage) in the basket provided with the system in use and soaked as before in the

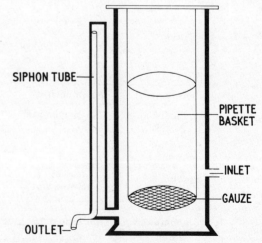

Fig. 2.7.　Diagram of pipette washer.

cleaning solution. After soaking, the basket is transferred to the washer, a diagram of which can be seen in Fig. 2.7. The washer alternately fills then empties by siphoning and the pipettes are rinsed. The loaded basket is then immersed several times in each of two tanks of distilled water. The pipettes can then be dried. This method is excellent for larger pipettes but less satisfactory for capillary pipettes.

PLASTICS

Most of the apparatus described in this chapter, as well as many other items of laboratory equipment, can now be manufactured in plastic. Table 2.2 gives an indication of the uses of some of the most frequently used plastics.

Table 2.2

Usual name	Typical laboratory applications	Comments
PTFE (polytetrafluoroethylene)	Stopcocks, stoppers, connectors, rigid precision tubing.	Almost completely inert. Autoclavable.
Polythene	(i) Conventional: bottles, jugs, tubing. (ii) Rigid: funnels, test-tube racks.	Very widely used in many forms.
Polypropylene	Test-tubes, staining jars, flasks.	More heat-resistant than others in this list except PTFE.
Polystyrene	(i) Conventional: boxes, storage racks for refrigerators. (ii) Expanded: packing material, light test-tube racks.	
PVC (polyvinyl chloride)	Flexible tubing, trays and dishes, instrument covers.	Versatile, can be clear or coloured, flexible or rigid.

3. Pure water, solutions and storage of chemicals

DISTILLED AND DEIONISED WATER

The vast majority of aqueous solutions required in the laboratory are made with some form of purified water. There are two ways of preparing such water, distillation and deionisation.

Distillation of water

Most readers will no doubt be familiar with the principle of boiling water, collecting the vapour and condensing it to produce pure water. This principle, with some refinements, is used in laboratory stills. There are many different designs of still available. A good electrically heated still should include the following features:

1. *Splash guard*. This is a device which prevents untreated water splashing over into the distillate.
2. *Safety cut-outs*. These switch off the power in the event of failure or reduction of water supply. Some stills also have a cut-out device that turns off the power when the collecting vessel is full. Stills without adequate safety cut-outs should not be left unattended.
3. *Ease of cleaning*. Stills, particularly in hard water areas, require frequent cleaning. They should therefore be easily dismantled and should be fixed in an accessible position. Many wall-mounted models are placed in such a position as to make their cleaning a gymnastic feat; this should be avoided!

The rate of production varies with the power of the elements and should be chosen with reference to the needs of the laboratory.

Testing distilled water

Distilled water should be clear, colourless, odourless and tasteless. There are a number of chemical tests that can be employed to determine its quality. These include:

(a) Test for chlorides. Add a few drops of 10% silver nitrate to a little of the water under test. No cloudiness should be visible.

(b) Test for sulphates. As above, using 10% barium chloride. Again no precipitate should be observed.

Cleaning stills

Stills should be frequently cleaned as the scale that collects reduces the efficiency of the heaters. The simplest method is to turn off the still, isolate it from the water supply and the collection vessel, and fill it with acid. A strong solution of acetic acid is convenient, the actual concentration being unimportant. After the scale is dissolved the still should be flushed out with tap water. After restarting the still the distillate should be run to waste for a while and then tested before collection begins.

Deionised water

Tap water is deionised by passing it through anion- and cation-exchange resins. These resins can be in separate columns or in a mixed bed. The cation-exchange resin contains exchangeable hydrogen ions. Cations such as magnesium and calcium present in the water are removed by the resin and replaced by hydrogen ions. Similarly the anion resin releases hydroxyl ions and removes such anions as bicarbonate and sulphate.

The resins will gradually become exhausted and after a time require regeneration. This can be done by passing hydrochloric acid through the cation resin, and sodium hydroxide through the anion resin and rinsing well with water. Some manufacturers give instructions for this procedure, other do their own regeneration and exchange resin cartridges on a one-for-one basis.

By passing distilled water through a deionisation column water of a very high degree of purity can be obtained equivalent for most uses to doubly distilled water. This process is more convenient in practice than the process of double distillation, and in addition has the advantage that the deionisation resins need less frequent regeneration than when they are used with tap water. Water of this degree of purity is sometimes required, as for example in some enzyme estimations, but is not necessary for most laboratory procedures.

Testing deionised water

Most deionisers incorporate a conductivity meter. Pure water has a very high resistance, and measuring this is a convenient method of monitoring the quality of the water produced. The purity required will depend upon the use to which the water is to be put, but in general a resistance of greater than about 1·5–2·0 MΩ per ml is suitable.

Storage of distilled and deionised water

Purified water should be stored in borosilicate glass or plastic containers. These containers should be kept stoppered to prevent contamination by fumes or dust.

CO_2-free water

For some purposes distilled water free of carbon dioxide is required. This is simply obtained by boiling distilled water. The water should then be bottled in a screw-cap bottle whilst still warm. Alternatively, the CO_2-free water may be stored under a CO_2 trap containing soda lime.

SOLUTIONS

Types of solution

Throughout this book references are made to a number of different types of solution. Definitions of these are given below.

1. Molar (M)

A molar solution is one containing one mole or gram-molecular weight of the solute in 1 litre of solution. Note that it is 1 litre of solution, not 1 litre of solvent. The term *molal* is used for a solution containing 1 mole in 1000 grams of solvent.

2. Normal (N)

A normal solution contains the gram-equivalent weight of solute in 1 litre of solution. The equivalent weight of a substance may be defined as the number of parts by weight which will combine with or displace 1 part by weight of hydrogen or 8 parts by weight of oxygen, or will react with that weight of an element which itself will react with these weights of hydrogen or oxygen. It should be noted that the equivalent weight of a substance can vary depending upon the reaction in which it

is involved. The use of 'normality' for chemical calculations is not favoured at present but is included here as the term will still be met occasionally. The term 'normal saline' should not be used for 'physiological saline' referred to below.

3. Isotonic

Isotonic solutions are those that exert equal osmotic pressures. The term isotonic when used in medical science usually means that the solution exerts the same osmotic pressure as blood serum. 'Isotonic' or 'physiological' saline is 8·5 g NaCl in 1 litre of aqueous solution.

4. Aqueous

Aqueous solutions are, of course, those using water as solvent. Where no solvent has been specified it can be assumed to be water.

5. Percentage solutions

Percentage solutions of solid solutes refer to grams per 100 ml of solution, percentage mixtures of liquids refer to ml of one to 100 ml of mixture. (E.g. 70% ethanol is 70 parts of ethanol plus 30 parts of water.)

6. Weight/volume and volume/volume

The abbreviations w/v and v/v are sometimes added after the strength of a solution. Thus trichloroacetic acid 10% w/v is a solution containing 10 g of trichloroacetic acid per 100 ml of solution, and 70% ethanol v/v is a solution containing 70 ml of ethanol per 100 ml of solution.

7. Buffer solutions

Buffers are solutions that *tend* to resist change in pH on the addition of *small* quantities of acid or alkali. Many buffer solutions are mixtures of either a weak acid and one of its salts or a weak base and one of its salts. Commonly used buffer systems include:

   (a) Acetate: Acetic acid + sodium acetate
   (b) Phosphate: Potassium dihydrogen orthophosphate (KH_2PO_4) + disodium hydrogen orthophosphate (Na_2HPO_4)
   (c) Barbitone (Veronal): Sodium diethyl barbiturate + HCl

(d) Citrate: Citric acid + sodium citrate

(e) Tris: Tris-(hydroxymethyl)-aminomethane + HCl.

Sources of error in preparation of solutions

The preparation of accurate solutions is of great importance in all laboratory work. Most analytical methods require at least one standard solution upon the accuracy of which depends the reliability of the results. Sources of error in the preparation of solutions are:

1. Impure chemicals.
2. Inaccurate weighing.
3. Inaccurate apparatus.
4. Inadequate technique.

1. Impure chemicals. Much reliance may be placed on 'analytical reagent' grade chemicals from reputable manufacturers meeting the stated specifications. It should be remembered, however, that no chemical is 100% pure although generally the impurities are present in quantities that do not affect most analyses. Great care should be taken to avoid contaminating stocks of chemicals. This contamination most frequently occurs when returning excess material to the container, and for this reason any excess analytical grade chemical removed from its container must not be replaced.

2. Inaccurate weighing. The balance, if used correctly, is capable of greater accuracy than any of the other techniques employed to prepare solutions. Do not waste this potential with poor technique. Comments on the use of balances may be found on page 25. The commonest inaccuracy in weighing is due to simple arithmetical error; it is advisable to write down all weights used and to check the arithmetic before proceeding.

3. Inaccurate apparatus. Glassware conforming to recognised standards (*see* Chapter 2) will be found to be satisfactory provided it is not damaged. Analytical balances should be periodically inspected and maintained by specialists.

4. Inadequate technique. Most errors will be due to inadequate techniques. Particular care should be taken in reading calibration marks on volumetric apparatus and in ensuring complete solution of solids and adequate mixing.

Preparation of a solution

What follows is an outline of the preparation of a standard solution; some variations will be necessary depending upon the substances involved and the type of solution required.

If the solid to be weighed is not a powder or small, readily soluble crystals it should first be ground in a clean, dry mortar. The powder is then transferred, using a spatula, to a pre-weighed (or tared, *see* p. 26) weighing boat or watch glass until the required weight is obtained. Filter paper should not be used in place of a weighing boat. The weighing boat should be handled with forceps; neither the chemical being weighed nor the weighing boat should be touched by the fingers. It is worth remembering that the molecular weight of a substance is usually printed on the manufacturer's label. The substance is then washed from the weighing boat into a beaker using a little of the solvent. Ensure that the volume of solvent used does not exceed the total volume of solution required, a common mistake! The substance is then dissolved by stirring and gentle heat if required. Normally the substance should not be transferred directly from the weighing boat to the volumetric flask, unless it is known to be very readily soluble in the amount of solvent to be used, as volumetric flasks should not be heated and are not convenient if the solution has to be stirred.

When all the solid has been dissolved and the solution has cooled it can then be transferred with care to the volumetric flask. The beaker, and any stirring rod used, should be washed with solvent at least three times and these washings added to the flask. The flask should then be made up to the graduation mark with solvent. Remember that the bottom of the meniscus must be on the line and it should be viewed at eye level. The flask is then stoppered and the solution mixed. The flask should be inverted and swirled at least six times, swirling or shaking alone is not sufficient.

The solution can now be bottled; it is a good idea to rinse the bottle with a little of the solution which is then discarded before the remainder is poured in. Finally the bottle is labelled.

Standardisation of solutions

After making a solution it may be necessary to standardise it against some other known solution. This may be done in one of several ways including spectrophotometry and titration. The technique of titration is less frequently used in medical laboratories than was once the case; however it is an extremely important technique and should be mastered. The description of this technique would be out of place in this book, but reference should be made to one of the standard textbooks on analytical chemistry.

Dilutions

1. Doubling dilutions

This technique is frequently used in clinical laboratories, particularly in serological methods. The technique described can, of course, be used for any volumes (*see* Fig. 3.1).

An equal volume of solvent is placed in each of a row of dilution tubes. The same volume of the solution to be diluted is added to the first tube containing solvent and mixed. This gives a dilution of 1 in 2. The same volume of this dilution is then transferred to the next tube and mixed to give a dilution of 1 in 4. This process is then repeated for each tube giving 1 in 8, 1 in 16, 1 in 32 and so on as far as required.

2. Diluting from one strength to another

A simple rule to remember when diluting from one strength to another is as follows. If x is the strength of the given solution and y is the required strength, take y parts of the given solution and make up to x parts with solvent. For example, a 6% aqueous solution may be obtained from a 20% solution by taking 6 ml of the 20% solution and making up to 20 ml with water.

If a definite volume of dilution is required use the formula:

$$\frac{yV}{x} = V_x$$

where V = volume required, V_x = volume of solution of concentration x to be diluted and y = concentration required.

Example. Given a 30% solution, prepare 500 ml of a 9% solution.

Substituting in the formula above

$$\frac{9 \times 500}{30} = V_x = 150$$

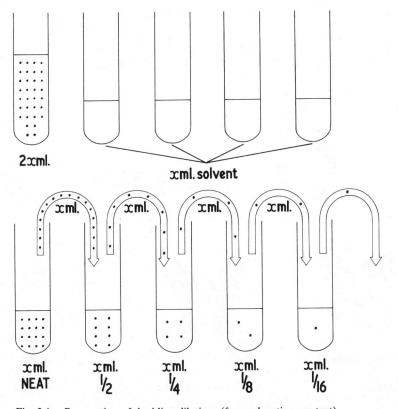

2$x$ml.

$x$ml. solvent

$x$ml. $x$ml. $x$ml. $x$ml.

$x$ml.	$x$ml.	$x$ml.	$x$ml.	$x$ml.
NEAT	½	¼	⅛	¹⁄₁₆

Fig. 3.1.   Preparation of doubling dilutions (for explanation see text).

Therefore take 150 ml of the 30% solution and dilute to 500 ml.

STORAGE OF CHEMICALS

1. Store rooms and cupboards

Store rooms containing bulk stocks of chemicals should be well ventilated and lit, and designed to reduce the risk of fire either breaking out or, having done so, spreading to other parts of the building. Fire-fighting equipment should be available just outside the room. Store rooms and cupboards should be locked to prevent unauthorised access. Bulk stores of flammable liquids should preferably be kept in a fire-proof and secure store away from buildings. Chemicals subject to Customs and Excise control, and radioactive substances, will require proper supervision as provided for in the relevant legislation. Stocks of substances included in the first schedule to the rules made under Section 23 of the Pharmacy and Poisons Act 1933 must be locked away in a separate cupboard and the key held by a senior member of staff.

2. Labelling

Any solution or chemical prepared in the laboratory must be labelled to show the nature and strength of the contents; the date prepared, particularly if the substance has a limited shelf-life; and any safety warnings applicable. Commercially prepared chemicals are normally well labelled as to content, purity, molecular weights and other data. In addition the label provides information on any potentially hazardous properties. The Council of Europe has recommended a number of warning signs and these are being increasingly used by manufacturers within the EEC. The signs, which are illustrated in Fig. 3.2, are printed in black on a bright orange or yellow background.

3. Storage

Before any chemical is stored consideration must be given to any warning information available, possible fire hazards, legal requirements (e.g. Dangerous Drugs Act), possible reactions with other substances, quantity involved and the duration of the shelf-life. A list of properties with the necessary precautions associated with them is given below. The first seven of these properties are those covered by the signs shown in Fig. 3.2.

Flammable. Such substances should be stored away from flames and combustible material, preferably in a special store. On commercially prepared substances details of the flashpoint will be given.

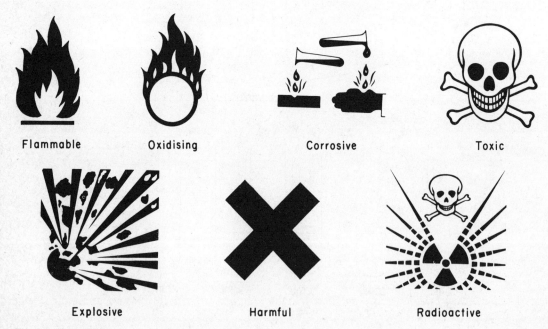

Flammable   Oxidising   Corrosive   Toxic

Explosive   Harmful   Radioactive

Fig. 3.2   Chemical hazard warning signs.

Oxidising. This is applied to those substances which give rise to exothermic reactions on contact with organic matter or other easily oxidised chemicals. It follows therefore that these types of substances should be stored well away from each other.

Corrosive. Defined as substances that can destroy living tissue; suitable precautions must therefore be taken to prevent such interaction.

Toxic. Poisonous substances. It should be remembered that the danger can be from inhalation of fumes, vapour or dust as well as from swallowing. Such substances must be stored in a safe place to prevent unauthorised access.

Explosive. Those substances liable to explode when dry or subjected to shock, friction or heat need special storage precautions relevant to the risk involved with each individual substance. Only a few such substances will be met with in clinical laboratories, for example picric acid, and mostly these are safe if kept moistened with water.

Harmful. Substances labelled harmful are those that can cause minor illness by being swallowed or by other types of contact.

Radioactive. The storage of radioactive substances is controlled by law. Normally a suitably qualified custodian is appointed and given the responsibility of controlling the storage and use of such material within an institution. Details of the requirements in the United Kingdom can be found in 'Code of Practice for the Protection of Persons against Ionising Radiations arising from Medical and Dental Use' and in the accompanying 'Guidance Notes'. These HMSO publications should be available in all laboratories using radioactive substances.

Volatile. Such substances should be kept cool and well stoppered.

Photosensitive. Substances that undergo change when subjected to light should be stored in dark glass or a cupboard.

Deliquescent, hygroscopic and efflorescent. Substances having one of these properties must be kept in well-stoppered containers.

A few further points should be borne in mind when considering the storage of chemicals. Always read the label before storing; in addition to the properties given above there may be some special requirements, as for

Table 3.1

Chemical	Special considerations
Chloroform	Avoid fumes. Toxic carbonyl chloride is formed on exposure to light.
Ethanol	Ethanol storage and usage is subject to Excise control.
Ether	Forms an explosive peroxide on exposure to light.
Formaldehyde (formalin)	Polymerises in cold. Formalin is 40% formaldehyde gas in water. Formalin should not be stored near hydrochloric acid because of the risk of forming a potent carcinogen bis-chloro-methyl-ether if HCl gas and formalin vapour mix even at very low concentrations.
Hydrogen peroxide	Store in polythene bottles in a refrigerator. H_2O_2 decomposes in glass, light and warmth.
Mercury	Avoid contact with skin. Clean up spillage as soon as possible. Mercury attacks lead and solder (beware of the effects of broken thermometers in the bottom of water baths, etc.).
Phenol	Oxidises and turns pink on exposure to light. Phenol is very corrosive; it also has the property of anaesthetising the skin so that very serious damage can occur before the victim is aware of contact.
Picric acid	Can explode when dry; store saturated with water and avoid gound-glass stoppers.
Sodium and potassium hydroxides	Do not use ground-glass stoppers. Solutions absorb CO_2.

example the necessity of periodic examination of closures or the possibility of pressure developing which can lead to the container bursting. Only those chemicals required for day-to-day use should be kept in the laboratory, all others being kept in the store room. Large containers such as, for example, Winchester bottles, should be stored low down or on the floor in trays, but not where they can be accidentally knocked or kicked.

A final point to remember is that whoever is responsible for ordering new stocks should be informed when stocks are getting low; do not wait until the bottle has been used!

4. Storage conditions for some individual chemicals

A short list of chemicals, frequently used in clinical laboratories, that require special consideration not necessarily covered by the foregoing precautions, is given in Table 3.1.

4. General equipment

Certain items of equipment are common to all medical laboratories and this chapter will deal with the care and use of some of these items.

BALANCES

The vast majority of weighing procedures necessary can be done on the following types of balance:

Analytical balance
'Top-pan' balance

A simple two-pan instrument for balancing centrifuge tubes is also required as mentioned in the section on centrifuges.

The analytical balance

An ideal analytical balance for most purposes is one that will take a maximum load of about 200 g with a sensitivity of 0·1 mg.

In the past, analytical balances worked on the principle of adding known weights to 'balance' the object being weighed. They were either two-pàn balances with a set of weights added by hand or single-pan having a system of weights added by a selection mechanism. One disadvantage of this system described above was that the sensitivity of the balance changed with differing loads on the beam. This disadvantage is overcome in more modern instruments by having the beam under constant load; the weight of the object being weighed is compensated for by removing an equal weight from the beam.

Most of these balances incorporate a partial release or pre-weighing device that speeds weighing and, by not exposing the fine balancing mechanism to sudden high loads, reduces wear and increases the life of the balance.

The advent of the microprocessor has led to the introduction of the electronic balance. This type of balance operates on the principle of automatic electromagnetic force compensation. Adding a weight to the balance pan causes a coil to move. This coil is suspended in the field of a permanent magnet and therefore movement of the coil will change the electrical current within it, leading to an equilibration of forces between the load on the pan and the electromagnetic force. The current flowing through the *compensating coil* produces a measuring voltage across a resistor connected in series and this measuring voltage is proportional to the load.

In analytical balances of this type there are built-in *substitution weights* added or subtracted by a motor.

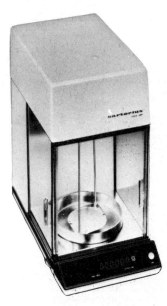

Fig. 4.1. An electronic analytical balance
(Sartorius Instruments Ltd.)

These are used to extend the weighing capability of the balance as the compensating coil operates over only a small range. The necessity for adding or subtracting the substitution weights is sensed by the *null indicator*. The signals from a control amplifier derived from the coil and null indicator are fed to the microprocessor which controls the substitution weight motor and computes the read-out data. Fig. 4.2 shows the design principle of the balance shown in Fig. 4.1.

25

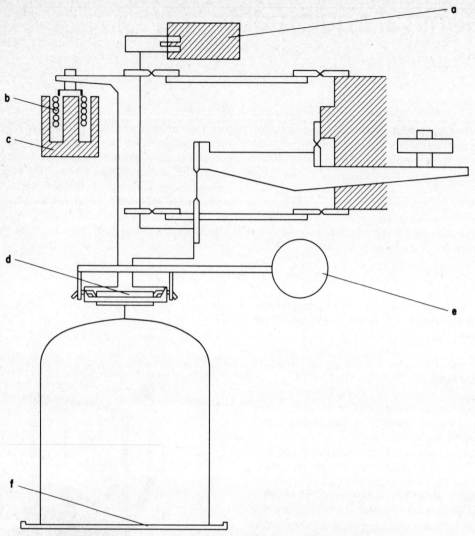

Fig. 4.2.   The mechanism of an electronic analytical balance (Sartorius Instru-
            ments Ltd.)
            (a) Null indicator; *(b)* compensating coil; *(c)* magnet; *(d)* substitution
            weights; *(e)* substitution weight motor; *(f)* balance pan.

Among the advantages of the electronic balance are the speed and ease of operation and the ability of the instrument to be interfaced with data-handling equipment.

Top-pan balances

These balances are particularly useful for weighing when less precision is required. They are quick to use and comparatively robust. Most models incorporate a *tare* device whereby the weight of a container can be compensated for and the instrument returned to zero so that the weight of the substance being added to the container can be read directly.

The specification of the balance chosen will vary according to the use envisaged, but an instrument with a capacity of 2 kg and a sensitivity of 0·1 g will be found generally useful.

Again electronic top-pan balances have been introduced. They have similar advantages over the mechanical type to those described under 'analytical balances'.

Some are particularly useful for weighing animals where the continual movement of the animal is a problem. The microprocessor can be programmed to do the equivalent of five weighings and then display the mean.

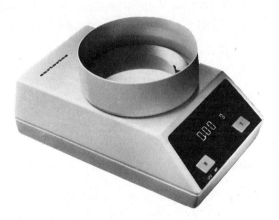

Fig. 4.3. An electronic top-pan balance (Sartorius Instruments Ltd.)

Do's and dont's in using balances

Do use a vibration-free bench. These are best constructed of slate with brick supports, but special trays are available to allow a balance to be used on a standard laboratory bench.

Do level the instrument before use; most instruments incorporate a spirit level.

Do use a fume-free environment, preferably in a separate room.

Do keep a constant temperature and allow objects to reach the temperature of the balance before weighing.

Do avoid draughts; analytical balances usually have a glass door that should be closed before reading weights.

Do use the mechanism in mechanical balances that keeps the beam and pan off the fulcrum when the instrument is not in use.

Do use forceps to handle weights, weighing dishes, etc.

Do keep pan surrounds dry with a desiccant.

Don't allow chemicals to come in contact with the balance. Keep a soft brush handy to brush off any chemicals that fall on to the pan, or on to the floor of the instrument.

When using mechanical balances:
Don't add weights while the balance is free to swing.
Don't move the balance without clamping the mechanism in the manner recommended by the manufacturer.

CENTRIFUGES

Centrifuges are potentially very dangerous items of equipment. In recognition of this many countries have introduced legislation concerning the design, maintenance and use of centrifuges. The most important safety consideration is the ability of a centrifuge to contain all the debris that results from disintegration of the rotor or a bucket becoming dislodged. Most small laboratory centrifuges have in the past been considered to be portable and have been moved from bench to bench; this is no longer considered acceptable and a fixed position for the bench centrifuge should be established and the instrument firmly fixed in that position. There should also be a locking device on the lid whereby the lid cannot be opened whilst the rotor is spinning nor the rotor set in motion whilst the lid is open.

The relevant standard in the United Kingdom is BS 4402 and all laboratory centrifuges should comply with its recommendations. In addition centrifuges must also comply with Electrical Safety Code for Hospital Laboratory Equipment.

For general purposes there are two main types of centrifuge:

angle head;
swing-out head.

The angle-head type, in which the buckets are kept at a fixed angle to the vertical axis of the head, is useful if it is desirable to remove almost all of the supernatant fluid (SNF). The angle-head centrifuge also gives a higher rate of sedimentation for a given speed than a swing-out head of the same radius. Angle-head centrifuges must have a stationary casing enclosing the head. They must not be used with infective material as aerosols are more likely to be produced than by swing-out heads. In addition angle-head centrifuges have the disadvantages of low capacity and inflexibility in that the number and type of bucket cannot be varied.

The swing-out head type of centrifuge is recommended for most purposes. The size of the bucket can be varied to take the required tubes.

Containers should be selected carefully; they should be either thick-walled glass or plastic tubes and should be inspected before use. For blood samples screw-topped disposable plastic tubes are recommended. It is important not to overfill containers, and they must be effectively capped or sealed; do not soil the rim of the container as this leads to droplet and aerosol formation during centrifugation. Tubes or bottles containing infective material must be centrifuged in sealed buckets. A suitable design of sealed bucket is shown in Fig. 4.4.

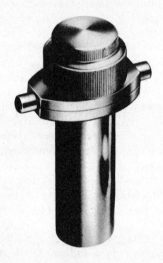

Fig. 4.4.   A sealed centrifuge bucket.

After centrifugation, open the buckets and screw capped bottles in an exhaust protective cabinet. Centrifuges should not be used in microbiological safety cabinets as they can adversely affect the air flow.

Method of use

1. Take the buckets from the centrifuge head and tip out any water in them.
2. Check that each bucket has the correct rubber pad in place.
3. Check that the tube or bottle to be centrifuged is not too big, so that it fits well within the cup and that it

will not be damaged on the head when the bucket swings out during spinning.

4. Place the bottle in a bucket which in turn is placed on one pan of a simple two-pan balance.
5. Place a similar bottle in a bucket on the other pan of the balance.
6. Add clean water with a Pasteur pipette to the lighter bucket until the two just balance. This is important to prevent vibration in the machine and to prevent damage to the bearing which would otherwise occur.
7. Place the two buckets in diametrically opposed positions on the head; repeat these manoeuvres with the other buckets if necessary.
8. Make sure that the buckets and trunnions are seated properly to prevent their flying off during use.
9. Close the lid, start the machine and gradually increase the speed to that required.
10. After a suitable time, switch off the motor and allow the centrifuge to come to a stop.

Cleaning

The entire centrifuge must be cleaned regularly and the buckets disinfected, to counter contamination, with a phenolic disinfectant such as 1% sudol or they can be autoclaved where practicable.

Should a breakage occur in the centrifuge it must be switched off at once. It is recommended that 30 minutes should elapse for the aerosol and droplets to settle before the centrifuge lid is opened, then the buckets, broken tube or tubes and contents, plus trunnions and head should be autoclaved if possible or immersed in disinfectant. Decontaminate the bowl with disinfectant (not hypochlorite, which is corrosive) allowing sufficient time for the disinfectant to act. Rinse the bowl and dry.

pH METERS

We owe our scale of measurement of acidity and alkalinity to the Danish biochemist Sörenson. Originally pH was defined as the negative logarithm of the hydrogen ion concentration. More recently, however, it has been shown that as so defined pH cannot in fact be measured, so that now the practical definition and basis of measurement depends on the differences in pH values between a primary standard and the solution being measured.

From the practical point of view the following points about pH are worth remembering:

1. The scale runs from 0 to 14. The pH of pure water is 7, values between 0 and 7 represent degrees of acidity and values between 7 and 14 degrees of alkalinity. (*N.B.* It is possible to have pH values outside the range 0–14.)

2. The scale is logarithmic. That is to say a change of 1 pH unit is equivalent to a tenfold change in hydrogen ion concentration.

filled with hydrochloric acid of known concentration *(b)*. Into this acid dips a silver wire *(c)*. This wire is coated with silver chloride. When the electrode is dipped into a solution a potential difference occurs across the fine glass wall. This potential difference is proportional to the pH of the solution. The electrode is connected to the instrument by means of a screened cable *(d)*.

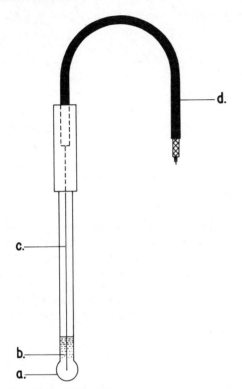

Fig. 4.5. Glass pH electrode
(a) Thin glass bulb; *(b)* HCl; *(c)* silver wire; *(d)* screened cable.

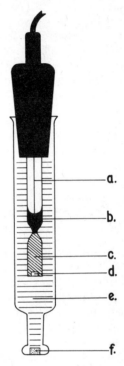

Fig. 4.6. Reference (calomel) electrode
(a) Platinum wire; *(b)* mercury; *(c)* KCl/calomel paste; *(d)* porous plug (inner tube); *(e)* saturated KCl; *(f)* porous plug (outer tube).

3. Since pH is considered as the negative logarithm of hydrogen ion concentration an increase in concentration (i.e. an increase in acidity) gives a decrease in pH value.

The basic principle of the pH meter is that two electrodes, one measuring, one reference, are immersed in the solution of which the pH is required and the e.m.f. of the resulting cell is measured.

Measuring electrodes

Glass electrodes are usually used. A diagram of such an electrode is shown in Fig. 4.5. The thin glass bulb *(a)* is

It is not possible to construct an accurate electrode to cover the entire pH range at every temperature. Therefore most manufacturers produce a range of electrodes, and it is important to ensure that an electrode is suitable for the desired application.

Note also that the glass membrane is quite thin and is easily broken; treat with care.

Reference electrodes

The commonest reference electrode for use in the measurement of pH is the calomel electrode (calomel is mercurous chloride). Fig. 4.6 represents such an electrode. A platinum wire *(a)* is in contact with mercury *(b)*; this arrangement serves as the electrode of the inner tube, the bottom part of which contains a paste of calomel and potassium chloride *(c)* and terminates in a porous plug *(d)*. The outer tube contains saturated potassium chloride solution *(e)* and again ends in a porous plug *(f)*. The KCl, by seepage through plug *(f)*, acts as a salt bridge between the solution being measured and the inner tube. The potential difference between KCl and many solutions is very small and can be kept stable. It is necessary that there is sufficient KCl in the outer tube, and a filling hole is located near the top. There are, of course, many designs of calomel electrode, but the one described is typical.

Combined electrodes

It is also possible to obtain electrodes in which both measuring and reference parts are included in one assembly. These electrodes are of particular value in the estimation of blood pH.

Method of measuring pH using pH meter

The method below is an outline guide and will vary in detail according to the instrument in use. It is assumed that separate glass and calomel electrodes are being used. Before using for the first time electrodes usually require soaking for a number of hours; details will be found in the manufacturer's instructions.

1. Switch on instrument and allow to 'warm up' for a few minutes.
2. Check that the correct electrodes are in place.
3. Rinse electrodes with distilled water and remove excess with a soft tissue, taking care not to touch the glass bulb.
4. Place electrodes in reference buffer solution, ensure that bulb is covered and adjust meter for correct reading.
5. Rinse as in 3 above.
6. Place in solution to be measured and take reading.
7. Rinse again and switch off instrument.

Note: Electrodes should not normally be allowed to become dry; glass electrodes are best kept in buffer solution of about pH 7 between uses and the calomel electrode kept in saturated KCl. If the electrodes are not going to be required for some time they should be rinsed, dried and stored carefully. They must be treated as new electrodes when brought back into service.

GAS CYLINDERS

Gases supplied for medical use must be in cylinders coloured to conform to BS 1319. Gases commonly used in the laboratory in this group are set out in Table 4.1.

Table 4.1

Gas	Colour	
	Cylinder	Neck
Oxygen	Black	White
Carbon dioxide	Grey	Grey
Nitrogen	Grey	Black (white spot = oxygen-free)
$O_2 + CO_2$	Black	White/grey quarters
Air	Grey	White/black quarters
Nitrous oxide	Blue	Blue

Other cylinder gases used in laboratories include hydrogen, propane and acetylene; these cylinders are usually red. Care must be taken to ensure that the correct gas is being used. Reliance on a colour code is not sufficient, especially for non-medical gases.

Cylinders should always be used with the reduction valves recommended as safe for that particular type of cylinder. Never use a hammer to tighten or release a valve. Always ensure that the cylinder cannot fall either by using a cylinder trolley or by chains, strapping or using a suitable metal ring to hold it against a wall or bench. Never use oil or grease to free a sticking valve.

Only those cylinders actually in use should be kept in the laboratory. Indeed it is preferable that no cylinders, particularly of inflammable gases, are kept in the laboratory but that the gases are piped from cylinders outside the building.

Gas cylinders must be periodically tested, usually every 5 years. The date of the last test is stamped on the shoulder of the cylinder and any cylinder due for retesting should be returned to the supplier.

WATER-BATHS

Water-baths can be used to maintain constant temperatures between ambient and about 90°C. Cooling devices can also be used for temperatures lower than ambient. A good water-bath will have a circulation device and a reliable thermostat. A false bottom that allows circulation of water below it serves two purposes. First, more efficient circulation is obtainable and, secondly, a greater depth of water can be used for a given tube size which increases the stability of the water temperature. A constant-level device is useful, particularly if the temperature required is high, as evaporation can be a problem. If a lid is fitted it should not be used if open tubes are being incubated. A useful means of keeping evaporation to a minimum is to use a layer of polythene spheres about 2 cm diameter as a 'carpet' on the surface of the water, these can be pushed aside to allow racks of tubes to be placed in the bath.

Footnote

There is an old cliché that says: 'When all else fails read the instructions'. A book of this nature can do no more than outline the care and use of instruments, many of which are expensive and vital to the working of the laboratory concerned. Most manufacturers issue very comprehensive instruction manuals; these should be read *before* attempting to use any unfamiliar instrument, not just after you have broken it!

5. Spectrophotometry

An understanding of the principles and practice of spectrophotometry is essential in medical laboratory technology.

THE BEER–LAMBERT LAWS

The fundamental laws of spectrophotometry are those described by Lambert (1760) and Beer (1852) long before the advent of photoelectric instrumentation. Both of these laws assume that the light used is *monochromatic*, that is to say of one wavelength.

Lambert's law

The proportion of light absorbed by a substance is independent of the intensity of the incident light, or to put it another way, each successive layer of equal thickness of the same homologous solution will absorb the same proportion of the light incident upon it. Lambert, then, kept the concentration of the solution constant, varied the light path and showed that the intensity of the transmitted light decreased exponentially as the light path increased arithmetically. Usually we maintain a constant light path size so that in practice Beer's law becomes the more important.

Beer's law

'The proportion of the incident light absorbed by the molecules in a solution is directly proportional to the number of absorbing molecules.'

If Beer's law is obeyed then as the concentration of absorbing molecules increases arithmetically, the intensity of the transmitted light decreases exponentially.

At this stage we should define some of the terms that are used to describe the absorption of light.

Transmittance. This is the ratio of the intensity of the transmitted light over the intensity of the incident light. This is usually multiplied by 100 to give percentage transmission.

Percentage transmission.

$$\%T = \frac{I_T}{I_0} \times 100,$$

where I_T is the intensity of the transmitted light and I_0 is the intensity of the incident light.

Absorbance (also known as extinction or optical density).

Without dealing with the mathematics we can say that absorbance (A) is related to transmittance in the following way:

$$A = 2 - \log_{10} \%T.$$

Thus if there is 100% transmission, then $A = 0$, that is to say the absorbance is zero.

Many photoelectric instruments are calibrated in both ways. For manual procedures we normally use absorbance since if Beer's law is obeyed, a plot of concentration against absorbance is a straight line and therefore much easier to handle than the exponential curve given by plotting $\%T$ against concentration. In automated procedures, however, $\%T$ is often used.

We can now derive the basic equation for photoelectric absorptiometry.

We have seen from Beer's and Lambert's laws that

$$A \propto C.L$$

where C = concentration and L = light path.

Therefore $\qquad A = K.C.L.$

where K is a constant.

If we consider two solutions containing the same substance, one a standard (S), of known concentration, and the other a test (T) solution of unknown concentration we can write:

$$(A)_S = K_S C_S L_S$$

and $\qquad (A)_T = K_T C_T L_T$

therefore $\qquad \dfrac{(A)_S}{(A)_T} = \dfrac{K_S C_S L_S}{K_T C_T L_T}$

32

By treating both solutions in the same way we can make $K_S = K_T$ and $L_S = L_T$, and our equation becomes:

$$\frac{(A)_S}{(A)_T} = \frac{C_S}{C_T}$$

Then

$$C_T = \frac{(A)_T}{(A)_S} \cdot C_S$$

i.e. Concentration of test

$$= \frac{A \text{ of test}}{A \text{ of standard}} \times \text{Concentration of standard.}$$

Note: C_T and C_S refer to the concentration of the measured substance in the cuvette, and therefore alteration to the above equation may be necessary to account for dilution factors and any differences in dilution factors between the test and standard solutions.

INSTRUMENTATION

It is, of course, not possible to describe all the instruments available. The notes that follow will describe the basic systems of the instruments with particular reference to practical considerations.

The five basic systems in a photoelectric absorptiometer are:

1. Radiation source (light).
2. Means of selecting the wavelength of the light used and focusing it on to the samples (monochromator and collimator).
3. Cells to contain samples.
4. Photosensitive detectors.
5. Means of measuring the current produced by the photosensitive elements and display of the result.

1. Radiation source

The type of light source used will depend upon the region of the spectrum required. For visible light the most common source is a tungsten-filament lamp, or more recently the higher powered tungsten–halogen (quartz–iodine) lamp. For measurements in the ultraviolet region, hydrogen or deuterium lamps are used.

Practical notes

(a) The current supplying the lamp should be constant. (This is usually controlled by the instrument, but can be a source of error particularly in older instruments.)

(b) The lamp must be correctly aligned with the optical system. When replacing a lamp, take note of the manufacturers' instruction to ensure correct fitting.

(c) Do not handle the lamp, always hold with a tissue when installing. Fingerprints can markedly affect the performance of a lamp.

(d) In instruments having more than one lamp ensure that the appropriate one is being used for the wavelength required.

(e) Allow sufficient time for the instrument to 'warm up' before use.

2. Monochromator and collimator

We have seen that the laws of photometry are based on light of one wavelength and part of the instrument that selects this wavelength is known as the *monochromator*. The light from the radiation source is split by one of the following methods.

(a) *Filters.* The cheaper instruments use filters as a means of selecting a band of wavelengths. These instruments are usually referred to as colorimeters. The simplest filters are either coloured glass or suitably dyed gelatin sandwiched in glass.

A more sophisticated form of filter is the interference filter consisting of two partially transmitting films of metal separated by a transparent spacer of low refractive index or of a piece of glass or silicon coated with different thicknesses of materials of various refractive indices. The filter is so constructed that only light of the required wavelength is allowed through; all other wavelengths being reflected or absorbed. Interference wedges act in a similar way to interference filters but are constructed so that one of a range of wavelengths can be selected depending upon which part of the wedge is in the light path. These wedges are not widely used as they are inferior in performance to diffraction gratings and are almost as costly to produce.

(b) *Prisms.* Prisms, made of glass for visible wavelengths, quartz or fused silica for the ultraviolet region, are mounted so that they can be turned to allow the required light to pass *via* the focusing optics through the sample. Prism monochromators are considerably more efficient than filters in that they allow for smaller bandwidths. (The bandwidth can be considered to be the range of wavelengths on either side of the desired wavelength that is allowed by the monochromator to pass to the sample.) However

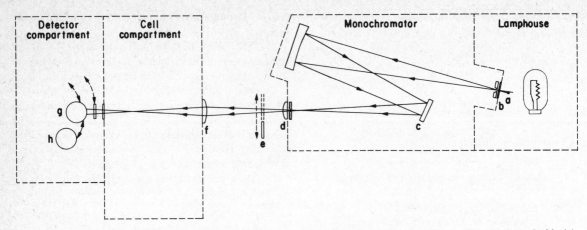

Fig. 5.1   Diagram of the optical system of the Pye-Unicam SP6–250/350 Spectrophotometer. (Pye-Unicam Ltd.) *(a)*
Tungsten lamp; *(b)* monochromator entrance slit; *(c)* diffraction grating; *(d)* monochromator exit slit; *(e)* filter
used to eliminate stray light between 270 and 410 nm; *(f)* cell compartment lens; *(g)* red-sensitive phototube; *(h)*
blue-sensitive phototube.

prisms are more expensive than filters and their characteristics require more advanced instrument design.

(c) Diffraction gratings. This is the method of
wavelength selection preferred in most modern spectrophotometers. The grating consists of a series of
finely etched parallel grooves on a highly polished
reflecting surface. The grating is placed at an angle to a
beam of light; this light is reflected off one surface of
the grooving, each groove acting as a very narrow
mirror. The reflected light from each groove overlaps
that from the neighbouring grooves and interference
occurs. However at a given angle the separation of the
grooves relative to the direction of the light will be a
whole-number product of the required wavelength; the
waves of this wavelength will be in phase with each
other and will be reflected without interference. Thus
the wavelength desired may be obtained by altering the
angle of the grating in the light beam. This is the
method of wavelength selection used in the Pye-
Unicam SP6 series of spectrophotometers (Fig. 5.1).
The grating is rotated and thus the wavelength selected
by movement of the wavelength control (Fig. 5.2).

The system of mirrors and lenses used to direct the
light from the source to the wavelength selector and
thence on to the sample is known as the *collimator.*

Practical notes

(a) Ensure that the correct filter or wavelength is
being used for the job in hand. (*See* below for choice of
wavelength.)

(b) Do not allow solutions, dirt, fingerprints or any
other contaminant to come into contact with any
optical component as this will greatly detract from its
performance.

(c) Avoid any rough handling of the instrument as
this may lead to malfunction. From time to time, and
always after moving, the instrument should be checked
to ensure correct working of the monochromator. The
wavelength selection can be checked by the method
described later in this chapter.

(d) Prisms and filters are to some extent affected by
changes in temperature. For this reason the instrument
should be switched on some time before required so
that all components reach a constant operating temperature.

3. *Sample holders*

A number of different sample holders are available for
manual, semi-automated and automated methods of
analysis.

(a) Test-tubes. These are used only in cheaper instruments. They should preferably be matched for transmission. Sometimes a mark is etched on them, and this
mark is lined up against a mark on the instrument to
ensure consistent optical path length.

(b) Cuvettes. These are rectangular cells with one
pair of opposite sides optically clear. The other sides
are usually ground (cuvettes with all four sides optically
clear can be obtained for use in fluorospectropho-
tometry). Cuvettes are of glass for use at visible
wavelengths and of silica or quartz for use in the
ultraviolet region.

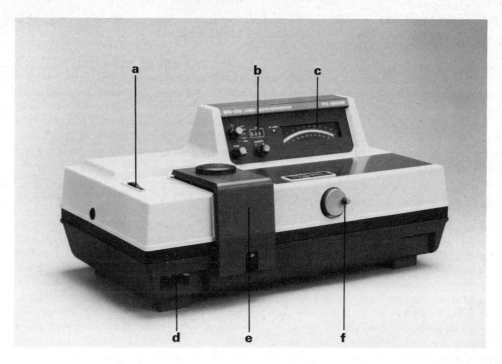

Fig. 5.2.   SP6–250 Spectrophotometer (Pye-Unicam Ltd.) *(a)* zero control; *(b)* wavelength indicator; *(c)* absorbance scale; *(d)* photocell selector; *(e)* cell compartment; *(f)* wavelength control.

(c) Flow cells. Various patterns of flow cell have been designed for use in automated or semi-automated equipment. These allow the sample to be changed without moving the cell.

Practical notes

(a) Cleanliness is of the utmost importance. No grease, dirt, dried solutions or fingerprints should be allowed to stay on the optical surfaces either inside or outside. A suitable method of cleaning cuvettes is to place them in a detergent solution overnight then rinse with water and transfer to dilute HCl in a small covered beaker. Before use rinse with distilled water, drain and dry outside surfaces with a soft tissue.

(b) Always rinse cells immediately after use and never leave them full of any sample.

(c) Handle cuvettes only by the ground edges, never by the optically clear faces.

(d) Avoid scratching cells; wipe only with soft tissue.

(e) If any solution gets on to the outside of a cell wipe it off before reading.

(f) If a number of cuvettes are to be used they should be matched; this can be conveniently done by filling with distilled water and checking that there is no significant difference between their optical densities at the wavelength to be used. The absorbance of one cell can be set to about 0·4 and used as reference; keeping the same setting of the instrument the other cells are read and differences of no more than 0·002 can be ignored. Greater differences should be taken into account when reading samples or, better still, sets of cuvettes should be made from those having similar absorbances.

4. Photosensitive detectors

The three common photosensitive detectors in use are: the barrier layer cell, the photoemissive vacuum tube, and the photomultiplier. All three types depend upon the release of electrons from photosensitive substances (e.g. selenium) when exposed to light and the subsequent collection of these electrons at an anode to produce a flow of current.

The barrier layer cell (photocell) requires strong incident light since the current produced cannot easily be amplified. For this reason it is usually used only in filter instruments where there is plenty of light energy available as the band pass width is wide. *The photo-emissive tube (vacuum phototube)* can be used at much lower light intensities since the current produced can be easily amplified.

The most sensitive detectors are *the photomultiplier* types. These can be employed in the most sophisticated instruments where the band pass of wavelengths can be made very small with consequent diminution of the amount of light energy available for measurement and particularly in double-beam instruments (see below) where a fast response is necessary.

Practical notes

(a) Detectors are subject to fatigue on prolonged exposure to light. They should be protected from light when not in use. A shutter is used to protect the detectors in many instruments, and this must be kept closed except when measurements are being made.

(b) Selenium barrier layers cells can be 'poisoned' by mercury and should not be allowed to come into contact with this metal or its vapour.

(c) Some instruments use different phototubes depending upon the wavelength of light in use (*see* Fig. 5.1); the correct one must, of course, be selected.

(d) Detectors are in part temperature-dependent, and this is another reason for employing a sufficiently long warm-up period before any readings are taken.

5. Display

The current from the detector is amplified and fed to a suitable measuring device. The read-out can be by means of a scale or a digital display. Often this result can also be fed to a suitable recorder.

The scale may be calibrated logarithmically to read directly in absorbance (i.e. 0, 0·1, 0·2, . . .) in $A \times 10$ (i.e. 0, 1·0, 2·0 . . .) or in $A \times 100$ (i.e., 0, 10, 20 . . .) and in addition may be calibrated with the linear percentage transmission scale. Some instruments allow the operator the facility of adjusting the read-out to give a linear response calibrated for true concentration of the substance being estimated.

Practical notes

(a) Be sure you know the type of calibration in use.

(b) In some instruments, since absorbance is a logarithmic scale, the divisions at the higher end of the scale are closer together than at the lower end. This means that a subdivision marked on the scale may

represent a greater change of A at the high end than at the lower end.

The spectrophotometer shown in Figs. 5.1 and 5.2 is used here to illustrate some of the points referred to earlier and some additional terms commonly used in spectrophotometry. The instrument shown in Fig. 5.2 is designed to operate between 325 and 1000 nm using a tungsten filament lamp. An alternative version is available that extends the wavelength range down to 195 nm; this is accomplished by the provision of a deuterium lamp for wavelengths in the ultraviolet region in addition to the tungsten lamp used for the visible region of the spectrum.

This is a *single-beam* instrument, that is to say the light from the lamp travels along only one pathway to the cell compartment (*see* Fig. 5.1) and all samples, both blank and test, are read in the same position. The alternative is the *double-beam* instrument. This type splits the light from the monochromator into two beams; one beam is used as reference, the other for reading. This method eliminates errors possible in single-beam instruments due to changes in source output, grating efficiency and sensitivity of the detector which occur with changes in wavelength. The double-beam instrument has a system of 'chopping' by which the detector is alternately exposed to the reference and the test beam. The signal going to the display is derived from the difference between test and reference beam intensities. The complications, of course, add to the price of the instrument and for many purposes a good single-beam instrument is perfectly adequate.

The SP6 series of spectrophotometers are examples of direct-reading instruments. Once the correct wavelength, light source and detector have been selected a cell containing the solvent blank is placed in the sample compartment and the absorbance set to zero using the zero control. The cell is now replaced by one containing sample and the absorbance read directly. Some older instruments used the *null balance* method of reading. The principle of null-balance operation is as follows. A solvent blank is placed in the light path and the meter is set to zero. The cell is then replaced by a similar one containing the test solution. The meter is then returned to zero by means of a potentiometer to give an electrical null. This potentiometer can be calibrated to give transmission or absorbance readings. This method is capable of a high degree of accuracy but direct-reading instruments are capable of quicker operation.

In the instrument illustrated the detectors are vacuum phototubes, one of which is blue-sensitive, the other red-sensitive. Phototubes produce a small output current even when no light is falling on them. This output is known as the *dark current* and is dependent on temperature. In practice this means that if the ambient temperature of the laboratory changes the zero control will need adjustment. Modern spectrophotometers are designed to minimise this problem and the SP6 series has a third photocell (not illustrated) which has its envelope permanently blackened so that no light can reach it. This third photocell is wired into the circuit with reversed polarity to compensate for any thermally induced dark current drift in the other cells.

Another cause of difficulty in spectrophotometry is *stray light*. A continuous spectrum of light enters the monochromator from the source but all that is required to emerge is a very narrow band of wavelengths. Ideally the unwanted radiation would be confined within the monochromator; however no monochromator is perfect and some unwanted radiation emerges from the exit slit and this is known as stray light. Stray light is usually most troublesome at the extremes of the spectrophotometer range and manifests itself in lack of linearity of absorption curves.

Choice of wavelength

To decide which wavelength or filter to use, the first step is to produce an absorption curve of the colour to be measured by plotting the absorbance against wavelength. Usually the wavelength giving the maximum absorbance is used; however, checks should be made to ensure that the following criteria are also observed:

1. Beer's law is obeyed over the range of expected values.
2. The degree of sensitivity is adequate. That is to say increases in concentration give suitable increase in absorbance. Instruments are often best used below an absorbance of 0·8, and a check of the method must be made to ensure that the required range of values can be read within this figure.

In instruments using filters it will usually be found that a filter of the complementary colour to that being read will be the most suitable (e.g. a blue filter for a red solution), but the criteria mentioned above should be satisfied as far as possible.

Checking the wavelength

The accuracy of the wavelength calibration of a spectrophotometer should be checked occasionally, especially after an instrument has been moved. This is best done by using one of the special filters available for this purpose. In the visible region of the spectrum the didymium-glass filter is used. This has a number of absorption peaks, the most useful of which are at 809, 586 and 573 nm. The precise checking and adjusting techniques for a particular instrument can be found in the manufacturer's handbook.

SOURCES OF ERROR IN COLORIMETRY

It is worth remembering the following list of possible causes of error in colorimetry.

1. *Faulty technique*, e.g. failure to mix solutions adequately (probably the most frequent cause of error); inaccurate pipetting.
2. *Beer–Lambert laws.* Errors can arise if these laws are not obeyed. A common error is to accept results that fall outside the range of standards tested where the method is no longer linear.
3. *Instrument errors.* Optical or mechanical faults in the instrument including excessive stray light or ambient light entering the instrument and inadequate warm-up time.
4. *Contamination* of reagents, standards or samples, including the use of dirty glassware, particularly cuvettes.
5. *Colour development.* Incomplete development or fading.
6. *Temperature* can have a variable effect on the results.
7. *Precipitation* within the cuvette. Some coloured complexes are particularly prone to precipitation.

Finally a spectrophotometer will only work efficiently if used properly. The manufacturer's instructions should be followed with care.

RECOMMENDED READING

1. Steward, J. E. (ed.) (1979). *Introduction to Ultraviolet and Visible Spectrophotometry.* Pye Unicam Ltd.

6. The microscope

This section is intended solely as a practical guide to enable the student to set up a microscope and obtain satisfactory results from visual examination by ordinary light. Settings and filter systems required for photography, fluorescence microscopy and other methods of illumination, together with explanations of the optical properties of lenses and other theoretical considerations, may be found in books such as *Modern Microscopy* by Culling[1] or *Hartley's Microscopy*[2], and from the instruction booklets supplied for individual microscope models by the better manufacturers.

ILLUMINATION

The light source may be either completely separate from, or built into, the microscope. The latter arrangement is becoming increasingly common and has the advantage of compactness and, in some cases, permanent alignment. The intensity of the light may be fixed, variable through a number of stops or continuously variable through a transformer. From its source the light may travel directly up through the condenser system or be deflected through it by a mirror system. Between the light source and the substage condenser and close to the former, it is advantageous to have a field diaphragm.

LENSES

1. Substage condenser

This is a lens system interposed between the specimen and the light source. It is used to concentrate and focus the light on the plane of the specimen. This is made possible by allowing the condenser to have a vertical movement. It may be fixed in position with regard to lateral movements or it may have centring screws allowing some adjustments. It has a diaphragm to limit the area of the cone of light which it passes and it usually has a filter holder on its underside. The focal length of the condenser governs the maximum diameter

of the cone of light emitted. In order that one condenser may be used with a variety of objective apertures it is usual that the top lens can be removed either by unscrewing or by swinging aside. This increases the focal length and thus the diameter of the cone of light.

2. Objectives

The variety of objectives available is very large both in quality and in magnifications. They should be matched to each other to ensure that they are parfocal. This enables the user to change from one to another without the need for refocusing. Flat-field objectives are now common, and for routine use a set consisting of ×4, ×10, ×40, and ×100 oil-immersion will meet most requirements.

3. Eyepieces

These are obtainable in a wide range of magnifications and ×10 is suitable for use with the objectives listed above. To take advantage of the flat field provided by modern objectives, eyepieces known as 'wide-field' are available and, as the name suggests, these cover a much wider field of view than the standard type. The microscope may be monocular or binocular. In the latter case one of the eyepieces should be of adjustable focus and their interpupillary distance should also be adjustable.

SPECIMEN STAGE

The stage supporting the specimen may have fixed or movable slide holders. The 'fixed' stage has two surface clips to hold the specimen steady, and movement from field to field with any degree of control is difficult. With a 'mechanical' stage the slide is held by side clips and may then be moved horizontally in both directions by means of control knobs on the side of the stage or underneath it. The whole of the specimen area can be slowly and steadily examined, and it is usual to have vernier scales for both directions of movement. These allow precise relocation of any given spot on the specimen.

FOCUSING

Focusing the specimen is achieved by altering the distance between the objective and the specimen. This may be done by moving the tube holding the objectives, but is more usually done by moving the stage holding the specimen. There is a coarse and a fine adjustment provided either by two separate controls or by a single combined knob. It is advisable that initial location and focusing of a specimen should be done by moving a low-power ($\times 4$ or $\times 10$) objective close to the specimen surface and then moving it slowly away while observing through the eyepieces.

SETTING UP THE MICROSCOPE

1. With separate light source

(a) Position the microscope lamp approximately 25 cm away from the microscope.

(b) Open the condenser iris diaphragm fully and raise the condenser to its topmost position.

(c) Using the plane side of the microscope mirror direct the light up the tube of the microscope to give the maximum intensity and evenness of light while observing through the eyepiece.

(d) Focus a specimen on the microscope stage using the $\times 10$ objective.

(e) Rack the condenser down until the light source is also in focus. Move the condenser slightly until the light source is just out of focus.

(f) Remove an eye-piece, look down the tube and adjust the condenser diaphragm to just fully illuminate the back lens of the objective. Replace the eyepiece.

2. With a built-in light source

Details of the procedure will vary slightly with different makes and models, and the manufacturer's instruction booklet should be carefully studied. A typical setting up is described here to illustrate the general principles involved and it should be followed in conjunction with Fig. 6.1.

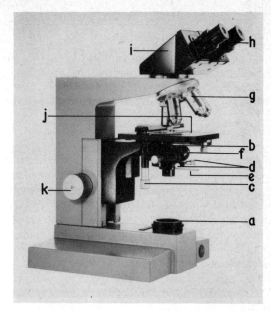

Fig. 6.1.   A standard binocular microscope (E. Leitz) (a) Field diaphragm and dust cover; (b) substage condenser; (c) condenser vertical adjustment; (d) condenser centring screws; (e) condenser diaphragm lever; (f) condenser top lens; (g) revolving nose-piece with objectives; (h) eyepieces; (i) binocular head; (j) specimen stage; (k) combined coarse and fine focusing knob.

(a) Centring and focusing the light source

Switch on the light. Place a frosted-glass filter or a piece of lens tissue paper over the dust glass and fully open the field diaphragm. Adjust the bulb position to give the smallest and brightest spot of light in the centre of the dust glass. Remove the frosted-glass filter.

(b) Adjusting the eyepieces

Place a stained section on the microscope stage. Swing the top lens of the condenser into the light path and raise the condenser to its topmost position. Using a $\times 10$ objective, focus the specimen. Open the condenser iris diaphragm fully. Set the interpupillary distance so that a single image is seen. Using the right eye at the right eyepiece focus the image sharply. Now with the left eye at the left eyepiece adjust this eyepiece by rotating its collar to give a sharp image. This procedure compensates for any differences in vision between the eyes.

(c) Centring the condenser and setting the field diaphragm

Close the field iris diaphragm until its image is visible and focus this sharply by lowering the condenser. Bring this diaphragm image to the centre of the field of view by means of the condenser centring screws. Open the field diaphragm until it just disappears from view. Raise the condenser to the top position. Remove one eyepiece from its tube and, looking down the tube, adjust the condenser diaphragm to just fully illuminate the back lens of the objective. Replace the eyepiece. For optimum performance the condenser should be adjusted in this manner for each objective. With experience this adjustment can be made without removing the eyepiece.

With the ×4 objective, the top lens of the condenser must be swung out and the condenser lowered to achieve even illumination. With the ×10, ×40, and ×100 oil-immersion objectives, the condenser remains at its top position with the top lens in the light path.

(d) Using the oil-immersion objective

As pointed out earlier the objectives should be matched for parfocality, and when changing from one to another only minimal, if any, focusing should be necessary. However, in the case of the ×100 oil-immersion objective it is necessary to connect the specimen to the objective with a drop of immersion oil. To do this the objective is separated from the slide enough to allow a drop of oil to be placed on the slide. While observing from the side, the objective and slide are slowly brought together until the objective is immersed in the oil. They are brought as close together as possible without being allowed to make contact. Looking down the eyepieces, slowly separate the objective and slide, using the fine focusing control, until the specimen appears in focus. After examination the objective lens and the slide preparation should be cleaned with a little xylene and lens-tissue paper.

REFERENCES

1. Culling, C. F. A. (1974). *Modern Microscopy; Elementary Theory and Practice*. London, Butterworth.
2. Hartley, W. F. (1979) *Hartley's Microscopy*, 2nd edn. Charlbury, Senecio.

PART TWO

Microbiology

7. Introduction to microbiology

The division of microbiology undertakes the investigation and assists with the control of diseases due to micro-organisms. These are classified biologically into four main groups, viruses, protozoa, bacteria, and fungi. Viruses are usually studied in a separate laboratory and fungi may be too. Hospitals with much tropical disease have a separate section to deal with parasites. Infected fluids, blood, excretions and discharges, and occasionally tissues, are received for examination. Swabs from throat, nose and other areas of the body are sent to the laboratory for culture whilst control of infection in the hospitals brings many other specimens such as dust and sterile supplies for examination. These specimens may be directly cultured on to culture media or examined microscopically with or without staining, or sometimes by animal inoculation. Investigation of antibodies in blood serum entails the mixing of serum with known cultures of organism or other antigens. This technique may be applied also for the investigation of particular types of organisms. Investigation of organisms in relation to their susceptibility or resistance to antibiotics is an important part of the work. Many laboratories do Public Health work, and this involves the examination of specimens such as water, dairy products and food.

Ideally when microbiological information is needed an appropriate specimen is taken from the right site, transported to the laboratory at once where it is processed immediately using the best tests which are correctly reported, and returned to the right place where results are properly interpreted at a time when the information is relevant. So it is most important that the results of the work done on a specimen in the laboratory are a true reflection of that specimen. For example in microbiology laboratories reports on cultures must indicate the presence of potential pathogens in the specimen, and if antimicrobial sensitivities are given they must be correct. It is known that there is variation in results between individual laboratories even when a divided specimen is examined by apparently the same methods in each. Reasons for failure to report an organism originally present in a specimen included delay in examination, the amount of specimen inoculated is insufficient, the amount of medium is insufficient, the medium is of doubtful quality or unsuitable for growth of the organisms present, the incubation period is too short or the wrong conditions are provided, too few colonies are examined or the organism is not recognised. Where possible, tests performed in reputable laboratories include internal standards whilst reagents and media are controlled by tests of performance using standard organisms and so on. The Public Health Laboratory Service provides a national scheme for microbiology quality control by providing simulated specimens through which participant laboratories can compare their results with others. In this way it is hoped that laboratories can be alerted to any inadequacy and their performance improved in consequence.

BACTERIAL CULTIVATION

One of the most notable activities of bacteria is reproduction; some growing under optimal conditions may divide as often as once every 20 minutes and some, such as vibrios, even more frequently. When a solitary bacterium multiplies on the surface of a suitable growth medium, such as after 18 hours' incubation at 37°C, the millions of bacteria produced become visible to the naked eye as a colony. Culture media must provide an adequate supply of energy and raw materials and be in an appropriate environment. Some organisms, e.g. *Mycobacterium leprae* and *Treponema pallidum*, are so fastidious that they can only grow in living tissue and will not grow in artificial culture media.

Energy

All pathogenic bacteria are chemotrophs, that is, they are able to derive energy from oxidation of chemical compounds. Of these, autotrophs can synthesise their own organic materials for their metabolism from inorganic sources. All parasitic bacteria with which we are mainly concerned are heterotrophs and require pre-synthesised material, although the quality of this may vary enormously.

43

Nutrition

Although there is great variation in the exact needs of various bacteria, it is fortunate that as a rule bacteria are very adaptable and are able to grow on a variety of media. Like higher forms of life, bacteria require water, a source of carbon, nitrogen, inorganic salts, metals, vitamins and other accessory growth factors. Nutrient materials provided artificially in a suitable form for growth are known as culture media (details of some commonly used media will be given later) and may be in the form of a liquid or a solid medium.

Oxygen requirements

Most bacteria will grow with or without free oxygen in their environment or under a wide range of oxygen tensions; these are called facultative anaerobes. Some species will only grow if oxygen is freely available; these are obligate aerobes. Others cannot grow in the presence of oxygen; these are obligate anaerobes. Other organisms will grow in the presence of traces of free oxygen and these are said to be micro-aerophilic.

Carbon dioxide

Carbon dioxide is needed in small amounts for the growth of many bacteria and larger amounts of 5–10% may improve growth. Additional carbon dioxide is essential for the isolation of *Neisseria gonorrhoeae* and *Brucella abortus*. These are described as carboxyphilic.

Hydrogen ion concentration

There is a narrow range of environmental pH for the growth of each species of bacteria, and for most of those which are pathogenic for man the optimum is between pH 6·5 and pH 7·5. The lactobacilli which are found in the vagina have an optimal pH of about 4·0 whilst *Vibrio cholerae* has an optimum pH of about 8·0, but these are exceptions.

Temperature

Bacteria have a range of temperature at which they prefer to grow. Most species parasitic on man have an optimal temperature of about 37°C, a range of growth between 25°C and 40°C and are said to be mesophilic.

Other bacteria grow best below 20°C and are called psychrophilic. Species flourishing at temperatures between 55°C and 80°C are thermophilic.

Light

The UV rays from the sun or from an artificial source are rapidly bactericidal. Bacteria are also sensitive to other radiations which may be used for sterilisation. Some bacteria produce a pigment in response to light and are called photochromogens.

Osmotic pressure

Most bacteria are tolerant of changes in the osmolarity of their growth medium because of the remarkable strength of their cell walls. Some food spoilage organisms are osmophilic and can grow in the presence of saturated solutions of salt or sugar. 'L' forms of bacteria, spheroplasts and mycoplasmas have much less tolerance because they have no cell wall.

INOCULATION

It is of primary importance that the laboratory study of micro-organisms is based on pure cultures. These cultures must be of a single clone or strain, that is, derived from the growth of a single organism. It is essential to avoid contamination by other organisms, therefore an aseptic technique is required during laboratory manoeuvres.

Plating out

Isolation of pure cultures from a mixture is generally done by plating the mixture out on a solid culture medium in a Petri dish using a wire inoculation loop. For most purposes this is achieved as in Fig. 7.1. Using a loaded inoculation loop or bacteriological swab, a primary inoculation is made over about a quarter of the surface of the plate.

If a swab has been used it is then discarded; if an inoculation loop is used it is now sterilised in a flame, allowed to cool, then a few parallel strokes made across a fresh part of the medium. The loop is then re-sterilised and cooled, and the procedure repeated using as inoculum the most distant part of the immediately preceding strokes. In this way the density of the inoculum is successively reduced so that eventually the organisms are separated and on subsequent incubation will give rise to individual colonies.

Inoculation for special purposes such as sensitivity testing is described elsewhere.

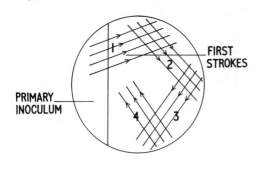

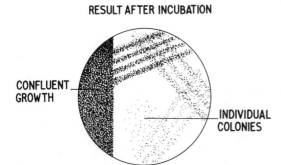

Fig. 7.1. Method of plating out to obtain separate colonies.

Inoculation of liquid media

Liquid media are dispensed in test-tubes with cotton wool plugs or some other form of cap, or in bottles such as bijoux and universal containers. Cotton wool plugs are removed from test-tubes before sub-culture or inoculation using the crook of the little finger of the hand holding the inoculation loop. The inner surface of the cotton wool plug must never be allowed to touch anything for fear of contamination, and may be lightly flamed before replacement. Pop-on and screw caps once loosened are held in the same way and not put down on the bench.

The mouth of the tube or bottle should be flamed momentarily after removing the top and again immediately before replacing. The inoculation is usually carried out using a Pasteur pipette, an inoculation loop or a swab. Once the cap has been removed, the exposed tubes are liable to contamination from air-borne particles which may be minimised by holding the tubes in an inclined position in the vicinity of the gas burner and by speed of working.

When liquid media are inoculated, particularly if from another liquid medium, it is essential that a purity plate is put up at the same time. To do this, solid medium of a suitable kind in a Petri dish is inoculated in the standard way.

Inoculation loops

Transfer of culture material and plating out is usually achieved using a wire inoculation loop or straight wire inserted into an aluminium handle. Inoculation loops may be made from Nicrome wire of 26 or 27 s.w.g. (standard wire gauge). The loops may be of different sizes for different purposes, but are generally between 1·5 mm and 5·0 mm internal diameter. The wire is wound round a rod of suitable diameter and, with a pair of scissors, one arm is cut leaving a loop. The other arm is cut some 50 or 60 mm from the loop, and the last 10 mm is bent back upon itself before this end is inserted into the wire holder. Platinum wire has been used in view of its toughness and resistance to repeated heating, but it is expensive and too soft. An alternative is to use a mixture of platinum (90%) and iridium (10%) which is much better. However, Nicrome wire is cheaper, more elastic and faster cooling, although it does not last as long. Disposable plastic loops in a limited range of sizes are now available and are useful and safer for purposes such as the plating out of faeces.

Wire inoculation loops are sterilised before and after use by holding nearly vertical in a gas flame where they are held until red hot. However, this can be dangerous because of spluttering, resulting in the dissemination of bacteria-containing particles. To overcome this, a hooded type of burner such as the Kampff burner should be used. Spluttering is also minimised if the loop is dipped into boiling water before being inserted into the flame. Loops must be allowed to cool before being used again to avoid thermal death of organisms on contact.

ANAEROBIC CULTURE

A number of methods have been described, but the most convenient for use in routine medical laboratories is that employing a modified McIntosh and Fildes jar. Air is removed from the jar and replaced with hydrogen. A cold catalyst in the jar then ensures the

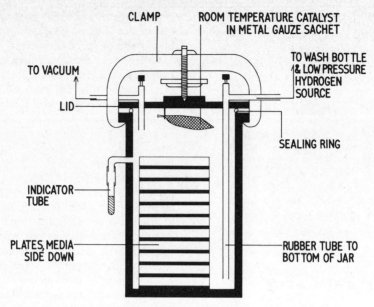

CLAMP   ROOM TEMPERATURE CATALYST IN METAL GAUZE SACHET

TO VACUUM

TO WASH BOTTLE & LOW PRESSURE HYDROGEN SOURCE

LID

SEALING RING

INDICATOR TUBE

PLATES, MEDIA SIDE DOWN

RUBBER TUBE TO BOTTOM OF JAR

Fig. 7.2.   Diagram of an anaerobic jar.

combination of any residual oxygen with the hydrogen resulting in anaerobiosis. The metal or polycarbonate jar is large enough to accommodate ten or more disposable polystyrene Petri dishes. The lid is usually fitted with two valves for connection to a hydrogen source and to a vacuum, and is secured by a clamp. There is a rubber ring-seal between the lid and the jar. A side-arm may be fitted to the jar which holds an external chemical indicator. The room-temperature catalyst consists of pellets of alumina coated with finely divided palladium which is enclosed in a metal gauze sachet (1 g per litre volume of jar). The use of a metal jar and a low-temperature catalyst minimises the risk of explosion which may occur when hydrogen combines with oxygen. The catalyst should be dry and changed after 30 anaerobic cycles.

Setting up an anaerobic jar (Fig. 7.2)

1. Place the cultures in the jar. If these are Petri dishes, place the pile so that the medium is lowermost. If they are placed as in an ordinary incubator with the medium uppermost there is a danger that the medium will flop when a vacuum is applied to the jar. If liquid cultures with screw caps are to be used, then the caps should either be loosened slightly or a No. 1 hypodermic needle, with the syringe end packed with sterile cotton wool, pushed through the top if there is a

suitable hole in the metal cap, to allow free flow of gases in and out of the bottle.

2. The lid is replaced and secured by the screw clamp.

3. One of the valves is attached by way of a gauge to a vacuum pump, and the jar is exhausted to a negative pressure of 300 mm Hg. The valve is then closed, if of the needle type, and the pump is disconnected. nected.

4. Carbon dioxide from a cylinder is passed into the jar until the pressure falls to minus 250 mm Hg.

5. The valve is connected to a low-pressure hydrogen source and the tap is opened to admit the hydrogen which at first is rapidly drawn into the jar. Then there is a short pause whilst catalysis occurs, then a further small volume of hydrogen is drawn into the jar to replace the gaseous hydrogen used up in combination with any residual oxygen which forms water; this takes about 10 min. The tap is then closed.

6. The jar is then placed in an incubator or hot-room, where any further catalysis continues.

It is important to see that the sachet containing the palladium catalyst is kept dry since the catalyst is inactivated by moisture. Whilst the jar is being incubated the Eh indicator (oxidation-reduction potential indicator) should change from a blue colour to colourless. The indicator most commony used includes methylene blue in its formula. This indicator can be obtained in sealed tubes or foil envelopes ready for use.

Another way of indicating that anaerobiosis has taken place is to include in the jar a culture of a strict anaerobe such as *Clostridium tetani*; this method is quite reliable if the indicator organism grows. Another indication of anaerobiosis is a change in colour from bright red to a much duller brownish-red of the commonly used blood agar plates due to reduction of their haemoglobin content.

Hydrogen source

Hydrogen can be obtained using a Kipp's or similar apparatus with hydrochloric acid acting on zinc, but it is much more convenient to use a cylinder of compressed hydrogen. Hydrogen cylinders must be fitted with a low-pressure or reducing valve and the gas must be delivered at not more than 0·5 p.s.i. A suitable low-pressure system incorporates either a football bladder or an aspirator system, both of which are filled from a cylinder. Another alternative is to use either the Gas Generating Kit (Oxoid) or the 'GasPak' system of disposable gas generator envelopes (Becton, Dickinson and Co., BBL). In these systems suitable chemical combinants are enclosed in a metal foil container and are activated by the addition of tap or distilled water to the container according to the instructions on the envelope, which then liberates hydrogen and carbon dioxide. In use, one of these is placed in the anaerobic jar with the culture material. Since some organisms grow better in an atmosphere containing 5% carbon dixode, and none is adversely affected by it, a mixture of 95% hydrogen and 5% carbon dioxide may be used with advantage. Cylinders containing this mixture can be obtained (British Oxygen Co. Ltd.), but the cylinders must be kept horizontal during use.

Opening the anaerobic jar

The external indicator is first checked to see that it is colourless, then one of the needle valves is opened; this should be accompanied by a hiss of in-rushing air which is evidence that the jar is air-tight. After removal of the cultures the jar is cleaned and dried, and should be stored in a warm, dry place.

Note: Anaerobic culture can also be achieved by using special media such as Robertson's cooked-meat medium and thioglycollate broth which contain reducing substances, but do not require incubation in an oxygen-free atmosphere.

Cultivation in carbon dioxide

This can be done in incubators produced commercially for the purpose which are designed to keep the level of carbon dioxide in the incubator between 5 and 10%. These use bottled gas as a source. Bottled gas may also be used together with an aerobic jar which is partially evacuated, after which the evacuated air is replaced by carbon dioxide from the cylinder as described for hydrogen. If bottled gas is not available, a simple method is to use a container, such as a biscuit tin, in which the cultures are placed together with a 100 ml beaker. A few marble chips, 1–2 g, are placed in the beaker, and before incubation about 10 ml (excess) of 2 M hydrochloric acid are poured on to the chips. The lid is then placed on the box and should be sealed on with adhesive tape. Another simple alternative often employed in the culture of *Neisseria gonorrhoeae* is to use a special copper container which holds a stack of Petri dishes on the top of which is placed a night-light. The night-light is lit and the top replaced before incubation. Carbon dioxide is one of the products of combustion.

Incubation

Inoculated media are incubated at a temperature which is about the optimum for the organisms being cultivated. For most pathogenic bacteria this will be 37°C. Solid media on plates are incubated in thermostatically controlled, electrically heated incubators or in a specially built warm room. Bacteria are usually incubated in the dark. Inoculated plates are placed media side up to prevent water of condensation from falling onto the medium and thus preventing the formation of discrete colonies. If incubation is to be prolonged then the Petri dishes should be sealed with adhesive tape or the plates placed in sealed containers or plastic bag, to prevent the drying-up of the medium. Liquid media in tubes or bottles should be placed in suitable racks and may be incubated in an ordinary incubator or hot-room. Alternatively they can be incubated in a water-bath at the desired temperature.

Preservation of stock cultures

Stock cultures are required for antibiotic sensitivity test controls, testing culture media, teaching and for comparison such as in the plate test for the identification of diphtheria toxin.

Lyophilisation

Freeze-drying preserves bacteria for very long periods and is the method of choice for long-term storage. A freeze-drying machine is required for this purpose. The organism is suspended in 30% glucose nutrient broth to which is added three volumes of sterile serum. Small volumes of this suspension are placed in glass ampoules which are sealed in a gas flame at the time of process whilst there is still a vacuum in the ampoule.

Ampoules of freeze-dried cultures from the National Collection of Type Cultures contain a piece of card with the code number on it and a piece of cotton wool to prevent contamination of the culture when the ampoule is opened. To open an ampoule a score is made round the tube, distal to the cotton wool, with a glass-marking diamond, and then the red-hot end of a piece of heated glass rod is applied to the score so that (it is hoped) a crack occurs along the score. The tip can then be pulled off. The freeze-dried deposit is then rehydrated aseptically, in a few drops of sterile distilled water, and both this liquid suspension and the piece of card with the code on it are transferred into some suitable liquid medium to rejuvenate before sub-culture.

Freezing

Many bacteria can survive for a long time when frozen as a suspension in sterile water or nutrient broth at −20°C in bijou bottles, or even longer in drops of broth in liquid nitrogen.

Drying

Bacteria in 10% serum or gelatin broth can be stored dried on cellophane discs in screw-capped bottles. The discs are dried in a vacuum-desiccator containing phosphorus pentoxide as the drying agent.

Sub-cultures

Most organisms can be maintained by serial sub-culture on suitable media, but care must be taken not to introduce contaminants and to minimise the risk of selection of a mutant by using an inoculum of several colonies each time, only incubating the new culture long enough to get the organism into the log phase.

Many organisms will survive for long periods in or on commonly used media such as Robertson's cooked meat in screw-capped bottles kept at room temperature in the dark. Haemolytic streptococci will survive for months on blood agar slopes in bijou bottles and enterobacteria and staphylococci last for years in agar stabs in bijou bottles. Many other bacteria will survive for long periods on Dorset's egg medium.

For organisms which are required frequently, such as the Oxford staphylococcus and the standard strain of *E. coli* used in sensitivity testing, the following is recommended:

Pure cultures of the organism are freeze-dried and kept in reserve. At the same time a stab culture in nutrient agar is made and incubated overnight before storage in a drawer. This is sub-cultured into broth each week for use and sub-cultured every month or so as another agar stab for maintenance.

8. Examination of specimens

APPARATUS

Containers

Strong, leak-proof, sterile containers of adequate size must be provided for the transmission of specimens from source to the laboratory. All medical specimen containers should conform to the relevant British Standards Specification, such as BS.4851:1972, *Medical specimen containers for Haematology and Biochemistry*, currently under revision, and have obtained the British Standards Kitemark. Standards pay particular attention to minimising the health hazard from leakage, fine spray, or spread of air-borne particles when opening a container holding a specimen. The following containers are in common use:

1. 6 ml glass 'bijou' bottle with a screw cap suitable for body fluids, transport media and bacteriological cultures.
2. 28 ml glass 'universal container' with a screw cap suitable for a wide variety of specimens including pus, exudate, skin scrapings, tissue, blood, CSF, urine and faeces. They are also used to contain culture media. Disposable plastic containers of this size are useful.
3. 300 ml glass 'honey jar' or similar plastic disposable bottle suitable for such specimens as complete early-morning urines, tissues and sanitary specimens.
4. Disposable plastic containers are available for special purposes such as holding sputum and faeces.

In general, plastic containers tend to leak more readily than glass containers. Screw-threaded caps appear the safest. Labels should be suitable for marking with a ballpoint pen, have sufficient space for name, address, date and nature of specimen, and have a moisture-resistant adhesive back. Any of the smaller containers selected for use from the large number on the market must be suitable for transmission through the post.

Swabs

Bacteriological swabs are made from a pledget of cotton wool attached to the end of a holder made of wood, plastic or metal, the whole of which is sterilised before use. These swabs are used for sampling where microbial infection or contamination is suspected. Material containing the microbes is taken up on the cotton wool, as in the swabbing of a throat or a wound. Most kinds of swab are available commercially either complete and sterile or as separate units which require assembly and sterilisation.

Swabs for most purposes can be made using commercially prepared wooden applicator sticks. Alternatively, aluminium wire of 15 gauge and 150 mm in length. One end is roughened by squeezing it in a small metal-working vice, or by rolling between two coarse rasps, one being fixed to a board and the other fitted with a wooden handle. Alternatively, a thin pledget of absorbent cotton wool is tightly wrapped round one end of the holder for 10–20 mm. The whole is then placed in a narrow thick-walled test-tube 125 × 12 mm and the top of the tube is plugged with cotton wool. Laboratory made swabs are best sterilised in an autoclave but hot-air ovens are used, although some charring of the cotton wool may occur, possibly liberating substances toxic to bacteria.

Much thought has gone into the problem of survival of bacteria and viruses on such cotton wool swabs, not only because of possible toxicity of the cotton wool but also because of the slow drying of the material on the swabs. The use of absorbent cotton wool has been challenged and the use of non-absorbent wool advocated; however, overheating of this material during sterilisation may release toxic substances. Serum-coated cotton wool swabs have also been recommended as prolonging the viability of organisms; these are prepared by dipping the cotton wool end of the swab into undiluted ox serum for about half a minute, drying, and finally sterilising in an autoclave at 121°C for 20 minutes. Activated charcoal has the power to absorb many substances which are toxic to delicate bacteria such as those of the genus *Neisseria*. This fact has been used in the preparation of 'charcoal' swabs which are made by dipping the cotton wool end of the swabs into a dense suspension of activated charcoal (Oxoid) in water and then sterilising the whole of the swab in a hot-air oven. These swabs are generally used only with Stuart's transport medium and are not suitable for use when microscopy is required.

Laryngeal swabs

Laryngeal swabs are used in the investigation of pulmonary tuberculosis when it is not possible to obtain sputum. Satisfactory swabs can be made using 15 s.w.g. aluminium wire in 300 mm lengths, one end of which has been flattened and roughened to take a pledget of nylon wool which is wrapped round the end in the same way as for ordinary bacteriological swabs. The nylon wool must have been washed in ether and dried before being attached to the wire. The wire is bent at an angle of 120° some 35 to 40 mm from the cotton wool end and then placed in a 200×28 mm boiling tube which is plugged with cotton wool. The protruding wire end is then bent back parallel with the boiling tube for convenience. Before use these swabs are sterilised in an autoclave at 121°C for 20 minutes. These swabs should only be used by trained personnel who will pass the swab to the larynx under the guidance of a laryngeal mirror. This procedure is not without danger since it initiates a reflex cough from the patient which may result in an aerosol containing tubercle bacilli.

Per-nasal swabs

These swabs are used for the collection of material from the nasopharynx and are an alternative to the use of cough plates for the diagnosis of whooping cough which is caused by *Bordetella pertussis*. Per-nasal swabs can be made in the same way as bacteriological swabs substituting a thinner wire such as 27 gauge Nicrome wire (used in the making of inoculation loops). Similar swabs with alginate wool tips are available commercially and are particularly useful in the investigation of whooping-cough.

Alginate wool (Medical Alginates Limited) can be used for all types of swab in place of the more usual cotton wool. It has the advantage that it is soluble in 'Calgen-Ringer solution'. The swabs are prepared using approximately 0·05 g of wool per swab and are sterilised by autoclaving at 121°C for 15 minutes. After sampling, the swab is aseptically broken or clipped off into a few millilitres of Calgon-Ringer solution and shaken vigorously for a minute or so, until the alginate dissolves, releasing all the organisms picked up. The suspension is then cultured in the usual way. However, there is some doubt about the ability of some organisms such as streptococci to survive on this type of wool, and this may be a contra-indication to its general use in bacteriological swabs.

Sterile capillary pipettes

Cutting glass tubing

To cut glass tubing a definite scratch is made on the surface of a piece of tubing with either a diamond-tipped glass-marking pencil, a glass-cutting knife or the edge of a triangular file. Holding the tubing with the scratch uppermost, the thumbs are placed on the under surface of the tubing, one on each side of the scratch, and gripping the tubing with the fingers both hands are jerked downwards and outwards using the thumbs as fulcrums.

Capillary pipettes (Pasteur)

These are usually obtained from commercial sources. They can be made from 200 mm lengths of 6 mm bore glass tubing which are heated in the middle by rotating them, always in the same direction in the hot part of a gas flame until the glass is melted. The glass is then withdrawn from the flame and, after a few moments, is drawn out into a thin capillary about 250 mm long. The hands are held steady maintaining just sufficient pull on the tubing to keep the capillary straight until the glass hardens. The capillary is then broken in the middle, producing two pipettes. These are finished off by rounding the wide end by holding in a flame and rotating slowly until the sharp edges just soften without the ends of the tubes becoming distorted. When cool, this end is plugged with cotton wool and the capillary end is sealed in a Bunsen flame. For sterilisation, they should be placed in a container such as a large test-tube with a cotton wool pad in the bottom, and closed with a cotton wool plug if it has no cap of its own before sterilising in a hot-air oven.

Measured-drop pipettes

Capillary pipettes can be prepared to give drops of a known volume. After the pipette has cooled, the capillary is inserted into the appropriate hole of a Morse drill gauge and pressed through it until it just fits. To make a '50 dropper' for water, that is 50 drops to the millilitre (each drop 0·020 ml), the hole used is Morse 59 (0·041 in diameter).

These pipettes must be standardised for each different

liquid used because of variations in surface tensions and viscosity. This can be done by counting the number of drops required to fill a 10 ml measuring cylinder, or it may be done by pipetting exactly 1 ml of fluid on to the surface of a watch glass which has previously been dipped in molten paraffin wax and allowed to cool. It will be found that the whole of this 1 ml can be taken up into the pipette if a suitable rubber teat is used; then the number of drops in 1 ml are counted. An alternative is to use a dropping pipette made of glass but which has a piece of platinum tube let into the end. These only require calibrating once for each liquid and can be used over and over again. A variety of calibrated micro-pipettes with disposable plastic ends are now available from commercial sources.

In the examination of clinical specimens for microbes it is important to look for the well known causes and at the same time to allow a reasonable chance of finding those which are less common or unusual.

BLOOD

Blood culture

1. CASTAÑEDA'S METHOD (aerobic)

Medium

Brain–heart infusion agar slope in bottle containing 45 ml brain–heart infusion broth ×2. Alternatively, Bacto Fluid Thioglycollate Medium (Difco) can be used in the same way but will support the growth of anaerobes as well as aerobes.

Procedure

(a) Add 5 ml of blood aseptically to each of two bottles of medium through the perforated cap.

(b) Mix and tip momentarily to cover the slope, then incubate at 37°C.

(c) Examine slope for growth after 18 hr incubation, repeat the tipping process and reincubate.

(d) Re-examine and tip every day for at least 2 or 3 weeks before discarding.

(e) Any colonies appearing on the slope are identified in the usual way.

Note: This method is good for isolation of brucellae if additional CO_2 is added to each bottle. Incubate cultures for brucellae for 6 weeks.

2. BROTH METHOD

Media

Aerobes—45 ml glucose broth ×2
Anaerobes—
  (i) 45 ml thioglycollate medium (Brewer's)
  (ii) 10 ml Robertson's cooked-meat medium usually one bottle of one of these in addition to aerobic culture.

Note: Sodium polyanethol sulphonate ('Liquoid') can be added to these media (0·05%) to destroy complement and help prevent coagulation but inhibits some streptococci.

Procedure

(a) Add 5 ml of blood to 45 ml volumes (2 ml to 10 ml) of medium aseptically through the perforated cap and mix.

(b) Examine for growth after 18 hours' incubation at 37°C.

(c) If there is growth in any bottle.
  (i) Gram stain
  (ii) Sub-culture on to
    Blood agar (aerobic)
    Blood agar (anaerobic)
    MacConkey's agar plus DCA or XLD
then identify in the usual way.

(d) Report to the pathologist any positive findings as soon as possible.

(e) If there is no visible growth after 18 hr incubation, then one of the bottles should be carefully sub-cultured as above and the bottle marked for identification.

(f) All bottles are then reincubated.

(g) Bottles are inspected daily for growth.

(h) If negative at the end of 2 weeks, sub-culture all bottles; if sub-cultures are negative, then discard and report 'No growth'.

Organisms

Staphylococcus aureus (may form a clot in the culture), *Staph. epidermidis* (possible contaminant from skin, but may be the infecting organism especially if obtained from more than one bottle).
Propionobacterium acnes from the skin
Brucellae
Streptococcus pyogenes, *Str. viridans*, *Str. pneumoniae*, *Str. faecalis*, enterobacteria including *Escherichia coli*, klebsiellae and salmonellae
Neisseria meningitidis

Pseudomonas aeruginosa
Bacteroides, clostridia.

Positive blood cultures must be reported to the pathologist at once. Any organism isolated must be fully considered before it is discarded as a contaminant.

Appropriate antimicrobial sensitivity tests must be undertaken.

Never keep inoculated blood cultures in a refrigerator, but incubate at once.

The majority of detectable bacteraemias will be discovered by the first three sets of blood cultures.

Bone marrow

Films
  Gram stain
  Ziehl-Neelsen stain
Media
  Blood agar
  Chocolate agar (5–10% CO_2)
  Two Lowenstein-Jensen slopes
Organisms
  Salmonella typhi, brucellae, *Mycobacterium tuberculosis*

CEREBROSPINAL FLUID

The specimen should arrive in at least three labelled bottles which are also numbered, 'first', 'second', etc. If a glucose level is required, one of the bottles should contain fluoride. Specimens for culture must be in sterile bottles such as universal bottles.

Procedure

(a) Note approximate total volume.

(b) Take the last part to be withdrawn, i.e. the second or third bottle.

(c) Note appearance:
  (i) whether turbid or clear
  (ii) colour, i.e. blood-stained or xanthochromic (yellow)
  (iii) presence or absence of a clot.

(d) Mix well and, using a sterile Pasteur pipette, aseptically transfer a small volume to a modified Fuchs-Rosenthal counting chamber.

(e) Perform:
  (i) total cell count
  (ii) total white cell count (red cell amount by subtraction).

If the specimen is heavily blood-stained or contains a large number of white cells, mix, then transfer a small quantity of the fluid aseptically to another tube. Dilute a known volume of this with white cell diluting fluid to lyse the red cells and stain up the white cells. Use a white blood cell counting pipette of the Thoma type, or another reasonably accurate method, to obtain a dilution of 1 in 10 or 1 in 20.

White cell diluting fluid contains 1% glacial acetic acid and a violet stain. It should be given a few minutes to work after the dilution has been made.

(f) Centrifuge the rest of the CSF in the second or third bottle at 2000–3000 rev/min for 5 min. This may require aseptic transfer of the CSF to a sterile centrifuge tube.

(g) Decant the supernatant CSF, noting its colour, into another bottle or tube for other investigations such as protein estimation or virology.

(h) Resuspend the deposit by gently tapping the tube then:
  (i) Culture on to
    blood agar
    chocolate agar
    Robertson's meat broth with 10% serum added
    two Lowenstein-Jensen slopes.
  (ii) Make three films on microscope slides:
    stain one with Gram's stain
    stain one with a Romanowski stain such as Leishman or Giemsa for a differential cell count
    stain one by the Ziehl-Neelsen method.

Colouring and turbidity in CSF are abnormal except when due to haemorrhage caused by the lumbar puncture. Turbidity begins when the white-cell count exceeds about 200 per μl. A red colour indicates blood mixed with the CSF either at the time of puncture or not more than 6 hours previously. A yellow colour, xanthochromia, results from mixture with blood more than 6 hours before the sample or when the permeability of the meninges to such substances as bilirubin, carotenes and lipochromes is increased as in meningitis or when the circulation is blocked by a tumour. CSF is normally sterile.

The Fuchs-Rosenthal counting chamber was designed for counting the cells in cerebrospinal fluid. The modified chamber (Fig. 8.1) has only 9 large squares instead of the 16 in the original.

The chamber is 0·2 mm deep and each of the smallest squares is $\frac{1}{16}$ mm^2. Each large square contains 16 of the small squares.

If the 4 large squares at the corners plus the middle one are counted (total: 5 large squares = 80 small ones) then, provided there has been no dilution, the number of cells counted in these 5 squares is the number per mm³ or microlitre (μl). If dilution has been necessary, then the number counted in 5 large squares is multiplied by the dilution factor to give the count per μl.

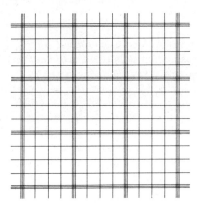

Fig. 8.1. Rulings of modified Fuchs–Rosenthal counting chamber.

For a dilution of 1 in 10 using a white-cell diluting pipette (Fig. 8.2), suck up the CSF (from the transferred portion) to the mark 1·0 on the pipette, wipe the end with a tissue, then fill to the 11 mark beyond the bulb. Mix by swirling so that the white bead moves around. Discharge the pipette into another clean tube and draw up and down a few times to mix. Transfer the fluid to the chamber using a thin-walled capillary tube. Dilutions of 1 in 20 are made in a similar way, but the

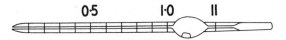

Fig. 8.2. White cell diluting pipette.

pipette is only filled up to the 0·5 mark with the CSF before filling the remainder of the pipette to the 11 mark with diluting fluid.

Organisms causing meningitis

Haemophilus influenzae is the most common cause in children under 5 years of age.

Neisseria meningitidis is common in children and is the most common cause in young adults and the elderly.

Streptococcus pneumoniae occurs mainly in the very young and the elderly.

Enterobacteria, *Pseudomonas* species, haemolytic streptococci, staphylococci and listeria tend to occur secondary to septicaemia and in neonates. *Mycobacterium tuberculosis* is not infrequent.

Leptospires and viruses usually cause transient meningitis, but viruses can also cause serious encephalomyelitis.

Very occasionally meningitis is caused by a yeast-like organism, *Cryptococcus neoformans* (demonstrated by an Indian ink preparation) and also very rarely by amoebae, e.g. *Naegleria*, seen in the counting chamber.

If there is a spidery clot, then culture part of this on Lowenstein-Jensen medium and stain the remainder on a microscope slide with Ziehl-Neelsen stain and examine for AFB.

Some properties of cerebrospinal fluid are given in Table 8.1.

URINE

Examination of early morning urine specimens for tuberculosis is described in the section on 'Routine

Table 8.1.   Cerebrospinal fluid

	Appearance	Cells	Protein	Glucose
Normal	Clear, colourless	0–4 lymphocytes per microlitre (μl)	0·2–0·4 g/l	0·3–1 mmol/l below blood level (2·5–4 mmol/l)
Bacterial meningitis	Turbid	Mainly polymorphs few lymphocytes	Raised (up to 4g/l)	Reduced
Tuberculous meningitis	Clear, opalescent or turbid	Mainly lymphocytes some polymorphs	Moderately raised	Usually reduced
Cerebral abscess	Turbid	Up to 1000/μl; mainly polymorphs some lymphocytes	Raised	Increased
Aseptic or viral meningitis	Clear or turbid	Increased; mainly lymphocytes	Slight increase	Normal

culture of mycobacteria' (p. 86). The diagnosis of urinary tract infections is based on the enumeration of bacteria in the urine. The presence of inflammation in the urinary tract is demonstrated by showing an increase in white cell excretion.

Collection of specimens

There is very little point in examining badly taken urine specimens, particularly from females, since the results are likely to be misleading. For the diagnosis of urinary tract infections, other than urethritis and prostatitis, it is usual to examine mid-stream urine. In the male this simply amounts to retraction of the foreskin if necessary, then passing the first part of the stream of the urine into the lavatory and catching the latter part in a sterile container.

In females it is more difficult, particularly when there is menstrual or vaginal discharge although the use of a vaginal tampon is helpful. The patients should be instructed to swab the vulva from before backwards whilst separating the labia with two fingers of one hand using a cotton wool or sponge swab soaked in sterile water, or if necessary, ordinary soap. Antiseptics must not be used. Keeping the labia separate, she passes the first part of the stream of urine into the lavatory and catches the second part in a sterile container. In babies and young children, clean catch specimens are difficult to collect and urine collected in adhesive bags is frequently contaminated. When diagnosis is urgent, percutaneous suprapubic aspiration of urine is undertaken by the doctor.

Catheterisation in order to obtain a specimen for culture is frowned upon because of the very real danger of initiating a urinary tract infection, but if catheterisation is being carried out for another purpose it is a good opportunity to culture the urine, when indicated.

Preservation of specimens

Urine should be examined within 1½–2 hours of collection; if this is not possible, then specimens can be refrigerated at 4°C for up to 48 hours without much change in the bacterial count, but the white cells may deteriorate rapidly, notably in alkaline or hypotonic urine. Where delay is unavoidable and refrigeration is not possible, such as when specimens are sent by post, the addition of 0·5 g of boric acid to a sterile universal container (28 ml), inhibits the multiplication of urinary pathogens without significant reduction in their numbers for up to three days. Alternatively by a dip-slide or dip-spoon method may be used.

Examination

1. Appearance

Normal freshly voided urine is clear and pale yellow in colour. Pus and crystals cause turbidity, and blood in small amounts gives the urine a smoky appearance, whilst fresh blood is obvious. Occasionally urine is an unusual colour, such as after taking certain drugs and dyes; an extreme example is the blue-green colour of the urine after taking proprietary backache and kidney pills containing methylene blue. Other causes of coloured urine are mentioned in the chemistry section.

2. pH

Urine pH varies with the nature of the food, intake of some drugs and the acid–base balance of an individual, so it is not a good indicator of tubular function in the uncontrolled situation, but may provide useful information to the clinician. pH affects the activity of some antimicrobial agents in the urine, for instance the aminoglycosides are much more effective in an alkaline medium, whereas the tetracyclines and mandelic acid are more effective in acid urine and hexamine will only work in an acid medium.

Knowing the pH of urine also aids in identifying crystalline deposits. Phosphates are deposited in alkaline urine whilst calcium oxalate, uric acid and some urates are found in acid urine. Organisms which split urea such as *Proteus* species and *Klebsiella* species cause the urine to be alkaline by the production of ammonia. The pH of urine can be determined accurately enough for routine bacteriological examination of urine, using indicator papers.

3. Protein

Easily detectable amounts of protein in the urine, that is, more than 0·2 g/litre, are abnormal. Persistent proteinuria is usually due to changes in glomeruli whilst intermittent proteinuria is more likely to be associated with disease of the lower urinary tract. It is better to test for proteinuria by precipitation either by boiling or by the addition of salicylsulphonic acid, than to use stick tests such as 'Albustix' which do not detect Bence-Jones (myeloma) protein. The results of tests for proteinuria are traditionally expressed in a semi-quantitative manner varying from a trace ($\pm$) to a heavy precipitate ($+ + + +$).

4. Sugar

Many Bacteriology Departments include a stick test for glucose as a screen for diabetes.

5. Microscopy

(a) White blood cells

White blood cells are excreted in normal urine and the average rate is about 50,000 white cells per hour with an upper limit of normal usually accepted as 200,000 per hour, whilst more than 400,000 per hour is definitely abnormal. It has been found that patients who excrete more than 400,000 white cells per hour have more than 10 white cells per μl in well-mixed urine from a mid-stream urine specimen and more than 3 white cells per high-power field when a centrifuged deposit is examined. In children and adults, 3 or less white cells per μl can be regarded as normal but in infants less than 10 white cells per μl is considered normal.

The white cell count is performed on well-mixed fresh urine using a modified Fuchs-Rosenthal counting chamber in the same way as for cerebrospinal fluid. The use of a centrifuged deposit in gauging the white cell content of urine is only useful when five or more white cells are seen per high-power field, when it can be safely assumed that there is a high urinary excretion of white cells. When there are three or less white cells per high-power field the white cell excretion rate may be normal or raised. However, a Gram stain of a drop of centrifuge deposit may be useful and provide early information about infection.

Useful results from white cell estimations can only be obtained from carefully collected uncontaminated specimens. In females with a purulent vaginal discharge it may be necessary to insert a vaginal tampon before swabbing the vulva in order to get a satisfactory specimen.

Persistently sterile pyuria in the absence of anti-microbial chemotherapy may be caused by renal tuberculosis, and if this is suspected three early morning urines should be examined.

(b) Red blood cells and casts

The rate of excretion of red blood cells is approximately the same as for white blood cells. Increased numbers may be of menstrual origin in females or from a lesion in the urinary tract.

Squamous epithelial cells are often present in small numbers in normal urine specimens. Large numbers are an indication of vaginal or vulval contamination. Parallel-sided casts of renal tubules are sometimes seen and are of three main types. Hyaline casts are transparent without any cells attached to their surfaces and are of no importance clinically.

Red cell casts are characterised by a diffuse orange-yellow colour which is haemoglobin, and these indicate that the red cells which they contain have originated in the kidneys and not lower down the urinary tract. Other cellular casts may be composed of the desquamated tubular cells. Granular casts are degenerated cellular casts. Spermatozoa when present are reported since the presence of semen in the urinary tract may account for an apparent increase in white cells and albumen. The presence of small amounts of mucus in urine is normal.

(c) Bacterial count

When urine is passed normally, some contamination of the urine by organisms of the urethra and vulva often occurs, although the effect of this upon culture is minimised by the use of mid-stream urine specimens. It is generally accepted that bacteria from this source will number less than 10^4 organisms per ml in freshly voided urine. On the other hand, if a single specimen of freshly voided mid-stream urine contains 10^5 or more bacteria per ml then there is an 85% probability of this being due to a urinary tract infection. A count of more than 10^5 organisms per ml on two consecutive occasions increases the probability of infection to about 99%.

When the number of organisms in the urine is between 10^4 and 10^5 per ml, particularly if there is a mixture of different bacterial species present, a poor collection technique is suggested, or delay in reaching the laboratory, or inadequate storage. Occasionally counts falling within this range are found in the early stages of infection, particularly in men, or they may be due to the lack of time for the organisms to multiply in the urine when an infection is present due to inhibitory substances in the urine. For these reasons, if a specimen gives a count between 10^4 and 10^5 organisms per ml it should be repeated, with a properly taken mid-stream urine. If all the specimens were collected properly and dealt with promptly only about 5% would fall into this category.

For special purposes a surface viable count is used, similar to those described in Chapter 15, which is better than a pour-plate method. Measured volumes of well-mixed dilutions of urine in sterile Ringer's solution are spread on well-dried blood agar plates and the colonies counted after overnight incubation at 37°C. It is assumed that each bacterium produces one colony in the inoculum and the dilution being known, the number of bacteria present per ml of urine can be calculated. In practice, one plate is inoculated with 0·1 ml of well-mixed undiluted urine and for another plate 0·1 ml of the undiluted urine is added to 9·9 ml of sterile Ringer's solution which is then mixed thoroughly, and 0·1 ml of the urine/Ringer's solution mixture is then spread on a plate so that each colony grown on this plate represents 1000 bacteria per ml of urine.

For routine purposes, surface viable counts are too time-consuming and so a semi-quantitative method is used. In these a standard method of inoculating the culture medium is used so that the number of colonies seen after incubation is proportional to the number of bacteria present in the urine. These methods are standardised against surface viable counts. Two semi-quantitative methods are in general use and these are described below.

1. *Filter paper test.* Pieces of filter paper (Postlip) 75 mm × 6 mm with a fold 12 mm from one end, are sterilised in a hot-air oven at 160°C for 1 hr, or can be obtained commercially ready for use (Mast Laboratories). In use one of the strips is dipped into the urine to a level just above the fold. It is held vertically for a few seconds with the folded end uppermost, then an impression of the 12 × 6 mm part is made on the surface of a well-dried MacConkey agar plate. Using another strip, a duplicate is made by the side of the first impression; up to eight such duplicate tests can be done on one plate.

The number of colonies in the area of each impression is counted and compared with a standard curve to give the bacterial count of the urine. Twenty-five colonies represents approximately 1000 organisms per ml, but this depends upon the nature of the paper used. In addition to the impression culture on MacConkey's medium a loop culture should be made on blood agar.

2. *Standard loop method.* In this method a particular size of inoculation loop is chosen which will result in a countable number of colonies. This can be made from either platinum wire welded to form a loop, or of Nicrome (nickel-chromium) wire which will have to be replaced more often to prevent inaccuracy due to distortion. Loops of 2, 3, 4 or 5 mm internal diameter are commonly used. The loop is dipped into the urine and removed vertically, then discharged by two or three strokes along a single diameter of the plate. This primary inoculum is then spread using the same loops across the whole surface of the plate by strokes at right-angles to the primary inoculum. One method is to use a 5 mm internal diameter 24 gauge Nicrome wire loop and to inoculate a blood agar plate for the count. This size of loop will deliver 0·005 ml ± 5% so that 50 colonies represents 10^4 organisms per ml. Standard loops can be obtained from commercial sources. All loops must be standardised before use.

The counts should be performed on blood agar, and it is advisable to use a medium such as MacConkey's agar in addition. This can be done conveniently using plastic Petri dishes with a central division, pouring blood agar into one compartment and MacConkey's agar into the other. With half-size plates a standard loop delivering 0·002 ml is used.

OTHER SPECIMENS

Ear swab

Film: Gram stain
Culture
    Blood agar (aerobic)
    Blood agar (anaerobic)
    Kanamycin agar (anaerobic)
    MacConkey's agar
    Sabouraud's agar
Organisms
Pseudomonas aeruginosa, staphylococci, *Streptococcus pneumoniae*, haemolytic streptococci, *Proteus* spp., coliforms, *Haemophilus* spp., corynebacteria, clostridia, *Aspergillus* spp.

Eye swabs

Film: Gram stain
Culture
    Blood agar (CO_2)
    Chocolate agar (CO_2)
Organisms
Staphylococci, *Haemophilus* spp., *Streptococcus pneumoniae*, *Str. viridans*, *Neisseria gonorrhoeae* (ophthalmia neonatorum), corynebacteria, coliforms and viruses such as *Adenovirus*.

Faeces and rectal swabs

Faeces are preferred to rectal swabs for all bacteriological examinations. If faeces are unobtainable then a rectal swab with visible faeces on it may be substituted. A mere anal swab is no use for this purpose.

Procedure

(a) Description. Describe the macroscopic appearance of the faeces such as whether formed or fluid; indicate the presence of blood, melaena, pus or mucus. Mention any other abnormality.

(b) Films

(i) Wet preparation, examine for red blood cells, white blood cells, Charcot-Leyden crystals, ova etc.

(ii) Concentration for parasites if required (for method *see* Parasitology).

(iii) Gram stained film if staphylococcal enterocolitis is suspected.

(c) Routine culture

(i) Desoxycholate-citrate agar (DCA) and xyloselysine-desoxycholate agar (XLD). These media are heavily inoculated.

(ii) Selenite F enrichment broth. 0·5–1·0 g of faeces is emulsified in the enrichment broth which is incubated at 37°C overnight before sub-culture on to the DCA and XLD media.

(d) If it is suspected that the cause is other than bacillary dysentery or salmonella food poisoning then one or more of the following media may be required in addition to DCA, XLD and selenite F.

(i) Enteropathogenic *Eshericha coli* in children under two years of age:
Blood agar
MacConkey's agar
(ii) *Salmonella typhi:*
tetrathionate broth
(iii) *Clostridium welchii* food poisoning:
Neomycin blood agar
Neomycin egg yolk agar
Robertson's cooked-meat medium or
Thioglycollate broth
(iv) *Staphylococcus aureus* enterocolitis:
Salt mannitol agar
(v) *Vibrio cholera*, El Tor vibrio:
TCBS
alkaline peptone water
(vi) *Campylobacter jejuni*
Skirrow's medium
(vii) *Vibrio parahaemolyticus:*
TCBS
salt mannitol agar
(viii) *Candida albicans:*
Sabouraud's agar

Examinations for faecal pathogens are described together with the general description of these organisms.

Fluids (including hydrocele, pericardial, peritoneal (ascitic), pleural and synovial fluids).

Procedure

If frankly purulent treat as pus, otherwise centrifuge and use the deposit.

Films:
Gram stain
Ziehl-Neelsen stain
Culture
Blood agar (aerobic)
Blood agar (anaerobic)
Kanamycin agar (anaerobic)
Chocolate agar (CO_2)
Robertson's cooked-meat medium
Two Lowenstein-Jensen slopes
Organisms
Streptococci, staphylococci, coliforms, gonococci, *Haemophilus* spp., mycobacteria, bacteroides and other anaerobes.

Gastric lavage

Treat as sputum for tuberculosis, *see* section on mycobacteria (p. 85).

Laryngeal swab

See section on mycobacteria (p. 85).

Nasal swabs

1. Anterior nares

Culture: Blood agar (aerobic)
Organisms
Staphylococcus aureus, Streptococcus pyogenes

2. Posterior nares

Culture
Blood agar (aerobic)
Chocolate agar (CO_2)
Tellurite agar
Organisms
Neisseria meningitidis and other (saprophytic) neisseria, *Corynebacterium diphtheriae, Haemophilus* spp.,

Streptococcus viridans, micrococci, *Staphylococcus epidermidis*, *Staph. aureus*, *Streptococcus pyogenes*, *Str. pneumoniae* and *Candida* sp. If the patient is on antibiotics, enterobacteria. Smears of curettings are stained by a modified Ziehl-Neelsen stain in the investigation of leprosy.

Pharyngeal, post-nasal and per-nasal swabs, cough plates

Culture
  Blood agar (aerobic)
  Chocolate agar (CO_2)
  Bordet-Gengou agar
  Tellurite agar (Hoyle or CST)
Organisms
Bordetella pertussis and the organisms found in the posterior nares.

Post-mortem specimens

1. Swabs

Treated in the same way as from the living body.

2. Tissues

These may be washed in peptone water or, if fairly large pieces, dipped momentarily in boiling water to remove contaminating organisms from their surfaces. Then treat as for other tissues and biopsies.

3. Blood and fluid

These should have been collected in an aseptic manner by the morbid anatomist and are treated as for other similar specimens.

Shortly after death the body is subject to invasion with bacteria such as the enterobacteria, and allowance for this must be made in interpreting the results.

Pus

A few ml of pus in a sterile bottle is much better than a swab.

Procedure

Description
Volume, colour and consistency, noting any granules etc.

Films:
  Gram stain
  Ziehl-Neelsen stain
Culture
  Blood agar (aerobic)
  Blood agar (anaerobic)
  Kanamycin agar (anaerobic)
  MacConkey's agar
  Robertson's cooked-meat medium
  or thioglycollate broth
If from a chronic source examine for mycobacteria as described in the appropriate section.
Organisms
Staphylococcus aureus, streptococci, anaerobic cocci, coliforms, *Proteus* spp., *Pseudomonas* sp., *Bacteroides* sp., *Haemophilus* spp., mycobacteria, actinomyces and many others.

Skin

1. Scrapings for fungal culture,

see Chapter 11.

2. Snip for erysipelothrix

Culture
  Blood agar (CO_2)
  Glucose broth

3. Swab

Culture
  Blood agar
  Salt-mannitol agar
if from perineal area, add MacConkey's agar.
Organisms
Staphylococcus aureus, *Staph. epidermidis*, *Streptococcus pyogenes*, *Candida* spp., coliforms, *Pseudomonas aeruginosa*, diphtheroids.

Sputum and bronchial aspirates

Description
Serous, mucoid, muco-purulent or purulent. Mention blood staining or other abnormality such as the 'red-currant jelly' appearance seen in severe *Klebsiella* pneumonia.
Films
  Gram stain
  Ziehl-Neelsen stain

Culture
   Blood agar
   Chocolate agar (CO_2)
   Sabouraud's agar if fungus is suspected.
The treatment of sputum and culture for mycobacteria is dealt with in the section on mycobacteria (p. 85). Sometimes a Romanowski stained film is examined for eosinophils associated with allergic conditions.
Organisms
Staphylococci, *Streptococcus pneumoniae* and other streptococci, *Haemophilus* spp., mycobacteria, *Neisseria*, *Klebsiella*, and other enterobacteria, *Pseudomonas* sp., *Candida* sp. and *Aspergillus* sp.

Tissues and biopsy specimens

These will frequently be seen by the pathologist who will describe them and prescribe the bacteriological procedures. It is important that the tissue has not been in formalin or other fixative and is quite fresh.

Procedure

For culture the tissue will need to be emulsified. If the specimen is large, then a Stomacher or other form of mechanical macerator can be used initially. Smaller pieces can be ground in a sterile Griffith tube. These procedures produce an aerosol which may contain dangerous organisms, so use an exhaust cabinet and hold the grinder in a wad of tissues in a gloved hand.
Films (impression smears or smears of the emulsion)
   Gram stain
   Ziehl-Neelsen stain
Culture
   Blood agar (aerobic)
   Blood agar (anaerobic)
   Kanamycin agar (anaerobic)
   Chocolate agar (CO_2)
   MacConkey's agar
   Robertson's cooked-meat medium
   Two Lowenstein-Jensen slopes
   Sabouraud's medium if fungus is suspected
Sometimes animal inoculation is required
Organisms
A great variety of organisms may be isolated including brucellae, pasteurellae, *Erysipelothrix*, mycobacteria and fungi in addition to more common organisms.

Throat swabs

Film: Dilute carbol fuchsin or methylene blue stain

Culture
   Blood agar (aerobic)
   Blood agar (anaerobic)
   Tellurite agar (quarter plate is sufficient for routine)
Organisms
Similar to posterior nares with the addition of Vincent's organisms and *Candida albicans*.

Wound swabs

Film:
   Gram stain
Culture
   Blood agar (aerobic)
   Blood agar (anaerobic)
   Kanamycin agar (anaerobic)
   MacConkey's agar
   Robertson's cooked-meat medium
Add Ziehl-Neelsen stained film and culture for mycobacteria if indicated
Organisms
Staphylococcus aureus, *Staph. epidermidis*, micrococci, *Streptococcus pyogenes*, anaerobic cocci, *Bacteroides* sp., enterobacteria and *Pseudomonas* sp., *Clostridium* sp.

Urethral swabs

One plain and one charcoal swab both in Stuart's transport medium are preferred.

1. Plain swab

Film
Gram stain (use neutral red as counterstain)
Wet preparation if *Trichomonas vaginalis* is suspected.

2. Charcoal swab

Culture
   Chocolate agar (CO_2)
   Blood agar
break swab in Feinberg's medium.

Vaginal, high-vaginal and cervical swabs

Preferably two swabs, one plain and one charcoal swab both in Stuart's transport medium.

1. Discharge

Film
  Gram stain
Preparation in saline
  Note presence of *Trichomonas vaginalis*,
Culture (charcoal swab)
  Blood agar (aerobic)
  Blood agar (anaerobic)
  Kanamycin agar (anaerobic)
  Chocolate agar (CO_2)
break swab into Feinberg's medium.

2. Puerperal (abortion and post-partum)

Film: Gram stain
Culture (charcoal swab)
  Blood agar (aerobic)
  Blood agar (anaerobic)
  Kanamycin agar (anaerobic)
  MacConkey's agar
break swab off into Robertson's cooked-meat medium
Organisms
Beta-haemolytic streptococci, anaerobic cocci, *Streptoccus faecalis*, clostridia, *Bacteroides* sp., enterobacteria and listeria. Also present may be lactobacilli, diphtheroids, streptococci, *Haemophilus* spp. and *Candida albicans*.

9. Preparations for microscopy

Examination of the morphology of micro-organisms is of considerable importance in their identification and much may be learned from fixed and stained films on microscope slides. It may be necessary to examine some micro-organisms in the living state, for example, to see if they are motile or when they are not readily stained.

Microscope slides

Glass slides $76 \times 25 \times 1$ mm are used and, when necessary, 22 mm square coverslips 0·1 mm thick. These are used once and then discarded. It is essential that the slides and coverslips are absolutely clean before use. Dirt and grease are removed by wiping and then passing several times through a Bunsen flame or by boiling in chromic acid made up as follows:

Concentrated sulphuric acid	60 ml
Potassium dichromate	60 g
Distilled water	100 ml

This mixture may be used repeatedly until it turns green.

After boiling, the slides are rinsed in running water and stored in 50% methylated spirit. For use, dry and polish with a clean, smooth piece of cloth or paper tissue. If a drop of water can be spread out on the surface of the slide it may be taken as clean.

All microscope preparations must be clearly labelled with a glass-writing diamond.

PREPARATIONS

Wet mount

(a) Take a clean, dry microscope slide.

(b) Place a small drop of the liquid to be examined in the centre. If the material is a solid, such a faeces, mix it on the slide with a small drop of liquid (normal saline, stain etc.).

(c) Place a clean coverslip upright to one side of the drop and lower the top edge over it so that no bubbles are trapped beneath the coverslip.

(d) To prevent evaporation and consequent turbulence, seal around the edges of the coverslip with nail varnish, beeswax or a mixture of equal parts paraffin wax and Vaseline on a bacteriological swab gently warmed over a low gas flame.

The hanging drop for motility

(a) Using Vaseline from a tube with a fine nozzle, make a ring in the middle of a clean microscope slide just less than the size of a coverslip.

(b) Lay a clean coverslip on the bench and place a small drop of a suspension of the organism in the centre.

(c) Pick up the slide and lower it gently on top of the coverslip so that the drop is surrounded by the Vaseline ring which sticks to the coverslip.

(d) Raise the slide and turn it over deftly so that the drop does not run.

(e) Press the coverslip down gently so that there is contact with the Vaseline all the way round to prevent evaporation and currents in the liquid.

(f) Using the microscope's ×10 objective with the diaphragm partly shut, focus on the edge of the Vaseline, then find the edge of the drop where the bacteria are most easily seen. Change to the ×40 objective to observe for movement.

(g) Discard into disinfectant solution after separating the coverslip and slide so that the organisms come into contact with the disinfectant.

This test is usually done on either a broth culture which is less than 18 hours old or on the condensation water from a 4–6 hour slope culture.

The use of a colony of organisms from a solid medium suspended in water or saline is not satisfactory. The temperature at which the culture has been incubated affects motility; for example *Listeria monocytogenes* are motile at room temperature but not at 37°C. True motility in which there is alteration of position in all directions must be distinguished from passive movement in the direction of currents in the suspending fluid and the oscillatory Brownian movements. Wet preparations should be examined soon after they have been made because the middle of the preparation rapidly becomes oxygen-deficient, and this affects the motility of obligate aerobes.

Smears for bacteriological examination

If bacteria are fixed on a microscope slide, they can be stained and examined using the high-power oil-immersion objectives of a microscope. Even simple stains enable more of the shape, arrangement and structure to be seen than in unstained preparations since bacteria have clear protoplasmic matter with a refractive index which is not very different from that of water. Valuable additional information can be obtained by the use of differential stains such as Gram's stain, the results of which have true biological significance. Staining is a biochemical test, the results of which may depend as much on the phase of growth, the growth medium, and the viability of the organisms as on species and method of staining. Films or smears for staining are made as follows:

(a) Take a clean microscope slide and label it with a glass-marking diamond.

(b) Smear a small amount of material on the slide. This may be an inoculating loopful of broth culture, part of a bacterial colony from solid media emulsified in a loopful of water on the slide, or a loopful of a specimen such as sputum. If the smear is to be made from a clinical swab which is to be cultured, then the slide must be sterilised in a gas flame and allowed to cool before use.

(c) Leave the slide on the bench to dry for a few minutes.

(d) Fix the smear to the slide by passing the slide, smear downwards, three times through a gas flame. This degree of heating does not kill all species of bacteria and the films should be regarded as infectious.

(e) Allow to cool before staining.

When it is necessary to examine patients' cells, such as those found in CSF, the smears for this are not heat-fixed, but are dealt with in the same way as blood films.

Microbiological smears are stained on racks over a sink and never in containers such as Coplin's jars to prevent carry-over from one smear to another. For the same reason, when blotting the smear dry at the end of staining, use a fresh piece of fluffless blotting paper. The stains are simply poured on to the slides or dispensed from a squeezy bottle, given time to react, then washed off with running tap water.

STAINING

Simple stains

These may be used alone to detect the presence of organisms and to show the nature of cells in exudates or as counter-stains, e.g. in the Ziehl-Neelsen stain and Gram's stain.

Methylene blue

(a) saturated solution of methylene blue in alcohol	50 ml
distilled water	950 ml

Mix thoroughly and filter before use.
Flood the slide with stain, leave for 30 sec, wash in running water and dry.

(b) Loeffler's methylene blue stain is less likely to overstain and is made as follows:

saturated solution of methylene blue in alcohol	300 ml
potassium hydroxide	0·1 g
distilled water	1000 ml

The films are stained for 3 min, then washed in running water and dried. A polychrome methylene blue, such as is used in McFadyean's reaction for the diagnosis of anthrax, can be made from Loeffler's methylene blue which is allowed to oxidise slowly forming violet compounds which will stain the granules in *Corynebacterium diphtheriae*. The oxidation is achieved by keeping the stain in a half-full bottle for a year or so and shaking it from time to time. Commercial preparations are available.

Malachite green

This dye may be used as a 0·1% aqueous solution in place of methylene blue in the Ziehl-Neelsen stain. The solution is applied for 30 sec, washed off with running water and the smear dried.

Gram's stain

Gram's staining method is the most important of all the stains used in routine medical bacteriology and is used at an early stage in the identification of bacteria. In this test, iodides appear to act as a mordant for dyes such as crystal violet and fix the dye in some species so that it is not washed out by alcohol or acetone treatment. These organisms appear dark blue or black in the final preparation and are described as being Gram-positive. Those organisms which do not retain the dye after treatment with alcohol or acetone are decolorised and are counter-stained with a red dye, such as neutral red, safranin or dilute carbol fuchsin. These are Gram-negative organisms. The mechanisms of the staining are complex and not totally understood. The Gram reaction is indicative of profound differences between bacterial species.

The original method of Gram has been subject to many modifications, and one which gives consistently good results is described below because it requires a minimum of practice and judgement in the decolorisation. In interpreting the results of a Gram stain it should be remembered that Gram-positive organisms from an old culture or those which have been damaged, for example by antibiotics, may appear Gram-negative.

Reagents

(a) Violet stain

methyl violet 6B	5 g
distilled water	1000 ml

The dye is dissolved in the water and filtered to form a stable solution.

(b) Iodine solution (Lugol)

iodine	10 g
potassium iodide	20 g
distilled water	1000 ml

The iodine and potassium iodide are put in a mortar and ground together. A few millilitres of the water are added to this mixture from time to time while grinding continues, until it is all dissolved when it is washed into the stock bottle with the remaining water. This solution remains stable for some months.

(c) Decoloriser

Acetone iodine solution (Preston and Morrell 1962).[1] This solution is made by adding 35 ml of strong iodine solution to 965 ml of acetone (100 ml of strong iodine solution is made from iodine 10 g, potassium iodide 6 g, distilled water 10 ml, and methylated spirit (74 OP) 90 ml). Alternatively, acetone may be used by itself or ethyl alcohol, but the latter requires practice for good results.

(d) Counter-stain

(i) Dilute carbol fuchsin

Ziehl-Neelsen carbol fuchsin	50 ml
distilled water	950 ml

(ii) Neutral red

neutral red	1 g
1% acetic acid	2 ml
distilled water	1000 ml

(iii) Safranin

safranin	10 g
distilled water	1000 ml

Procedures for smears

(a) Place the slide with fixed smear uppermost on a staining rack.

(b) Flood the slide with violet stain for about 30 sec.

(c) Rinse in running tap water and drain off excess.

(d) Flood slide with iodine solution for about 60 sec.

(e) Rinse in running tap water.

(f) Wash the slide with acetone iodine solution, leave the slide flooded and allow to act for 30 sec. Then rinse thoroughly in running tap water.

(g) Counter-stain with dilute carbol fuchsin for 30 sec, or neutral red or Safranin for 3–5 min.

(h) Blot carefully and dry.

The smear is now ready for examination using the oil-immersion lens of the microscope.

If acetone by itself is used as a decolorising agent, the slide should be flooded with acetone which is washed off almost immediately in running tap water, the period of contact between the smear and the acetone being no longer than about two seconds. This operation requires some skill and practice but is easier and quicker than differentiation with alcohol. Thick films take longer to stain and differentiate than thin films.

Ziehl-Neelsen stain

This staining method is used for the demonstration of mycobacteria and a few other organisms which are difficult to stain using ordinary techniques. It employs a very strong stain, concentrated carbol fuchsin, which is usually heated to aid penetration. Once they have been stained mycobacteria are difficult to de-stain and resist acid and often alcohol, whereas most other bacteria are decolorised by any of these agents. Those organisms which resist acid are termed 'acid-fast' (AFB), those which will resist decolorisation with both alcohol and acid are termed 'acid- and alcohol-fast bacteria' (AAFB) and these are stained red by this method.

A blue or green colour is chosen as the counterstain for staining the background and other organisms so that the red acid-fast or acid- and alcohol-fast organisms stand out against the blue or green background, and are consequently more easily detected when scanning a film. When scanning a ZN-stained film, it is convenient to use the ×50 oil-immersion objective of a microscope which should be wiped clean of oil in between slides to prevent carry-over of acid-fast bacilli from one slide to another.

Reagents

(a) Ziehl-Neelsen (strong) carbol fuchsin stain

basic fuchsin	10 g
crystalline phenol	50 g
95% alcohol	100 ml
distilled water	1000 ml

The basic fuchsin and phenol are dissolved in the alcohol in a litre flask which is heated on a boiling water-bath. When these are dissolved the distilled water is added. The mixture should be filtered before use.

(b) Decolorising agent

For mycobacteria: 20% sulphuric acid

For Nocardia and leprosy: 1% sulphuric acid

alternatively acid/alcohol mixture: for tubercle bacilli

methylated spirit or isopropyl alcohol 970 ml

concentrated hyrochloric acid (SG 1·19) 10 ml.

(c) Methylene blue or malachite green.

Procedure for smears

(a) Place the slide with the fixed smear uppermost on a staining rack.

(b) Flood the slide with the concentrated carbol fuchsin.

(c) Heat the slide until steam just begins to rise, using a burning swab. One of these may be easily made using wire and cotton wool on to which methylated spirit has been poured before lighting. The carbol fuchsin should not be allowed to boil or to dry, but should be heated from time to time for 3–5 min. A metallic-looking sheen is seen on the surface of the dye at the end of this operation if it is done properly.

(d) Rinse in running tap water.

(e) Flood the slide with the decolorising agent for 2 or 3 min. Wash off with running tap water and replace with fresh decolorising agent. This may need to be repeated and the decoloriser should be left in contact with the film until no more pink colour runs from it, that is, for 10–20 min.

(f) Counter-stain for 3–5 min.

(g) Wash well with water, blot carefully using a fresh piece of blotting paper, and dry. The film is now ready for examination.

Auramine stain

This stain is used for the detection of *Myobacterium tuberculosis* in sputum by fluorescence microscopy. The bacilli appear as bright luminous yellow rods against a dark background, and it is because they are so easy to see that this method is suitable for use when screening large numbers of sputa. Since auramine is carcinogenic, it is better to buy a commercially prepared stain than make it up in the laboratory. This method is not suitable for staining fast-growing non-chromogenic (Group IV) mycobacteria.

Reagents

(a) Auramine phenol (Lempert's) stain (obtained from Gurr or Raymond A. Lamb)

This contains auramine O which is a fluorochrome dye.

(b) Decolorising agent

sodium chloride	5·0 g
concentrated hydrochloric acid (SG 1·19)	5·0 ml
75% methylated spirit	995·0 ml

(c) Counter-stain

0·1% aqueous potassium permanganate solution or thiazine red diluted 1 in 10 for use from a 1% stock solution.

Procedure for smears

(a) Place the slide with fixed smear uppermost on a staining rack.

(b) Flood the slide with Lempert's auramine phenol (undiluted) for 10–15 min.

(c) Rinse in running tap water.

(d) Flood the slide with decolorising agent for 2·5 min, wash off and replace for a further 2·5 min.

(e) Rinse well in running tap water.

(f) Counter-stain for 0·5 min with potassium permanganate or for just a few seconds with thiazine red.

(g) Rinse in running water, drain and allow to dry in air. Do not blot.

(h) These films are examined using a fluorescence microscope and a suitable ×50 oil-immersion lens, a ×40 high or a ×25 dry objective.

Albert's stain (for staining corynebacteria)

A characteristic of organisms of *Corynebacterium* species is that their protoplasm contains volutin (meta-chromatic) granules. Using Albert's stain the granules appear a bluish-black colour and the rest of the organism is green. Before this stain test is applied the test organism should be grown for 18–24 hours (absolute minimum of 4 hours) on a Loeffler serum slope, after which time corynebacteria usually have a characteristic appearance.

Reagents

(a) Solution I

malachite green	2 g
toluidine blue	1·5 g
glacial acetic acid	10 ml
95% ethyl alcohol	20 ml
distilled water	1000 ml

Dissolve the dyes in alcohol, then add to the water and acetic acid. Allow to stand for one day, then filter.

(b) Solution II (iodine)

iodine	2 g
potassium iodide	3 g
distilled water	300 ml

Procedure

(a) Prepare film and fix by heat.
(b) Apply solution I for 3–5 min.
(c) Wash in water and blot dry.
(d) Apply solution II for 1 min.
(e) Wash in running tap water and blot dry.

The film is now ready for examination using the ×100 oil-immersion objective.

Capsule demonstration

Use is made here of a negative staining technique using either Indian ink or nigrosin. In the Indian ink method the capsule displaces the colloidal carbon particles of the ink and appears as a clear halo around the micro-organism. In wet unstained preparations the capsule may be more clearly differentiated from the body of the organism if phase-contrast microscopy is used. In dry stained preparations the organisms appear coloured with a colourless halo, the capsule, against a dark black background.

Reagents

(a) Nigrosin

nigrosin	10 g
distilled water	100 ml

The nigrosin is dissolved in the warmed distilled water by stirring it from time to time for about one hour, and finally filtering the solution. Formalin 0·5% may be added as a preservative. Alternatively Indian ink may be used. Pelikan Indian ink (Gunter Wagner, Hanover, Germany) is recommended, since not all Indian inks are suitable for this purpose. When Indian ink is used, a negative control of ink alone should be put up each time because the ink may become contaminated by micro-organisms and give a false result.

(b) Violet stain.

As used in Gram's stain.

Procedure (wet mount)

(a) Place a small drop of the Indian ink or 10% nigrosin on a microscope slide.
(b) Mix into it a small loopful of bacterial culture or suspension.
(c) Carefully place a coverslip on the drop, avoiding air bubbles.

Examine with a high-power, preferably phase-contrast, lens.

Procedure (dry film)

(a) Make a suspension of the organism in 5% dextrose at one end of the microscope slide.
(b) Add to this suspension a loopful of nigrosin and mix.
(c) Using the edge of another microscope slide, spread the drop to make a film in a similar way to making a blood film, and allow to dry.
(d) Fix the film by flooding with methyl alcohol for about 2 min.
(e) Wash in running tap water.
(f) Flood the slide with methyl violet stain for a few seconds then wash again in tap water. Do not blot, but stand the slide on its end on the bench to dry. The organisms are stained purple with the capsule showing as a colourless halo against a black background.

Spore stains and flagella stains are not described because they are seldom required in a routine bacteriology laboratory.

REFERENCE

1. Preston, N. W. and Morrell, A. (1962). Reproducible results with the Gram stain. *J. Path. Bact.,* **84,** 241.

10. Identification of common bacteria of medical importance

INTRODUCTION

In medical microbiology there are two principal requirements:

To distinguish between potentially pathogenic and generally non-pathogenic organisms.

To determine whether an outbreak of infection is due to a series of simultaneous infections caused by different organisms, or is due to the spread of a single organism.

The criteria used for these two types of classification differ since a much finer identification is needed for the latter than for the former.

Classification of bacteria leading to identification is based on the following:

1. Microscopy indicating morphology, Gram-staining reaction and whether acid-fast, motile, capsulate or sporing.
2. Cultural requirements and the colonial appearance of the organism on artificial culture media.
3. Biochemical tests of their metabolism.
4. Bacteriophage sensitivity.
5. Serology.
6. Occasionally virulence and pathogenicity tests in animals.

Nomenclature

Living things are classified in a systematic way, hence there is the plant kingdom and the animal kingdom followed by divisions or phyla, then classes and in turn, orders, families, genera and species. The scientific name of a species consists of two parts, the generic and the specific. The name of the genus is always spelt with a capital letter, e.g. *Bacillus* and is always a noun. The specific name is spelt with a small letter and must agree with the generic name in both gender and number. It is descriptive of the organism itself, of the person who first described that organism or the disease which it produces, e.g. *Neisseria meningitidis*—a common cause of meningitis. Occasionally species are divided into a number of varieties, e.g. *Streptococcus faecalis,* var. *zymogenes*, but a more common practice is to describe

serological types, phage types and bacterocine types when describing different strains within a species.

Morphology and Gram staining

There are two classes of bacteria, lower bacteria (eubacteria) which are simple, independent, unicellular organisms which do not form a mycelium; and higher bacteria which are filamentous and may branch and form mycelia. It is the lower bacteria which are most commonly found in pathological material. These may be simply classified depending upon their shape:

Cocci—spherical or spheroidal.
Bacilli—rod shaped, and generally straight.
Vibrios—curved rods and Spirilla—spiralled, non-flexuous rods.
Spirochaetes—thin, spiralled, flexuous filaments.

The cocci and bacilli are further sub-divided on the basis of their Gram reaction so that we have Gram-positive cocci, Gram-negative cocci, Gram-positive bacilli and Gram-negative bacilli. As can be seen from the chart, this simple procedure already divides the bacteria into a number of easily recognisable categories. Using the atmospheric requirements of bacteria, most of these categories can be further sub-divided into those organisms which are aerobes and those which are anaerobes. For the Gram-positive cocci however, it is more convenient to divide them on the basis of the simple catalase test which divides them into the two major groups, namely streptococci and micrococci. The anaerobic Gram-positive cocci are difficult to classify.

We are now in a position to consider ways of identifying the various genera, species, and possible strains within species (Table 10.1).

Cultural requirements

The particular media on which organisms grow or do not grow may be relevant in their classification, e.g. some will only thrive in the presence of certain accessory factors such as haematin (X-factor) and diphosphopyridine nucleotide (V-factor) in the case of

66

Haemophilus influenzae. Some media contain substances which are less poisonous for certain groups of bacteria than others, i.e. selective media such as crystal violet in streptococcus selective media. Note whether the organism grew in the presence of oxygen (aerobic), or in the absence of oxygen (anaerobic) or both, and whether it required additional carbon dioxide for growth (carboxyphilic). The temperature at which growth occurs may be noted in special instances where cultures are incubated at differing temperatures. The length of incubation required to produce a visible colony may also give a clue to the identity of an organism, e.g. some of the atypical or opportunistic mycobacteria will produce colonies within a week whilst *Mycobacterium tuberculosis* requires about three weeks.

Table 10.1.   Lower Bacteria
(non-branching, non-filamentous)

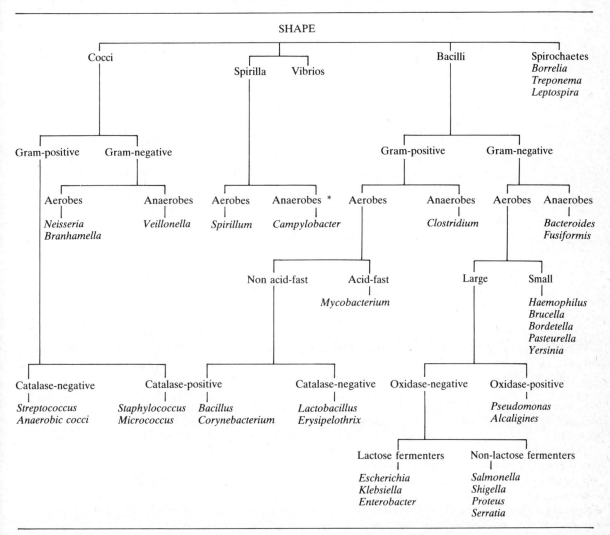

A scheme of the relationships of commonly encountered genera which may be used in their identification. This in not intended as a taxonomy.

* Most of those isolated in medical bacteriology are microaerophilic.

Colonial appearances

Surface colonies on solid media are often characteristic of particular species of bacteria and may be described as follows:

Size: note the diameter of the colony in millimetres and also the diameter of any zones of change in the medium such as haemolysis.

Shape: looking from above, colonies may be discrete and roughly circular with edges as described in the diagram, or sometimes they may be effuse (poured out appearance) or be spreading and have no well-defined edge. Viewed from the side, discrete colonies may have a flat, low-convex, high-convex, plateau or an umbonate elevation (Fig. 10.1).

Surface: this may be rough or smooth, dull or glistening.

Biochemical tests of metabolism

The metabolism of different species of bacteria varies and differing genera, and even species such as those of the enterobacteria, can be differentiated and identified according to the presence or absence of particular enzymes and enzyme systems. This is done by biochemical tests which use specific substrates such as glucose, and test for particular end products such as acetyl methyl carbinol in the Voges-Proskauer test. Gram-negative anaerobic bacteria are often partly identified by gas–liquid chromatography of their products of glucose metabolism to detect the amounts of short-chain fatty acids produced. Another example is the production of indole from tryptophan contained in the peptone used in the medium. For further information on individual tests, *see* the section on biochemical tests.

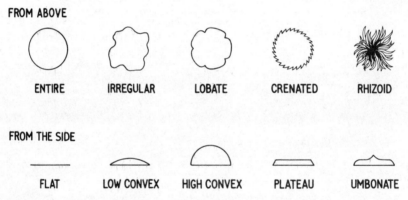

Fig. 10.1.   Shapes of bacterial colonies.

Opacity: they may be transparent, translucent or opaque.

Consistency: this may be butyrous, viscid or granular.

Colour: note the colour if any of the colony and whether any pigment diffuses into the surrounding medium.

Odour: whether present or absent or characteristic, e.g. the smell of pyocyanin characteristic of *Pseudomonas aeruginosa*.

Growth in broth is occasionally characteristic but the appearance is generally of uniform turbidity; however, the growth may be flocculent or principally at the surface, with or without pellicle, absent in the top few millimetres, or there may be a deposit at the bottom of the culture.

Several commercially produced kit systems are now available for the identification of micro-organisms, such as the API Laboratory Products 'API 20E', Roche 'Enterotube', Becton Dickinson 'Minitek', Warner 'Pathotec' and Flow Laboratories 'r/b Enteric' systems for the Enterobacteriaceae, 'API Strep' for streptococci to species level, Flow Laboratories 'N/F' (non-fermenter) system for pseudomonads and 'Unit-Yeast-Tek' for clinically important yeasts. These systems are quite different from one another and the reader is referred to their makers' literature. It has been usual to use batteries of standardised biochemical tests with tables or flow diagrams to work out what the results mean on a 'best fit' basis. This is necessary because micro-organisms are found to be variable in their biochemical activity. Even the primary tests may not be reliable indicators. For example, the oxidase test is variable with *Haemophilus* and *Brucella* species. Naturally there has been a temptation to increase the number of tests performed for each identification but this can make it very difficult to interpret the results, particularly where the significance of the result of each test must be weighted differently. It is also expensive and time-consuming. For many years organisations such as the National Collection of Type Cultures have used computers to aid identification with standardised biochemical tests and a results probability matrix. This matrix is made by performing a battery of relevant biochemical tests on a very large number of previously identified organisms of each type or taxon and examining the results statistically. This information is stored in a computer so that the reaction pattern of the battery of tests for an unknown organism can be compared with that of other known organisms and the mathematical probable identification found. The computer may also list other possible but less likely identities for the organism and some will suggest the most relevant further tests to improve the identification. API, Roche and others have each devised a simple method of converting the pattern of results from the use of one of their kits, like the API 20E and Enterotube, into numerical codes or profile numbers. To obtain the identification it is a simple matter to look up this number or code in a computer-based identification code book (which API call an 'Analytical Profile Index') provided by the makers of the system or to feed it in to a computer with a suitable program.

Bacteriophage sensitivity

Viruses that are parasitic on bacteria are called bacteriophages. These viruses are particularly host-specific, and a strain within a species may be recognised by the particular phage or phages which attack it. This form of identification is especially useful in epidemiology where recognition of the source and manner of spread of the organism is investigated.

Serology

Serology is used to detect structural antigens such as those in the cell wall. Serum from animals or people who have been immunised with a particular organism will produce antibodies to that organism. In the laboratory these sera have an observable effect upon the organism such as agglutination or fluorescence. Sero-logical tests can be made specific and an unknown bacterium can be identified by demonstrating its reaction with one out of a number of standard known antisera. In some of these tests such as in Lancefield's Grouping Tests for streptococci, only part of the organism is used as the antigen, in this case the carbohydrate in the cell wall. In this way a number of different serotypes within a species can be identified. Alternatively, using known bacteria with defined antigens a search may be made of a patient's serum for antibodies to those antigens. This is a useful aid to diagnosis and is used frequently for such diseases as salmonellosis and brucellosis.

Virulence tests

Some organisms produce characteristic lesions in laboratory animals, and an inoculation test may provide a method for identification of either the organism itself or for the demonstration of a toxin which may be produced by that organism, such as the exotoxin of diphtheria. Animal pathogenicity and virulence tests can be controlled using specific neutralising antisera, consequently the organisms can be identified with a high degree of specificity.

GRAM-POSITIVE COCCI (Tables 10.2, 10.3)

Streptococci

Streptococci are widely distributed and very common bacteria. The aerobic streptococci are classified according to their haemolytic effect on horse-blood agar.

Alpha-haemolytic organisms, i.e. *Streptococcus viridans* and *Str. pneumoniae* have a greenish zone around their colonies of blood agar, but this may be more obvious on chocolate agar.

Beta-haemolytic organisms have a larger clear haemolysed zone around their colonies, in which the red cells have been destroyed by a soluble haemolysin. These include *Str. pyogenes*, and some strains of *Str. faecalis*. Other streptococci produce no haemolysis and are sometimes rather strangely called gamma-haemolytic streptococci.

Streptococcus pyogenes

Beta-haemolytic streptococci are responsible for most of the primary streptococcal infections in man which are usually exogenous. The cell walls contain a group-specific carbohydrate called C antigen and using specific typing sera in a precipitation technique seventeen different groups designated by A–H and K–S are distinguished. This immunochemical method is called Lancefield grouping. About 90% of human infections with streptococci are caused by beta-haemolytic *Str. pyogenes* Lancefield Group A organisms, the majority of the remainder are caused by groups B, C, D, and G (Table 10.2).

Str. pyogenes frequently gains entry into the body either by way of the mucous membrane of the upper respiratory tract leading to pharyngitis and tonsillitis; lower respiratory infections or otitis media may follow. Alternatively the organism can enter by way of broken skin, wounds and the placental site producing skin infection, erysipelas, wound infections and puerperal pyrexia.

These infections can spread locally, producing cellulitis, or into the blood stream causing septicaemia. About 2% of Group A streptococcal infections are caused by strains that produce an erythrogenic toxin which is responsible for the widespread red skin rash of scarlet fever. *Str. pyogenes* is also responsible for sterile non-suppurative (no pus) complications which may follow the acute infection including acute rheumatic fever and acute glomerular nephritis. Further serotyping of *Str. pyogenes* mainly for epidemiological purposes is based on the specific protein M and T antigens. Acute glomerular nephritis is usually caused by T (Griffiths) types 12 or 49. *Str. pyogenes* produces several exotoxins. One of these, streptolysin O, is produced in the patient during an infection, consequently the patient produces antibodies to it which can be demonstrated later and provide evidence that the patient has had a streptococcal infection when the organism is no longer available for culture, such as when acute rheumatic fever develops. This organism as a cause of human disease has diminished in importance since the introduction of sulphonamides and penicillin; *Str. pyogenes* is always sensitive to benzyl penicillin.

However, it is still capable of producing epidemics of sore throats and wound infections; indeed much of our knowledge about the spread of infection has come from the numerous investigations into the spread of this organism in hospitals where it was a very serious cause of cross-infection until the 1940s. Some of the other Lancefield groups of beta-haemolytic streptococci sometimes cause infections in man but more often are found as commensals. The enterococci, the streptococci found in faeces and belonging to Lancefield's Group D are also sometimes beta-haemolytic. Group B streptococci are often found in the normal human vagina, and in recent years their role in neonatal infections particularly meningitis and pneumonia has become clear. Other groups are mainly associated with animals.

Culture

Str. pyogenes grows well on horse-blood agar incubated aerobically and even better when it is incubated anaerobically. A selective medium, horse-blood agar containing 1 ppm crystal violet may sometimes be useful. The organism does not grow on MacConkey's medium.

Bacitracin-sensitivity

The majority of strains of Lancefield's Group A streptococci are more sensitive than the other groups to bacitracin and this is tested by using a disc containing 0·1 unit of bacitracin which is placed on an inoculated blood agar plate in the first set of streaks away from the pool. This screening test can be used on the primary or subsequent cultures, but is no substitute for proper grouping.

Grouping

Beta-haemolytic streptococci have a complex antigenic structure. Rebecca Lancefield divided them into the groups already mentioned, in 1933, on the basis of specific carbohydrates present in their cell walls. These C carbohydrates can be extracted from the isolated streptococci by various means and the group identified by immunochemical methods using specific antisera in the Lancefield Precipitin Test, by immunodiffusion, or immunoelectrophoresis. These methods are laborious and time-consuming, but a simpler slide method where an enzyme extract containing C carbohydrate is reacted with specific antibody-coated latex particles which agglutinate in the presence of the homologous carbohydrate antigen is available in kit form as Streptex. Another more rapid method has been devised based on co-agglutination where extraction is not required. Specific antibodies against groups A, B, C, and G are bound to protein A on the cell wall of pre-treated staphylococci. These reagents are mixed individually on slides with a suspension of the streptococci being tested. When the streptococcus cell wall carbohydrate C meets its corresponding antibody attached to the staphylococci binding occurs to form a heavy coagglu-

Table 10.2. *Features of catalase-negative, Gram-positive cocci (streptococci)*

Gram film	Appearance on blood agar (18 hr)	Name	Haemolysis on horse-blood agar	Serology	Bacitracin	Optochin	Other features
1 μm, spherical, arranged in chains (especially from pathological material and broth culture). Divide in one plane only	1–2 mm, low-convex entire, colour-less or grey, matt or shiny surface	*Str. pyogenes*	Beta (clear colour-less zone)	Lancefield group A	Sensitive	—	Further serology based on T and M protein antigens
				Lancefield groups B–Q	Resistant	—	
		Str. viridans	Alpha (green zone)	—	—	Resistant (negative)	Not bile-soluble. Many types
		Non-haemolytic streptococci	None	—	—	—	May be facultative aerobes or strict anaerobes
		Str. faecalis (enterococci)	Sometimes Beta	Lancefield group D	—	—	Small, heat-resistant compared with other streptococci. Magenta colonies on MacConkey's agar. Aesculin-positive. Different kinds differentiated biochemically
1 μm, in long axis. Slightly elongated and often in pairs and chains. Sometimes a capsule can be seen	1–2 mm, Plateau becoming draughtsman on further incubation. Sometimes 2–4 mm, mucoid (type 3)	*Str. pneumoniae* (pneumococcus or diplococcus)	Alpha (green zone)	Quellung type reaction, three types common	—	Sensitive	Bile-soluble. Further tests not usual but sero-typing by agglutination and 'capsule swelling' tests can be done

tination lattice which is visible to the naked eye within 1 minute. The Streptosec and the Phadebact Strepto-coccus Test use this principle and are available as kits.

Alpha-haemolytic streptococci

Two distinct groups of streptococci produce alpha-haemolysis. These are the *Str. pneumoniae* (pneumococ-cus) and *Str. viridans*. *Str. viridans* is a blanket term for a number of *Streptococcus* species and, since it is difficult to distinguish them and seldom necessary to do so, their identification will not be discussed further. They are found as commensals in the upper respiratory tract, mouth, bowel, vagina and sometimes other sites

such as the urethra. Their importance is that they are the most common organisms isolated in sub-acute bacterial endocarditis (SBE). This occurs when dam-aged heart valves become infected, commonly the mitral valve after rheumatic heart disease. Organisms from the infected vegetations can be isolated by blood culture in many instances.

Str. viridans are not necessarily sensitive to penicil-lin, and organisms which are isolated from SBE should not only have a range of sensitivities to antimicrobial agents tested, but the bactericidal levels required of the drugs that the patient is receiving should be deter-mined. It may be necessary to test for bactericidal combinations of drugs in a search for a suitable ther-apy. *Str. pneumoniae* is sometimes called diplococcus because it is usually found in pairs or chains, or pneumococcus because of its association with lobar pneumonia. The pneumococcus is also frequently incriminated in other acute and chronic respiratory infections, in meningitis, otitis media, conjunctivitis, sinusitis and peritonitis in children.

Culture

Str. pneumoniae grows well on horse-blood agar where most strains produce a flat colony 1–2 mm in diameter after a day or so's incubation. Others resemble *Str. viridans*, and still others produce a highly mucoid colony (serotype 3). Two characteristics which distinguish *Str. pneumoniae* from *Str. viridans* are optochin-sensitivity and bile-solubility.

Optochin test

Optochin is ethylhydrocuprein hydrochloride. Discs containing 5 μg are placed on the streaked part of an inoculated blood agar plate in the same way as for the bacitracin test. Sensitivity is indicated by a zone of inhibition several millimetres wide after overnight incubation.

Bile-solubility test

(a) Inoculate 20 ml of a 5% serum broth with the suspect organism and incubate overnight.
(b) Add two drops of phenol red indicator and neutralise to pH 7·0 (bile salts are precipated below pH 6·5).
(c) Add 9 ml of culture to each of two test-tubes.
(d) To one of the test-tubes add 1 ml of 10% sodium taurocholate in saline and incubate both tubes at 37°C for 30 min. Smooth strains of *Str. pneumoniae* are bile-soluble, which is indicated by clearing in the tube containing the bile salt compared with the cloudiness in the control tube.

Pneumococci are always sensitive to penicillin, but some are resistant to tetracycline.

Streptococcus faecalis

Str. faecalis is another name often, but incorrectly, used to describe a number of different species which in many ways resemble one another and are distinct from other streptococci. These organisms are sometimes called enterococci because they are part of the normal flora of the human intestine. *Str. faecalis* is one of the organisms which cause urinary tract infections and also sub-acute bacterial endocarditis.

Culture

Enterococci grow like other streptococci on blood agar, but some strains are beta-haemolytic. Unlike other streptococci they grow well on MacConkey's agar as small, often magenta-coloured colonies easily distinguished from the much larger colonies of *Escherichia coli*. Enterococci are distinguished from other streptococci by a heat-resistance test and aesculin hydrolysis. They are distinguished from one another by biochemical tests if necessary.

Heat-resistance test for Streptococcus faecalis

An overnight nutrient broth culture of the suspect organism is sub-cultured on to half a blood agar plate. The broth culture is then incubated at 60°C in a water-bath for 30 min and a sub-culture made in the same manner on to the other half of the blood agar plate which is then incubated at 37°C overnight. Growth will occur on both halves of the plate if the organism is *Str. faecalis*, otherwise it will only occur on the half which was inoculated before the heating.

Aesculin hydrolysis test

Plates of aesculin agar or MacConkey/aesculin agar are prepared and the area of the plates divided into segments by drawing on the back with a fibre-tip pen. A suspect colony is streaked into one of the quadrants which is labelled appropriately. About six tests can be accommodated on one plate. After incubation at 37°C overnight blackening occurs in the region of colonies of *Str. faecalis* produced by products of aesculin hydrolysis reacting with iron citrate in the medium.

Enterococci are sometimes very resistant to antibiotics.

Staphylococcus aureus (*see* Table 10.3)

Staph. aureus or *Staph. pyogenes* is a common commensal of the nasal vestibule and the skin, notably the groin, perineum and axilla. Infections are either autogenous by way of damaged skin and mucous membranes or by cross infection. Most frequently these are minor such as pustules, boils, styes, impetigo, neonatal ophthalmia, paronychia and stitch abscesses. More serious infections are common and include wound infection, breast abscesses in nursing mothers, pemphigus neonatorum, staphylococcal pneumonia occurring both post-operatively and post-viral infection, and

Table 10.3   Features of catalase-positive, Gram-positive cocci

Gram film	Name	Blood agar appearance	Coagulase etc.*	Novobiocin 5 µg disc	Mannitol acid	Glucose O and F test	Phage typing
1 µm diameter spherical cocci in irregular groups, like bundles of grapes, because they divide in different planes	Staphylococcus aureus	2–4 mm. Cream to yellow colonies. Low convex. Entire. Sometimes a zone of beta-haemolysis. Aerobe, facultative anaerobe	Positive	Sensitive	Positive	Fermentation	Useful
	Staph. epidermidis (albus)	2–4 mm. White to cream (rarely yellow and pink). Low convex. Entire. Aerobe, facultative anaerobe	Negative	Sensitive	Negative	Fermentation	Experimental only
	Micrococcus spp.	2–4 mm. White to cream usually, but some spp. yellow or pink. Low convex. Entire. Aerobe	Negative	Mainly resistant	Positive or negative (by oxidation only)	Oxidation	Not done

* The ability to produce coagulases is closely associated with the ability to produce DNase and phosphatase, both of which can easily be tested for.

deep-seated infection following a bacteraemia or septicaemia such as osteomyelitis and perinephric abscess. Staphylococci can spread from a primary lesion by way of the blood stream to form metastatic abscesses in the brain, lung, kidney and elsewhere. Some strains of *Staph. aureus* when growing on food can produce an enterotoxin which produces food poisoning shortly after the food has been eaten.

Strains of staphylococci first found in hospitals but now with a more general distribution are commonly resistant to penicillin, tetracycline and other antibiotics. This is surely due to natural selection in an antibiotic-laden environment. Penicillin-resistant staphylococci are of two kinds, those which are naturally highly resistant and those which are able to produce penicillinase (beta lactamase) which destroys most forms of penicillin. Penicillinase-resistant penicillins, such as flucloxacillin, are very useful but cannot be used successfully against the naturally resistant strains of *staphylococcus* which, although rare in this country, are nevertheless being found from time to time and are a potential threat. *Staph. aureus* can be responsible for epidemics of wound infection and neonatal infection in

hospitals. Exact identification of strains recovered is necessary for the investigation of epidemics, for the tracing of sources, and for following the spread of the organism. *Staph. aureus* is susceptible to attack by bacteriophages. These are viruses which are parasitic on bacteria and have a high strain specificity. A number of different strains of bacteriophage, all of which are parasitic upon *Staph. aureus*, have been collected and each strain is designated by a number. The majority of strains of *Staph. aureus* isolated are attacked by one or more of the phages in the collection, for example, a well-known hospital strain is attacked by phages 80 and 81, another by 47/53/75/77. These numbers represent the phage type of the strain. The technique of phage typing is quite complex, and should only be done in large centres and reference laboratories.

Staphylococcus epidermidis

Staph. epidermidis is also known as *Staph. albus* and is essentially part of the normal flora of human skin, although occasionally it infects prostheses such as artificial heart valves and artificial vein grafts. Certain strains have been incriminated in urinary tract infections, particularly in young women, that are resistant to novobiocin; these strains are now called *Staph. saprophyticus*.

Micrococcus species

These are common saprophytes found in air, water and soil, and frequently in food. Apart from the urinary tract disease already mentioned they are very rarely pathogenic for man.

Culture

Staphylococci and micrococci are easy to culture, and grow well on nutrient agar and blood agar. Growth on MacConkey's medium produces small pink colonies which are characteristic, being often larger and lighter in colour than the enterococci, but smaller and drier than coliforms. Staphylococci will also grow in the presence of high concentrations of sodium chloride and a 10% salt broth or 7% salt agar is highly selective for them. A combined indicator and selective medium for *Staph. aureus* is readily made by adding mannitol and phenol red indicator to 7% salt agar. After incubation on this medium, coagulase-positive staphylococci produce a yellow coloration. *Staph. epidermidis* and most *Micrococcus* species are surrounded by pink medium.

The most fundamental difference between the genus *Staphylococcus* and the genus *Micrococcus* is in the DNA base composition. Staphylococci have a guanine and cytosine (G and C) content of about 30–40% and micrococci of about 50–75%. This estimate is far too difficult for the majority of laboratories and other methods must be used if they are to be distinguished. *Staphylococcus* species ferment glucose anaerobically whereas *Micrococcus* species will only produce acid from glucose aerobically (oxidation) using the oxidation/fermentation medium. A test using novobiocin-impregnated discs in a sensitivity test where staphylococci are sensitive to the amount of novobiocin used and micrococci are resistant, is less satisfactory.

Coagulase tests

Two forms of coagulase occur, a 'free' coagulase which is detected by the coagulase tube test and a 'bound' coagulase which is detected by a slide test.

Tube coagulase tests

0·5 ml of a 1-in-5 dilution of citrated rabbit plasma is placed into each of two small tubes. One of the tubes is heavily inoculated with a 24-hour culture of the organism, then both tubes are incubated at 37°C in a water-bath. Complete or partial coagulation in the inoculated tube after an hour or so is interpreted as positive. The test should be observed at intervals for up to 24 hours and not left for this period before examination since, in a small proportion of cases, the clot after being formed is lysed. Typical strains of *Staphylococcus aureus* are coagulase-positive whereas typical strains of *Staph. epidermidis* and micrococci are coagulase-negative. Plasma from outdated human bank blood should not be used for this test since some human blood contains inhibitory factors and, in addition, there is always the possibility of the human blood containing Hepatitis B virus or other infectious agents.

Slide coagulase test

This measures the 'bound' coagulase or clumping factor. Using a clean microscope slide, a fairly thick emulsion of growth from solid medium is made in a drop of saline. To this emulsion an inoculation loopful of plasma is added and mixed in thoroughly for approximately 5 seconds. If the reaction is positive, easily visible white clumps will immediately appear; if no such clumping appears immediately, the reaction must be regarded as negative and should be checked by the tube test.

Controls of known coagulase-positive and coagulase-negative strains should be used in both the slide and the tube test. The 'Oxford' *staphylococcus* used as a control in antibiotic sensitivity tests can be used as a weak positive control in either type of coagulase test.

Anaerobic cocci

Anaerobic Gram-positive cocci are widely distributed among the normal human bacterial flora of the skin, mouth, upper respiratory tract, intestine and female genital tract. Nevertheless they are often found in anaerobic infections, frequently with other anaerobes like *Bacteroides fragilis*, and facultative bacteria like *Escherichia coli* and streptococci. There is no doubt that they are pathogens and may be the predominant organisms in diseases, such as dental abscess and puerperal pyrexia.

These bacteria are isolated on blood agar incubated

anaerobically and there are a number of different kinds. Many attempts have been made to classify them, but no method has been generally agreed as being satisfactory. However, it is possible to divide the bacteria into two main groups: those which resemble micrococci, called *Peptococcus*, and those more like streptococci, called *Peptostreptococcus*. A simple test to distinguish the two main groups uses a 5 µg novobiocin disc to which *Peptococci* are resistant and *Peptostreptococci* sensitive. They are sensitive to antibiotics including penicillin, tetracycline, erythromycin, chloramphenicol, clindamycin and metronidazole.

GRAM-NEGATIVE COCCI (Table 10.4)

Neisseriaceae

Members of the family Neisseriaceae are Gram-negative cocci which occur in pairs or masses. They may be found in the mouth, pharynx, the intestine and the genito-urinary tract of man and other animals. All species are parasitic, but only two of the species within the genus *Neisseria* are well recognised as being pathogenic to man. These are *Neisseria meningitidis* and *N. gonorrhoea*, both of which are seen intracellularly in pus cells as Gram-negative diplococci. The former *N. catarrhalis* is now classified as *Branhamella*.

Neisseria meningitidis

This organism, often called the 'meningococcus', has as its normal habitat the human nasopharynx and it is carried by many people without symptoms. However, in closed communities such as army barracks, there is an increase in the rate of throat carriage of meningococci before an epidemic of meningitis which it may cause in these circumstances. Outbreaks in families are also well known. In a susceptible person the meningococcus gains access to the central nervous system either by way of the blood stream or by extension from the sinuses through the lymphatics or bones. A suppurative infection of the meninges then occurs producing a syndrome of bacterial meningitis or of meningo-spinal fever. The blood stream invasion may result in an early petechial rash on the limbs and trunk of the patient which is characteristic. Occasionally massive adrenal haemorrhages, which are usually fatal, occur in this infection (and sometimes other severe infections) producing the Waterhouse-Friderichsen syndrome.

Isolation

The organism is isolated from cerebrospinal fluid, the nasopharynx, blood and from petechiae in the skin. Material from such sources is streaked on to chocolate agar plates and incubated in an atmosphere containing 10% CO_2 at 37°C. A positive-oxidase test on the

Table 10.4.   *Features of Gram-negative cocci*

Cultural requirements	Colonial appearance	Name	Fermentation*	Serology
Aerobic, fastidious temperature range 35–38°C. Improved by 5% CO_2. Grow on protein-enriched media only	1–2 mm, shiny, semi-translucent, discrete, circular, non-chromogenic. Oxidase-positive	*Neisseria meningitidis*	Acid from maltose and glucose	Typing by agglutination tests
		N. gonorrhoeae	Acid from glucose only	Immuno-fluorescent and coagglutination slide identification tests
Aerobic, temperature range 23–45°C. Grow on ordinary media	1–2 mm, smooth or rough, opaque, non-chromogenic Oxidase-positive	*Branhamella catarrhalis*	No carbohydrate fermentation	—
	1–3 mm, smooth or rough, opaque, chromogenic, often yellowish. Oxidase-positive	Other species	Variable	—
Aerobic. Grow on ordinary media	Minute, some species haemolytic on blood agar. Oxidase-negative	*Veillonella* spp.	Variable	—

* Commonly used carbohydrates are: glucose, maltose, lactose and sucrose.

colonies and a Gram stain showing Gram-negative cocci is presumptive evidence of the presence of the organism. Identification is achieved by inoculation of serum agar carbohydrate media containing, respectively, glucose, maltose or sucrose, and by serology. Using a slide agglutination test, *N. meningitidis* can be classifed into a number of serotypes, the most common of which are A, B, C, X, Y and Z. About 60% of the infections in the United Kingdom are group B, about 30% group C, and the majority of the rest—group A. Recently isolated strains may be inagglutinable, but this can be overcome by heating the suspension of the organisms for 10 minutes. Group A are sometimes associated with epidemics. There is an increasing tendency for the *Neisseria* to become sulphonamide resistant.

Neisseria gonorrhoeae (Fig. 10.2)

The gonococcus is a Gram-negative diplococcus in which the paired cells have flattened adjacent walls. Like the meningococcus, this organism is fastidious and requires enriched media such as chocolate agar for its

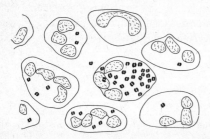

Fig. 10.2.   Appearance of *Neisseria gonorrhoeae* or *N. meningitidis* in a Gram-stained smear of exudate, showing pus cells with intracellular Gram-negative diplococci.

cultivation. It is an obligate human parasite and causes a number of human infections including urethritis, sometimes leading to epididymitis in males and cervicitis sometimes going on to salpingitis in females, vulvovaginitis in female children and conjunctivitis leading to ophthalmia neonatorum in babies. Proctitis and arthritis may also occur. More rarely, oral infection and meningitis are seen.

If acute gonorrhoea is not treated the disease can become chronic. Chronic urethritis in the male leads to urethral stricture, and chronic salpingitis in the female leads to stricture of the tubes with consequent sterility. In general, *Neisseria* are very sensitive to antibiotics although recently there has been an increase in the

resistance of *N. gonorrhoeae* to penicillin, particularly in the Far East, and some beta lactamase producing strains are now seen. Pathogenic *Neisseria* are generally sensitive to the penicillins, amino-glycosides, tetracyclines and sulphonamides, as well as other groups of antibiotics.

In males with a urethral discharge, a presumptive diagnosis of gonorrhoea can be made by examination of a smear of the discharge which is stained by Gram's method, using neutral red as counter-stain. In gonorrhoea the film shows large numbers of pus cells, some of which will contain large numbers of Gram-negative diplococci. In females suspected of having gonorrhoea the situation is much more difficult because of the presence of organisms resembling *Neisseria* in the genito-urinary tract, so in females culture is always required. The best results are obtained when both a urethral and a cervical swab are examined, and it is often helpful to examine a rectal swab in addition. Diagnosis of gonorrhoeal proctitis in either sex requires culture.

Gonococci are very delicate organisms and isolation from clinical material requires great care. The best results are obtained if the clinical material, for instance, on a swab, is plated immediately on to previously warmed chocolate agar and then placed in an atmosphere containing 10% CO_2 and incubated at 37°C for 24 or 48 hours. If it is impossible to culture the specimen immediately it has been taken, then it is advisable to use a transport medium such as Stuart's transport medium. Particularly when trying to isolate this exacting organism from cases of proctitis where large numbers of faecal bacteria may also be expected, it is useful to use a selective medium such as that described by Thayer and Martin. This medium is a chocolate agar which usually contains the following: a polymixin, vancomycin and nystatin. Identification of the gonococcus is based on its morphology in the Gram stained film, on the oxidase reaction, its fermentative characteristics and serology. An immunofluorescent identification test applied to slide smears of isolates of *Neisseria gonorrhoeae* takes a relatively short time and is sometimes used in lieu of the carbohydrate fermentation tests which take 18 hours or more. The Phadebact Gonococcus Test is a rapid, specific coagglutination test.

Veillonellae

Organisms of this genus are anaerobes. Microscopically they appear as Gram-negative cocci in pairs or masses

Table 10.5. *Features of genera of Gram-positive bacilli which are catalase-positive and not acid-fast*

Gram film	Name	Culture	Other tests
Large, brick shaped *bacilli*, often in filaments. Size 1–1·5 × 4–8 μm. Spores may be seen, often without bulging	*Bacillus* spp.	Grow well on ordinary media. Colonies 2–3 mm dia after 24 hr. Aerobic or facultative anaerobe. Wide temperature range, some thermophilic. Colonies usually large, whitish yellow or brownish colour, opaque, dry, occasionally moist	Most are motile (anthrax is an exception)
Slender, sometimes slightly curved or club-shaped. Size 0·3 × 3 μm with some variation. Involution forms occur in cultures. Irregularly staining. Arranged in palisades (Chinese letters). Non-sporing, non-capsulate	*Corynebacterium* spp.	A wide range of colonial morphology on ordinary media, but those which cause diphtheria produce small, dull whitish opaque colonies about 1 mm dia. The different varieties have characteristic appearances on tellurite media. Aerobic or facultative anaerobes	Non-motile. Volutin granules are seen in films of growth on Loeffler's serum medium stained by Albert's method of some species, including the diphtheria bacillus
Straight or slightly curved. 0·5 × 2·0 μm, arranged in pairs and filaments. Non-sporing, non-capsulate	*Listeria monocytogenes*	Grows on ordinary media but is often barely visible after 24 hr incubation. Later forms tiny droplet-like colonies which are smooth and translucent. Small black glistening colonies on tellurite medium with zone of alpha-haemolysis	Only feebly motile at 37°C, but has typical tumbling motion at 25°C. Further identification by biochemical and agglutination tests

which are slightly smaller than the *Neisseria*. They are parasitic and occur in the respiratory, intestinal and genitourinary tracts of man and animals. They are occasionally isolated from blood cultures and from deep-seated abscesses.

AEROBIC GRAM-POSITIVE BACILLI

Bacillus species (Tables 10.5, 10.6)

Organisms of the genus *Bacillus* are rod-shaped, Gram-positive, spore-bearing bacteria. They are common inhabitants of water, soil, animal and plant surfaces and the intestines of animals. They are generally saprophytic. *Bacillus anthracis* is the principal pathogen of the forty or so species within this genus; however, *B. cereus* is being incriminated more and more as a cause of bacterial food poisoning. In medical microbiology there is little need to distinguish between the various aerobic spore-forming species other than to be able to recognise *B. anthracis*, which causes anthrax, and *B. cereus*, since the majority of strains encountered will be contaminants.

The two most common saprophytic species encountered routinely in laboratories are *B. subtilis* and *B. cereus*. On nutrient agar, colonies of *B. subtilis* are flat, dull and rough with a typical ground-glass appearance, colonies of *B. cereus* may vary from small, smooth, shiny, compact colonies to the large, feathery, spreading type, and it will grow on a salt-mannitol agar used for the isolation of staphylococci.

B. anthracis is seldom encountered in the average hospital or Public Health Laboratory, and suspect material and cultures should only be handled in specially equipped laboratories by experienced personnel. Anthrax in man occurs in three forms:

1. Cutaneous anthrax—the lesion consists of a localised cutaneous necrosis described as a malignant pustule which appears most commonly on the hands or forearms. The lesion is not malignant in the usual sense of the word. The bacilli are readily recognised in the sero-sanguinous discharge from the pustule.

2. Pulmonary anthrax, commonly called wool sorters' disease, in which the bacilli are found in large numbers in the sputum of the patient who has pneumonia. This form readily progresses to fatal septicaemia during which the organisms can be demonstrated in the blood by McFadyean's reaction or by culture.

Table 10.6.   Differentiation by Bacillus anthracis from other Bacillus species

	Film	Culture	Motility	Special tests
Bacillus anthracis	1–1·5 × 4–8 μm. Oval central spores which do not deform the bacilli seen in films from cultures. Capsules may be seen in films of pathological material but no spores. Often in long chains giving a 'bamboo' appearance	Temp. range 12–45°C for growth, 25–30°C for spores. Colonies 3 mm dia, opaque, whitish, with 'medusa head' appearance and irregular outline. Aerobic or facultative anaerobe. Little or no haemolysis on blood agar	None	'W' phage-sensitive. Animal virulence: tests positive with small inoculations. Gelatin stab: thin 'inverted fir tree' formed (slow liquefaction). Tissues: Ascoli test positive. Animal blood: McFadyean's test positive. Biochemical: Carbohydrates fermented, nitrate reduction
Other *Bacillus* spp.	Similar size or smaller. Spores may be a similar size or may distend the organisms, be central, terminal or sub-terminal. No capsules seen	Abundant growth on ordinary media. Large colonies usual, whitish yellow or brownish in colour. Opaque and dry, but occasionally moist. Aerobic or facultative anaerobes. Many are haemolytic on blood agar	Most	'W' phage: resistant. Animal virulence: tests negative with small inoculations. Gelatin stab: no 'inverted fir tree' formed or a thick one (rapid liquefaction). Tissues: Ascoli test negative

3. Violent enteritis is the most severe and rare form in which the organism may be isolated from the stools. This disease is usually fatal.

The pathogenicity of an organism suspected of being *B. anthrax* can be determined by injecting 1 ml of a centrifuged and washed 24-hour broth culture intraperitoneally into a guinea-pig, or smaller amounts into each of several white mice. The animals die in 2–4 days after inoculation. Death is by septicaemia and the organism is readily recovered from heart blood, spleen, liver and lungs of the animal.

Ascoli test

This is a precipitin test used to diagnose anthrax in dead animals and to determine whether hides have been removed from infected animals. The antigen is prepared by boiling a small piece of spleen or hide in 5–10 ml of normal saline for 15 minutes. This is cooled and filtered to clarify, 1 ml of the filtrate (antigen) is then layered carefully over an equal volume of anti-anthrax serum which has been raised in rabbits against the encapsulated anthrax organisms in the same way as in the Lancefield grouping test for streptococci. A positive reaction is recognised by the formation of a ring of precipitation at the interface of the two reacting substances.

It is said that the best way to identify anthrax bacilli is to spot W phage on lawns of the organism on nutrient agar.

McFadyean's reaction

Heat-fixed blood films from infected animals stained with polychrome methylene blue show chains of large square-ended bacilli with the remains of their capsules forming pink-coloured debris between the ends of adjacent organisms.

Corynebacterium (Table 10.7)

Organisms of the genus *Corynebacterium* are Gram-positive, non-sporing, mainly non-motile rods. They are often club-shaped and frequently banded or striped with irregularly staining granules. In films, they frequently exhibit characteristic arrangements resembling Chinese letters or palisades. They are mainly aerobic, but some microaerophilic and anaerobic species do occur. They are widely distributed in nature, some are plant and animal pathogens whilst others are part of the normal flora of the skin and upper respiratory tract in man. The type species is *C. diphtheriae*; this produces a powerful exotoxin which causes diphtheria in man.

Diphtheria is a disease which was formerly endemic in all large centres of population and still occurs sporadically, and in small epidemics in susceptible populations. This disease was largely wiped out in the United Kingdom by the immunisation programme. The triple vaccine which is used to immunise the majority of children in their first year of life is designed to give immunity to diphtheria, whooping cough and tetanus.

Table 10.7. Differentiation of commoner Corynebacterium *species from human sources*

Name	Appearance on tellurite medium	Glucose	Sucrose	Starch	Urea	Albert-stained film of 6-hr Loeffler slope culture
Corynebacterium diphtheriae var. *gravis*	Colonies 1–2 mm dia with raised centre and broken edge, rough mat surface, 'daisy head' appearance due to radial striations in older cultures. Greyish black. Difficult to emulsify in saline	Acid	–	Acid	–	Relatively short bacilli, often barred or beaded with polar metachromatic granules. Chinese-letter arrangement
C. diphtheriae var. *intermedius*	Colonies 1 mm dia with domed centre and irregular edge, dull surface. Black colour	Acid	–	–	–	Typically shorter than mitis and larger than gravis with barring or beading
C. diphtheriae var. *mitis*	Colonies 1–2 mm dia, convex with entire edge. Smooth, shiny surface. Dark grey colour	Acid	–	–	–	Long slender bacilli with barring and often polar metachromatic granules
C. ulcerans	Colonies resemble gravis in appearance	Acid	–	Acid	+	
C. xerosis	Colonies 1–2 mm dia, flat with serrated edge. Rough, mat surface. Grey colour	Acid	Acid	–	–	May resemble *C. diphtheriae* and must be differentiated on biochemical grounds

Note: The microscopical and cultural appearances described are for typical strains and can only be used as a guide to identity. Identification is based on biochemical tests and sometimes differential haemolysis tests. Examination of exotoxin may be required.

In susceptible populations diphtheria occurs mainly in children under 10 years, characteristically as a localised inflammation of the throat with an adherent grey-coloured exudate producing a false membrane. In its most typical form it occurs on the tonsils, the fauces, uvula, and soft palate; sometimes it occurs in the larynx and even in the nose. The bacilli are present in large numbers in the membrane and throat secretions where they remain and produce a diffusible toxin. This toxin has an affinity for nerve tissue, which may lead to paralysis, and for heart muscle, so death can occur from heart failure. Wound infections and conjunctivitis also occur.

It is alleged that the most severe forms of diphtheria are caused by the 'gravis' and 'intermedius' types. The 'mitis' type is said to be associated with mild infection, except when it involves the larynx and trachea where there is danger of death by obstruction of the airway. Following the disease a proportion, approximately 5–10%, will continue to carry the organism in their throats, or noses and throats.

Diagnosis of diphtheria must be made on clinical grounds and antitoxin administered at once without waiting for bacteriological confirmation. Cultures of the diphtheritic membrane will not be available until the next day when a report of the morphology and cultural appearances of isolated organisms may be given. Positive identification and evidence or otherwise of toxin production by the strain isolated will take a further few days. Antibiotic therapy should be started at the same time as the antitoxin is given, penicillin or erythromycin being satisfactory both for this purpose and for the elimination of diphtheria bacilli from carriers.

The Schick test is used to decide whether or not a patient is susceptible to diphtheria toxin. A very small quantity of the toxin is injected intradermally into the forearm. In a susceptible person a reddening occurs after a few days, and persists for a week or so. If the patient is not susceptible, that is, his blood contains enough antitoxin to neutralise the injected toxin, then no reaction occurs.

Culture

Material for culture should be plated on to blood agar and tellurite agar (Hoyle and CST). These are examined after 24 and 48 hours incubation at 37°C for typical colonies. Suspicious colonies should first have a Gram stain made of them to check the morphology of the organisms. *C. diphtheriae* appears as slender, sometimes slightly curved or club-shaped bacilli, possibly with palisading. They are weakly Gram-positive compared with staphylococci. If diphtheria still remains a possibility after the Gram staining, then the remainder of the colony is sub-cultured on to a moist Loeffler's inspissated serum slope which is incubated with the top loosened for at least 4 hours and preferably rather longer, say 18–24 hours. At the end of this period an emulsion of the growth from the surface of the serum slope is made in the condensation water within the tube.

A film on a microscope slide is then prepared and stained by Albert's method. In general, 'mitis' strains appear as long slender bacilli with polar metachromatic granules, 'gravis' strains are much shorter and fatter but also have polar metachromatic granules, whilst 'intermedius' strains have barred staining. The morphological appearances of the bacilli depend to a very large extent upon the nature of the medium, and films of growth on blood agar or tellurite blood agar will give misleading results, and even on Loeffler's serum slopes there is considerable variation. When the culture has been examined from a case of suspected diphtheria then the presence of organisms resembling *C. diphtheriae* should be reported to the physician at once. Biochemical confirmation is obtained by sub-culturing from the Loeffler's slope into a set of buffered serum water media containing glucose, sucrose, starch and urea.

Diphtheria toxin

In patients with clinical diphtheria there is no doubt that the organism is toxigenic; however, if the organisms are isolated from a suspected carrier who may himself be immune, it is essential to find out whether the strain is toxigenic or not. Toxin production by diphtheria bacilli is related to their infection with a phage which, when present, stimulates the organism to produce the toxin. This is an example of lysogeny. *C. ulcerans* is able to produce diffusible toxins causing clinical diphtheria, but this is very rare. Tests of toxin production are sometimes called virulence tests.

Plate method

The original method was described by Elek, but a modification, Jameson's method, is described below because it is more sensitive.

Take a Petri dish containing Elek's medium with additional horse serum, dry the plate and place in the middle a piece of sterile filter paper 5 mm × 75 mm which has been soaked in diphtheria antitoxin, 500 units per ml. Using a swab or a large inoculation loop, inoculate the plate from the Loeffler culture in the shape of arrow-heads as in Fig. 10.3. The size and position of the arrows can best be kept standard by using a pattern on which to stand the Petri dish whilst

the inoculation is being carried out. The test must include a non-toxigenic control, a toxigenic control and, if possible, a weakly toxigenic control. The antitoxin diffuses from the filter paper into the agar and away from the strip. Toxin produced by the culture diffuses from the bacteria and into the agar. Where the toxin meets the antitoxin in roughly equivalent amounts they react in the agar to form a precipitate which is visible and can be seen as a white line. Where

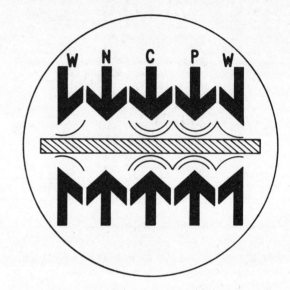

Fig. 10.3. Plate test of toxin production (after Jameson) *C* = toxigenic control; *W* = weak toxigenic control; *P* = positive test with reaction of identity; *N* = negative test.

the lines produced by the toxigenic control and the lines produced by the test strain, if any, are identical, then it may be said that the test strain is toxigenic. This test requires experience in its performance and prior knowledge of the efficiency of the particular batch of medium, antiserum and the control strains.

Guinea-pig inoculation

(a) Subcutaneous test. This is a reliable test which is used when only one organism is to be tested and is the easiest to interpret by those with little experience of diphtheria.

Two adult guinea-pigs of approximately equal size are selected, and one is given an intraperitoneal injection of 1000 units of diphtheria antitoxin which is absorbed quickly, giving that guinea-pig protection. The growth from an 18-hour culture of the bacilli on a

Loeffler's serum slope is emulsified in about 2 ml of peptone water so that it becomes opalescent. 1 ml of the suspension is injected subcutaneously into the right thigh of each of the two guinea-pigs. The unprotected guinea-pig will die in 2–4 days, and at post-mortem will have characteristic haemorrhages in the adrenals and a blood-stained pleural effusion. The protected guinea-pig should be unaffected.

(b) Intradermal test. For this test two adult white guinea-pigs of about equal size are selected and the hair is shaved from the flanks of both of them. One of the guinea-pigs is protected against diphtheria toxin in the same way as for the subcutaneous test, by injecting 1000 units of diphtheria antitoxin intraperitoneally about 24 hours before the test. Using a solution of red dye and a swab, the shaved area is divided into squares, one for a positive control, one for a negative control, and one for each of up to 10 tests. 0·2 ml of a suspension of the organisms as prepared for the sub-cutaneous test is injected intradermally using a tuberculin syringe and needle, and the position of each injection is noted both on the test and control guinea-pigs. The test guinea-pig is then injected with antitoxin at the rate of 1/50 of a unit per gram of body weight, say 5–10 units, which is enough to protect the guinea-pig from death but not enough to inhibit the skin reaction. The guinea-pigs are examined daily for 3 days for skin reactions. A positive result is a well-defined red area about 15 mm in diameter in the test animal but not in the control. In the positive test, after a few days there is an area of necrosis at the site of injection.

Non-toxin-producing strains produce no visible effect in either animal; a reaction in both guinea-pigs casts doubt upon the purity of the isolate injected or its identity.

Diphtheroid bacilli

Diphtheroid bacilli are morphologically similar and sometimes difficult to distinguish from diphtheria bacilli.

C. ulcerans is sometimes isolated from ulcerated tonsils and pharyngitis. Very occasionally it is responsible for clinical diphtheria. It differs from *C. diphtheriae* in that it splits urea and fails to give a reaction of complete identity in the plate toxigenicity test.

C. xerosis closely resembles *C. diphtheriae* microscopically and is isolated from the conjunctiva and vagina from time to time, but is probably not a pathogen.

C. hoffmani (C. pseudodiphtheriticum) occurs in the normal throat and is not pathogenic.

C. haemolyticum is occasionally isolated from patients with a sore throat and an irritant rash.

There are a large number of different diphtheroid bacteria which have not been described here, some of which produce disease in animals, others in plants, and some are found in milk and foods. Many of these diphtheroid bacteria are difficult to classify and may not be true members of the genus *Corynebacterium*.

Listeria monocytogenes

L. monocytogenes is a non-sporing, Gram-positive bacillus which is responsible for an acute highly fatal form of meningoencephalitis in neonates and sometimes in adults. It has also been incriminated in repeated abortions and still-births. It was originally isolated from rabbits with a disease characterised by a great increase in the circulating mononuclear leucocytes, but does not have any aetiological relationship with infectious mononucleosis in man.

Listeria can be cultivated on blood agar and also on tellurite agar which should be incubated at 37°C for 1 or 2 days. Enrichment can be carried out in contaminated material such as the products of conception by keeping the material in the refrigerator at 4°C for up to a month. This works because *Listeria* continues to reproduce at 4°C whilst most other organisms do not. Broth cultures from the dew-drop-like colonies on blood agar should be incubated at 22°C (room temperature) if motility is to be tested, since they are motile at this temperature but only feebly so at 37°C. The Craigie tube method of testing motility may be useful with this species. When these organisms are seen to be motile they exhibit a characteristic tumbling motion.

If it is necessary to demonstrate the pathogenicity of an isolate suspected of being *L. monocytogenes* the ocular test of Anton is used. Two or three drops of an emulsion of an overnight culture suspended in 5 ml of distilled water are instilled into the conjunctival sac of a rabbit or guinea-pig. A purulent conjunctivitis develops in a few days which eventually heals completely.

The demonstration of *Listeria* agglutinins in the patient's serum with a rising titre during the infection is often helpful.

Erysipelothrix rhusiopathiae (E. insidiosa)

This is a non-sporing, non-capsulated, non-motile Gram-positive bacillus with a tendency to form long filaments.

The organism causes erysipelas in pigs (diamonds) and is sometimes present on fish scales. It is the cause of erysipeloid in man which results from infection of skin abrasions when handling infected pork or fish. The infection in man appears as a painful erythematous swelling in the region of the injury surrounded by dusky discoloration of the skin. A biopsy of the edge of the lesion or tissue fluid is more likely to yield the organism on culture than is a swab.

The specimen is cultured on blood agar, 1% glucose broth or thioglycollate broth. The blood agar is incubated at 37°C in 5–10% CO_2 for 24–48 hours, when a small dew-drop-like colony with surrounding alpha-haemolysis in the agar is seen. The broth culture is sub-cultured on the blood agar as above after 24 hours' incubation. The organism is further identified by biochemical tests.

Lactobacilli

Lactobacilli are catalase-negative, Gram-positive, non-motile, non-sporing bacilli which metabolise carbohydrates to produce lactic acid alone or lactic acid, carbon dioxide and alcohol. The genus includes a large number of very different types of bacteria; for example, some are thermophilic, some are aerobic, some micro-aerophilic, some anaerobic. *Lactobacillus acidophilus* occurs as a commensal in man in the saliva, in the bowel, in the vagina (Döderlein's bacillus), and in milk. Others such as *L. bulgaricus* are used in cheese manufacture and yoghurt making. There is seldom any requirement for isolation and identification of these organisms.

A species of *bifidobacteria* formerly called *L. bifidus* is found in the faeces of breast-fed infants and, as its name suggests, is sometimes seen as a Y-shaped bacillus in films.

ANAEROBIC GRAM-POSITIVE BACILLI

Clostridia (Table 10.8)

The clostridia are Gram-positive, anaerobic, spore-bearing bacilli. Most are obligate anaerobes but some are microaerophilic. Characteristically, the spores cause a swelling of the bacterium and they may be central, subterminal or terminal in position. However, the spores are not often seen in clinical material. Clostridia are widely distributed in soil, dust and water,

and are common inhabitants of the intestinal tract of animals, including man. Consequently they often find their way into wounds, particularly those occurring on farms and in gardens, and also into war-wounds. The spores find a suitable environment for germination in the warm, moist nutritive reducing conditions of the necrotic centres of dirty wounds; this is one reason why wounds must be cleaned and all the dead tissue removed, so reducing the possibility of infection. The spores of some species can germinate in food both in improperly prepared home-canned produce and badly prepared meat products like reheated stew, and may be the cause of food-poisoning symptoms.

Gas gangrene is caused by clostridia. It is an acute, rapidly spreading myositis with gas formation from fermentation of carbohydrates and, if not treated, ends in a rapidly fatal septicaemia. It most commonly occurs after severe accidents and only rarely in surgical operation wounds, other than amputation for obliterating arterial disease. It is also a cause of puerperal pyrexia and septic abortion where, presumably, the source of the organism is in the vaginal flora. In the case of severe accidents the source of the infection is likely to be spores in the soil and so on, but in the case of the infected amputation stump, it is more likely that the source of infection is the skin in the neighbourhood of the anus.

The gas-gangrene-producing clostridia include *Clostridium welchii (perfringens)* type A, *Cl. oedematiens (novyi)*, *Cl. septicum*, *Cl. histolyticum* and a few others. These organisms are seen in Gram stained smears as large Gram-positive bacilli. Cultivation from tissue, pus or swabs must be done as soon as possible, preferably on to pre-reduced media. Suitable solid media include blood agar, neomycin-blood agar and egg-yolk agar. Suitable liquid media include Robertson's cooked-meat medium and Brewer's thioglycollate medium.

Clostridium welchii (perfringens)

Cl. welchii can be divided into six types, depending upon the exotoxin that it produces. It is type A which is responsible for gas gangrene and food poisoning in man. Type F has, on rare occasions, been known to cause a severe necrotising enteritis. Type A *Cl. welchii* from wounds is seen as colonies about 3 mm in diameter with a zone of beta-haemolysis after 24 hours incubation. Some food-poisoning strains are not haemolytic. The test used to differentiate Type A *Cl. welchii* from the other serotypes is called the Nagler reaction. The alpha-toxin of *Cl. welchii* is a lecithinase.

Table 10.8. Some features of the more common clostridia

Name	Microscopy	Blood agar	Cooked meat	Litmus milk	Lecithinase	Glucose	Lactose	Maltose	Sucrose	Indole
Clostridium tetani	Slender 2–5 × 0·5 μm. Round terminal spores— Drum stick' appearance	Less than 1 mm dia, grey, Translucent with spreading projections. Spreading growth difficult to see. Haemolytic	No action at first. Slight blackening, digestion later. Pungent smell	No change at first, small clot later	−	−	−	−	−	+
Cl. welchii	Thick, brick-shaped 4–6 × 1 μm. Spores usually absent (oval, central). Capsule may be seen in tissues (non-motile)	Large colonies —about 3 mm dia. Slightly opaque, flat, circular with regular outline. Haemolytic (except some food-poisoning strains)	Reddening and gas	'Stormy Clot' Acid Gas	+	+	+	+	+	−
Cl. oedematiens	Similar size or slightly larger than *Cl. welchii*. Spores not often formed (oval, sub-terminal)	1–3 mm dia, transparent, irregular spreading colonies. Haemolytic under colonies	Reddening and gas	Gas, clot later	Variable	+	−	Most + − (not D)	−	D only
Cl. septicum	Large 3–10 × 0·5–1 μm. Oval sub-terminal spores	1–4 mm dia. Transparent, spreading irregular with projecting radiations. Becomes grey and opaque later. Haemolytic	Reddening and gas	Weak acid, clot later	−	+	+	+	−	−
Cl. histolyticum	Similar size to *Cl. welchii*. Oval sub-terminal spores	Small 1–2 mm dia at first, regular and transparent, becoming greyish and spreading later. Haemolytic	Blackening, digestion H$_2$S smell. White tyrosine crystals formed later	Digestion	−	−	−	−	−	−
Cl. botulinum	Pleomorphic 4–6 × 1 μm. Oval sub-terminal or central spores	Large 2–3 mm dia colonies. Semi-transparent, greyish, with fimbriate edge. Haemolytic	Variable some serotypes only— blackening, digestion and gas	Variable	+	+	−	+	−	−

Serum contains lecithin and egg yolk, lecitho-vitellin. If an exotoxin-producing *Cl. welchii* is cultured on a plate of serum agar or, better still, egg-yolk agar, then where the exotoxin diffuses from the colony into the medium a zone of precipitation is seen. The exotoxin is antigenic and specific antisera can be prepared which will inhibit the activity of the toxin. In Nagler's reaction a plate of egg-yolk medium is prepared by smearing a few drops of specific alpha-antitoxin over half of it with a sterile bacteriological swab. The suspect culture is streaked in a single line diagonally across the plate from the plain side to the smeared side. After anaerobic incubation overnight, on the plain side the streak is surrounded by an area of whitish precipitation, whereas in the case of a type A *Cl. welchii* there is no zone of precipitation on the smeared side because the exotoxin has been inhibited. If the *Clostridium* is not type A, no inhibition occurs. *Cl. welchii* is sensitive to penicillin, and treatment of gas gangrene requires large amounts such as 10–20 mega units per day.

Clostridium tetani

Tetanus is the state of intoxication produced by the exotoxin of *Cl. tetani* called tetanospasmin. Early in the disease there is spasm of masseter muscles causing lock-jaw, although the first spasms may be seen in the proximity of the wound. Tetanus most commonly occurs in association with deep wounds contaminated with soil or foreign bodies, or where there is extensive tissue destruction. The spores need to be in a situation of reduced oxidation-reduction potential (Eh) before germination, and presence of the spores alone in the tissues is not enough for this. They must be present together with some other agent such as soil, or calcium salts which can cause tissue necrosis before they will germinate. Tetanus can be very largely prevented by previous active immunisation and a suitable antigen is included in the Triple vaccine given to children but it is also available on its own. Patients with large wounds generally get appropriate treatment in hospital, and so it is that the majority of cases of tetanus follow relatively small puncture injuries caused by rusty nails and thorns etc. Formerly, before adequate sterilisation of surgical materials, such as cat-gut, was universal, tetanus was an occasional complication of surgical operations.

Cl. tetani is present in the intestinal tract of herbivores, notably horses, and is therefore present in farm land and gardens. The spores can also be found in the dust of streets and even hospitals. It is an occasional inhabitant of the human gut. Microscopically, tetanus bacilli when sporing have a characteristic drum-stick appearance (so do one or two non-pathogenic species). *Cl. tetani* is a strict anaerobe, is motile and will spread over a surface of moist solid media to produce a thin film which may not be readily visible. Isolation of tetanus bacilli from material containing a number of organisms can be achieved by heating the material at 80°C for 30 minutes and then inoculating the bottom of a blood agar slope with it. The culture is then incubated anaerobically, and a pure culture of tetanus bacilli is harvested from the top of the slope.

Unfortunately it is usually impossible to give bacteriological confirmation of clinical tetanus because so few of the bacilli are present in the wound. However, a search should be made for drum-stick bacilli and the material should be cultured. *Cl. tetani* is identified by its motility, its lack of saccharolytic activity and, if need be, by virulence tests using mice, half of which are protected by antitoxin.

Clostridial food-poisoning

1. Poisoning by Clostridium welchii (perfringens)

Some strains of this organism can withstand 100°C for 1 hour, and if such spores are present at the centre of a piece of meat they may not be killed during the normal cooking process, and if the food is allowed to cool slowly, particularly if it is kept warm before serving, the spores will germinate. Characteristically this disease presents with abdominal cramps 8–12 hours after ingestion of the meal, followed by mild diarrhoea, nausea and headache which may last 12–24 hours. In the investigation of such an outbreak any remnants of food are examined, stools from patients and those at risk are also examined. If the outbreak is very large it is permissible to examine the stools of only a proportion of the patients for the heat-resistant *Cl. welchii*.

Culture

A search for food-poisoning clostridia is made by macerating samples of the food then plating on to blood agar containing 70 μg to 200 μg of neomycin sulphate per ml, or neomycin egg-yolk agar, and into Robertson's cooked meat medium, or thioglycollate broth (inoculation of other media for other causes of food-poisoning is described elsewhere). The inoculated solid media are incubated anaerobically and examined at 24 and 48 hours. Remember that some food-poisoning strains of *Cl. welchii* are not haemolytic. This examination can be made quantitative by placing weighed amounts of the macerated food into known volumes of broth, e.g. 1 g in 10 ml, and then carrying out a Miles and Misra type count on neomycin egg-yolk agar. Stool specimens are plated directly on to neomycin blood agar which is incubated anaerobically. Secondly, about 3 g of faeces are emulsified in Robertson's cooked-meat medium which is then placed in a steamer for 1 hour, incubated overnight at 37°C and then subcultured on to two blood agar plates, one of which is incubated anaerobically, and the other aerobically (for *Bacillus* species).

In an outbreak, heat-resistant *Cl. welchii* should be isolated from about 70% of patient's faeces if the results are to be significant. Apparently non-heat-resistant *Cl. welchii* can also cause food poisoning.

2. Botulism

Botulism is an intoxication by the exotoxin of *Cl. botulinum*, which is one of the most toxic substances known to man. Fortunately it is very rare in the United Kingdom. The source of the toxin is usually home-preserved meat or vegetables which have been contaminated with soil or animal faeces containing the spores of *Cl. botulinum*. This usually fatal disease manifests itself 12–36 hours after the meal with a pharyngeal palsy and other symptoms such as double vision, the investigation of botulinus intoxication is a serious matter and includes both culture and demonstration of the toxin, and it should be carried out in a specialist food laboratory.

MYCOBACTERIA

Organisms of this genus, of which the type species is *Mycobacterium tuberculosis*, are aerobic, non-motile, non-sporing, Gram-positive bacilli. They are to a greater or lesser extent acid-fast and some species are also alcohol-fast. Their cell walls contain waxy substances and mycolic acids. Some of them have not so far been cultured, and others are among the slowest-growing of bacteria.

Distribution is extremely widespread; some species are soil, dust or water organisms and many of them are opportunist pathogens for a variety of animals. Others are strictly parasitic, sometimes with remarkable host specificity.

For practical purposes they can be divided into four groups:

1. *M. leprae* which causes leprosy in man.
2. *M. tuberculosis* and *M. bovis* which cause human tuberculosis.
3. The 'Atypical' or 'Opportunistic' mycobacteria which can cause disease in man.
4. *M. smegmatis* and *M. phlei* which are saprophytes and are not known to cause human disease.

Mycobacterium leprae

These organisms appear from time to time in bacteriology laboratories in curettings where they are seen as weakly acid-fast bacteria within the tissues. The organism cannot be grown on artificial culture media. The laboratory diagnosis of leprosy depends on finding acid-fast bacilli in smears, scrapings and biopsies from the nasal mucous membrane, and from skin nodules. The organisms are usually present in large numbers, notably inside mono-nuclear cells (lepra cells).

Mycobacterium tuberculosis

M. tuberculosis is responsible for the great majority of human tuberculosis. The infection is nearly always acquired by inhalation of dust or droplets containing the bacilli. The primary form of the disease usually occurs in childhood and consists of a single focus of infection in the lung with secondary involvement of the hilar lymph glands. This is called the primary complex. In the majority of cases there is spontaneous cure and the disease progresses no further, but in a very few cases the infection spreads to produce progressive forms of the disease such as miliary tuberculosis, bronchopneumonia, meningitis or isolated foci of infection in bones, joints or kidneys.

In secondary tuberculosis the infection may be a reawakening of the bacilli in lesions or may be a reinfection by tubercle bacilli from elsewhere. Most commonly this appears as pulmonary tuberculosis characterised by a lesion near the apex of the lung which may progress to caseation, cavitation, fibrosis and destruction of lung tissue. *M. bovis* causes only a very small proportion of cases of tuberculosis at the present time, and the most important source of infection is cows' milk. Cows suffering from tuberculous mastitis excrete large numbers of organisms in their milk. If this milk is not pasteurised or sterilised and is drunk by a susceptible child, the bacilli may infect the cervical lymph glands by way of the pharynx and the abdominal or mesenteric lymph glands by way of the intestines.

Laboratory diagnosis

M. tuberculosis is demonstrated by microscopy of smears and tissue sections, culture and animal inoculation. The greatest care must be taken when dealing with material suspected of containing tubercle bacilli, and all manipulations must be carried out in a Class 1 exhaust protective cabinet in Category B1 accommodation.

Microscopy

Films of sputum, pus, etc. are stained by Ziehl-Neelsen's method and examined for acid-fast bacilli. These appear as slender red bacilli on a blue or green background. If the auramine method is used they appear as bright yellow rods against a dark brown background. Virulent *M. tuberculosis* is seen as beaded bacilli often lying side-by-side, the so-called 'cording'. *M. tuberculosis* resists decolorising both by acids such as 20% sulphuric acid and by alcohol. It is therefore acid- and alcohol-fast (AAFB). In some material such as pus from a cold abscess, acid-fast bacteria may be very numerous, but it is more often the case that only a very few are seen. Consequently such preparations as sputum smears must be examined very carefully, and not less than 200 high-power fields looked at before a negative result is reported. It has been said that there must be 50,000 AFB/ml or more to be certain that they will be seen. If acid-fast bacilli are seen, this fact is reported to the clinician. The presence of acid-fast bacilli in sputum usually indicates pulmonary tuberculosis, but occasionally is due to the presence of opportunistic or atypical mycobacteria which may or may not be causing disease. Acid-fast bacteria seen in films of pleural fluid, CSF and pus from enclosed abscesses are most likely to be *M. tuberculosis*, but in urine, saprophytic acid-fast bacilli are seen from time to time.

Culture

Specimens such as cerebrospinal fluid, pleural fluid, ascitic fluid and tissues, such as biopsies or lymph nodes, which can reasonably be expected not to contain any micro-organisms other than those causing infection can be cultured without any special treatment. Fluids are centrifuged, with great care, for a few minutes in sealed buckets which are opened in the exhaust cabinet and the deposit used for culture. Tissues must be ground up with the greatest of care in a cabinet before culture. The material is inoculated directly on to Lowenstein-Jensen slopes. In some laboratories any material remaining is inoculated into a liquid medium such as that of Kirchner. This method undoubtedly increases the number of positive cultures, but liquid cultures are dangerous to handle.

Sputum, early morning urine deposits, and other specimens which are likely to contain bacteria other than those causing the infection, must be treated first in such a way as to remove these extra organisms without eliminating all the mycobacteria. Fortunately, mycobacteria are relatively resistant to various chemical agents such as caustic soda, consequently they can be treated with such substances prior to inoculation of culture media. Although the majority of mycobacterial species will grow at 37°C, there are a number which will not do so readily on primary isolation, and for this reason a temperature of between 32° and 35°C should be chosen for incubation.

Mycobacteria are strict aerobes and many of them, including *M. tuberculosis* and *M. bovis*, will not grow on ordinary media but require special media such as that of Lowenstein and Jensen. These media are usually in the form of slopes in screw-capped bottles. After incubation, colonies appear on Lowenstein-Jensen slopes any time from 10 days to 8 weeks, depending upon the inoculum. Mature colonies of *M. tuberculosis* are not pigmented but often slightly buff coloured, and have the appearance of bread crumbs. This good growth is called eugonic; *M. bovis* on the other hand grows relatively poorly as pale, much finer colonies, described as dysgonic growth.

Routine culture of mycobacteria

Sputum

Reagents

(i) Sodium hydroxide   2 g
Sodium citrate   1·45 g
Distilled water   100 ml
Sterilise by autoclaving at 121°C for 15 min then, before use, add 0·5 g *N*-acetyl-L-cysteine (NAC).

(ii) M/15 phosphate buffer pH 7·0.

Method

(i) Pool three early morning specimens of patient's sputum into one or two disposable universals.

(ii) Add an equal volume of NAC/NaOH reagent and, after mixing well, leave to stand for 10 min.

(iii) Centrifuge at 3000 rev/min for 15 min in sealed buckets which are opened in a class 1 safety cabinet.

(iv) Tip off supernatant and resuspend in phosphate buffer.

(v) Recentrifuge as above and culture on Lowenstein-Jensen slopes.

Alternative method

Reagents

(i) Fungizone solution 500 u/ml
(ii) Oxalic acid solution (sterile) 5%
(iii) Sodium citrate solution (sterile) 5%.

Method

(i) Two sterile swabs are moistened in the Fungizone.

(ii) In a safety cabinet, they are both dipped into the sputum and vigorously rotated.

(iii) Place the charged swabs into a sterile 20 × 120 mm glass test tube.

(iv) Two-thirds fill the test tube with 5% oxalic acid and leave for 35 min.

(v) Remove from the oxalic acid and place in a similar test tube two-thirds filled with 5% sodium citrate. Leave for 10 min.

(vi) Inoculate a Lowenstein-Jensen slope with each swab, taking care to transfer most of the material to the medium by firm rubbing and rotation of the swab.

(vii) The swabs are then discarded into strong phenolic disinfectant for at least 24 hr.

Urine

Method

(i) Three complete early morning urines are allowed to stand in a refrigerator for at least 24 hr.

(ii) Decant the top halves of the urine and pool the rest in universal containers.

(iii) Centrifuge the urine at 3000 rev/min for 15 min in sealed buckets which are opened in a class 1 safety cabinet.

(iv) Resuspend the deposit in a small amount of 5% oxalic acid and leave for 30 min.

(v) Add a large volume of phosphate buffer to the specimen and mix well.

(vi) Recentrifuge as above and culture the deposit.

Body fluids

Method

Decontamination is not required. If a clot is present it should be cultured on an L-J slope. If no clot is present, centrifuge at 3000 rev/min for 15 min in a sealed bucket and culture the deposit.

Tissue

Method

(i) Grind up the specimens in a Griffith's tube using 5% oxalic acid and a little sterile sand.

(ii) After 15 min neutralise with sodium hydroxide solution using two drops of phenol red as indicator.

(iii) Centrifuge at 3000 rev/min for 15 min in a sealed bucket and culture the deposit.

Swabs, including laryngeal swabs (cotton or nylon wool)

Method

(i) Pour 5% oxalic acid into the swab tube to completely immerse the swab and leave for 15 min.

(ii) Neutralise with N sodium hydroxide and phenol red, and culture.

Swabs (alginate wool)

Method

Dissolve swab in Calgon/Ringer solution then treat as for normal swabs, using an equal quantity of 5% oxalic acid.

Further identification tests other than to check the acid-fast nature of the culture are not usually carried out in routine medical laboratories because of the danger of technical staff contracting the disease, but are carried out in special centres with experienced staff and suitable facilities.

The niacin test can be carried out safely in ordinary laboratories if desired. This test is positive only with the human *M. tuberculosis*. Animal pathogenicity tests could distinguish *M. bovis* from *M. tuberculosis*. Both organisms will produce a fatal disease after intramuscular injection of 0·1 mg of the organism into a guinea-pig. Injection of 0·001 mg intramuscularly into a rabbit causes a similar disease in the case of bovine tuberculosis, but not with the human tubercle bacillus. Sensitivity tests to antituberculous drugs should be carried out in the special centre at the same time as identification tests. They will include streptomycin, isoniazid (INAH) and para-aminosalicylic acid (PAS).

Niacin test (nicotinamide) using Bacto-TB niacin test strips.

Method

For the test organism and known positive control

(i) Add 1·5 ml distilled water to a well-grown culture on Lowenstein-Jensen medium, cutting the medium with the pipette to help liberate the niacin.

(ii) Autoclave at 15 p.s.i. for 15 min with the medium horizontal and covered with the water.

(iii) Cool and stand upright for 10 min to allow the particles to settle.

(iv) Place 0·6 ml of the fluid in a 7·5 mm × 12 mm test tube.

(v) Set up a negative control tube containing 0·6 ml of distilled water.

(vi) Using forceps so as not to touch the strips, place a Bacto-TB niacin test strip, arrow downwards, into each of the three tubes in a rack and stopper the tubes.

(vii) Shake gently without tilting immediately, after 5 min, and again after 10 min.

(viii) After 12–15 min, but not more than 30 min, compare the colours of the extracts. A positive reaction is indicated by a yellow colour in the extract of the test and positive control not seen in the negative control.

Mycobacteria can be divided conveniently into four groups on the basis of their cultural characteristics. This is often known as Runyon's classification, and depends upon the rate of growth and production of yellow or orange pigment before or after exposure to light. It allows division into the following groups:

Photochromogens which produce pigment only after exposure to light
Scotochromogens which produce pigment in the dark
Slow-growing non-chromogens
Fast-growing non-chromogens.

Although Runyon's criterion of a 'fast grower' is an organism producing good growth from minimal inocula on egg media within 7 days incubation at 25°C, a much more useful criterion for the routine laboratory is 'good growth after 3 days incubation between 32° and 37°C'. Speed of growth refers to sub-cultures, not primary cultures in which the lag phase may be long. There are approximately 30 species of mycobacteria, some 10 of which are pathogenic for man and belong in category B1 for laboratory safety purposes. A few examples are given below:

Photochromogens: *M. kansasii, M. marinum (balnei)*
Scotochromogens: *M. marianum (scrofulaceum), M. xenopi*
Slow-growing non-chromogens; *M. tuberculosis, M. bovis, M. ulcerans, M. avium*
Fast-growing non-chromogens: *M. smegmatis, M. ranae (fortuitum), M. phlei*
Non-culturable: *M. leprae, M. lepraemurium.*

Identification of species may be very simple or very difficult, depending on the species involved. In general, methods of species identification can be put under a series of headings:

(a) Cultural: colonial morphology, microscopic appearance of stained smears, growth on various inhibitory media, sensitivity to the various antimycobacterial drugs.

(b) Biochemical: ability to utilise certain substrates such as sugars and salts of organic acids, amidases, nitrate reductase, arylsulphatase, catalase and various other enzyme activities. Production of nicotinamide (niacin) and by lipid chromatography.

(c) Pathogenicity for experimental animals: guinea-pigs, rabbits, chickens and mice.

(d) Serological methods such as agglutination and immunodiffusion.

Mycobacterium kansasii

This photochromogen is often associated with pulmonary tuberculosis, but is itself capable of causing a chronic fibrosing lung disease.

Mycobacterium marinum

This organism has been cultured from swimming-bath and tropical fish tank water where it is the cause of a granulomatous condition of the skin of elbows, knees and other parts likely to be abraded.

Mycobacterium marianum

This scotochromogen has been isolated from infected neck glands in children (scrofula).

Mycobacterium ulcerans

This is the causal organism of Buruli ulcer which is a serious ulcerative condition of the skin and superficial tissues occurring in central Africa.

Mycobacterium avium

This organism causes tuberculosis in chickens, but a close relative, commonly called the Battey bacillus and also known as *M. avium-intracellulare*, is responsible for a rare pulmonary disease indistinguishable from that caused by *M. tuberculosis*.

Tuberculins and purified protein derivatives

These are substances obtained from heated culture filtrates and they depend on 'tuberculoprotein' for their activity. Tuberculins and PPDs of this type produced from different species of mycobacteria have only limited specificity.

Delayed hypersensitivity responses are elicited by these substances in those who have encountered mycobacteria although not necessarily as infecting agents. They may be used for indirect assessment of immunity and in the diagnosis of mycobacterial disease.

The Mantoux, Heaf and Tine tests utilise the intradermal inoculation of tubercule protein which produces an indurated red reaction at its maximum after three days at the site of injection as evidence of delayed hypersensitivity.

In the differential tuberculin reactions the effect of equal doses of tuberculin prepared from different species, administered at different sites at the same time, are compared with one another.

Lepromin is a suspension of whole killed organism prepared from high-count tissue obtained from cases of lepromatous leprosy. It is in no way analogous to the tuberculins, and reaction to it reflects the ability to react to leprosy bacilli rather than hypersensitivity to an antigen.

PSEUDOMONAS AND ALCALIGENES

Pseudomonadaceae

The pseudomonads are Gram-negative, motile bacteria which are oxidase-positive; some produce water-soluble pigments, pyocyanin and fluorescein. They have a very wide distribution and are found both in soil and water. Many are plant pathogens, but the principal pathogen in man is *Pseudomonas aeruginosa* although infections with others such as *Ps. pseudomallei* are increasingly being recognised.

Ps. aeruginosa is occasionally isolated from the skin and faeces of normal individuals but most human infections are exogenous. This organism is to be found lurking in any moist situation such as wash-basins, drains, mop buckets, humidifiers of respirators and babies' incubators, bottle corks, pharmaceutical products, such as eye drops and ointments, and even in weak disinfectants. *Ps. aeruginosa* is an opportunist and causes serious infections of burns, wounds, ulcers, the urinary tract, and it occasionally causes meningitis, pneumonia and septicaemia. Pus from a wound infected with *Ps. aeruginosa* is often a blue-green colour with a distinctive smell of pyocyanin (Table 10.9).

Table 10.9.   Large oxidase-positive Gram-negative motile bacteria

		Blood agar	MacConkey agar	Cetrimide agar	Pigment	Glucose O–F test	Penicillin	
Pseudomonas spp.	1·5–3·0 × 0·5 μm, non-sporing	2–4 mm dia, moist, translucent convex colonies with irregular, spreading edge. Often haemolytic	Growth. NLF	Growth	Green fluorescent or none	Oxidation	Resistant	Green pigment (pyocyanin) produced best at room temperature and has a characteristic sweet musty smell
Alcaligenes spp.	Non-sporing	Smaller, smooth colonies, semi-translucent, whitish. Sometimes haemolytic	Growth. NLF	Poor or no growth	None	No action	Usually sensitive 5 μg disc	

This organism is resistant to the commonly used antibiotics and particularly liable to cause super-infections during antibiotic therapy. Its presence in specimens does not, however, always indicate infection; for instance, it is often isolated from the sputum of patients on ampicillin for a chest infection caused by another organism and in this situation is just a saprophyte. Infections with *Ps. aeruginosa* are difficult to treat. Burns can be treated topically with such agents as silver nitrate whilst systemic treatment is with an aminoglycoside such as gentamicin and/or another drug such as ticarcillin, cefotaxime or a polymyxin. Some strains are resistant to one or more of these antibiotics.

Culture

Ps. aeruginosa will grow on most of the media used in medical laboratories and frequently produces the characteristic green pigment called pyocyanin which diffuses through the medium and has a distinct musty smell. Colonies on nutrient agar are usually of 2–4 mm diameter with a tendency to spread. A selective medium can be made by the addition of 0·1% cetrimide (cetyltrimethyl-ammonium bromide).

Alcaligenes species

Alcaligenes faecalis is often part of the normal human gut flora but has been incriminated in cases of septicaemia, meningitis, and urinary tract infections. They are catalase-positive and oxidase-positive, although the reaction may be weak or delayed. It grows as non-lactose-fermenting (NLF) colonies on MacConkey's agar, but is easily distinguished from salmonellae and shigellae by its lack of action on peptone water sugars.

ENTEROBACTERIA (Table 10.10)

The members of the family *Enterobacteriaceae* are Gram-negative bacilli which are generally motile, glucose-fermenting and oxidase-negative. These organisms are found in the intestine of man and animals, in

Table 10.10.   *Differentiation of large oxidase-negative bacteria (enterobacteria)*

Size: 5 × 0·5 μm	Motility	Lactose (acid)	Glucose (gas)	Mannitol (acid)	Dulcitol (acid)	Sucrose (acid)	Indole	Urea	Notes
Escherichia coli	+	+	+	+	−	−	+	−	Serological typing—O and K antigens
Klebsiella spp.	−	+	+	+	Varies	+	−	+	Biochemical—MR, VP, KCN, Malonate Serological typing O and K antigens
Enterobacter spp.	Varies	+	+	+	−	+	−	−	Biochemical into species
Salmonella typhi	+	− (acid only)	−	+	−	−	−	−	Serological confirmation—O, H and Vi antigens. Phage typing
Salmonella spp.	+	−	+	+	+	−	−	−	Serological typing—O, H and Vi antigens. Biochemical variants occur
Shigella spp.	−	±**	−* (acid only)	+ except *dysenteriae*	−	−	−	−	Serological typing—O antigens *The Manchester and Newcastle strains of Flexner type 6 produce small amounts of gas. **Sh. sonnei* ferments lactose late
Proteus spp.	+	−	+	− except *rettgeri*	−	+	+ except *mirabilis*	+	Biochemical into species
Serratia marcescens	+	Varies	Varies	+	−	+	−	−	Biochemical confirmation. Some strains produce red pigment in a proportion of their colonies on nutrient agar, the remainder are white

the soil and on plants. Many are parasites, others are saprophytes and a number of them are pathogenic for man, producing a spectrum of disease from mild diarrhoea to fatal septicaemia, which includes wound infections and urinary tract infections. Classification within this family is complex and only a few of the more important genera will be described. They are distinguished from one another by biochemical reactions and further classification within the species is frequently by serology.

To facilitate the identification of enterobacteria using their biochemical characteristics a number of commercially produced systems have been devised; some, like the API 20E and Roche Entero-tube, using computer-based codes for classification.

Escherichia coli

These organisms are part of the normal bowel flora of both man and animals. *E. coli* is the most common cause of acute urinary tract infections particularly in young women and is also found in urinary tract infections of babies and children, bacteriuria of pregnancy and pyelonephritis. About a dozen serotypes are known which are enteropathogenic for infants up to about two years of age in whom these serotypes sometimes cause an enteritis, producing vomiting and diarrhoea resulting in severe fluid loss, often requiring hospital treatment. There have been disastrous outbreaks in baby nurseries which are difficult to control. *E. coli* has also been blamed for travellers' diarrhoea often given picturesque names like 'The Aztec two-step' and 'Malta dog'. Neonatal meningitis is commonly caused by *E. coli* which also causes some wound infections and septicaemias including the bacteraemic shock syndrome.

Antimicrobial sensitivity is unpredictable so that sensitivity tests should be carried out. Antimicrobials commonly used against the Gram-negative organisms include sulphonamides, cotrimoxazole, nalidixic acid, nitrofurantoin, tetracycline, ampicillin and amoxycillin, cephalosporins and aminoglycosides like gentamicin. Some are naturally resistant to one or two of these, whilst others may be multi-resistant owing to the infectious R factors which carry genetic material for the inheritance of resistance to one or several antimicrobials from one Gram-negative bacterium to another.

E. coli are Gram-negative, non-sporing, actively motile bacilli. Microscopy fails to reveal a capsule which is demonstrated by serology since it contains the K antigen.

Culture

E. coli are aerobic or facultative anaerobes which grow well on ordinary media at 37°C. Colonies on blood agar are of 2–4 mm diameter, convex, smooth and opaque with entire edges. Some stains are haemolytic. Since they ferment lactose they produce pink colonies on MacConkey's agar which are not characteristic, but are the same as those produced by a number of different enterobacteria which also ferment lactose and are collectively known as coliforms.

Enteropathogenic E. coli

The specimen, e.g. faeces, is plated on to MacConkey's agar and the plate incubated overnight at 37°C. Using a clean microscope slide and an inoculation loop, organisms from one colony are emulsified in a drop of saline on the slide. The inoculation loop is flamed and is then used to transfer a loopful of polyvalent antisera to the saline suspension with which it is mixed. The slide is gently rocked for a few moments and then examined for evidence of agglutination. If agglutination occurs, then the test should be repeated using, in turn, each of the monovalent antisera of which the polyvalent serum is made up. Both types of antiserum are available commercially (Wellcome). If the first test is negative, then other polyvalent antisera should be used until all the possibilities have been exhausted (for example, three polyvalent antisera may contain antiserum against all the common enteropathogenic *E. coli*). This performance must be repeated if negative until at least 5 colonies have been tested.

Should agglutination occur, then the remaining portion of the colony is sub-cultured on to blood agar which is incubated overnight at 37°C and the test repeated. If the test is still positive, a suspension from the blood agar plate or a broth culture of the organism is placed in a boiling water-bath or steamer for 30 minutes, and tube agglutination tests carried out to determine if the organism is agglutinated by the antiserum at a titre given by the manufacturer. If so, then the organism is reported as belonging to a particular serotype, e.g. 0–26. A culture of the faeces of a baby with enteritis will contain very large numbers of enteropathogenic *E. coli*, and these will be readily detected by the method described. Symptomless carriers are much more difficult to detect; the colonial appearance of enteropathogenic *E. coli* may be indistinguishable from others in the specimen and they may constitute only a very small proportion of the total numbers.

The slide test using live *E. coli* detects the K antigen (sometimes designated B antigen) see Fig. 14.1. In most cases a particular K antigen is associated with a particular O antigen, but this rule does not always hold good and it is the O antigen which is more closely associated with enteropathogenicity. The K antigen, being on the outside, masks the O (somatic antigen) and must be inhibited or removed by heat before the O antigen can be detected. The commercially available antisera are O–K antisera.

The dozen or so serotypes of enteropathogenic *E. coli* such as O–26, O–111, O–118 often cause enteritis, but may also be present in the absence of enteritis; conversely, serotypes not previously known to be enteropathogenic can cause outbreaks of enteritis. This fact must be borne in mind when investigating an epidemic of diarrhoea in babies and infants where no known enteropathogenic *E. coli* has been demonstrated.

Klebsiella

The genus *Klebsiella* consists of non-motile capsulated, Gram-negative bacilli which ferment lactose and split urea. Klebsiellae are isolated from urine in some urinary tract infections and from sputum, particularly patients on broad-spectrum antibiotic therapy. Klebsiellae can also cause septicaemia, meningitis, wound infections, peritonitis and, very rarely, a necrotising form of lobar pneumonia and severe enteritis in children. They are a cause of cross-infection in hospitals, notably in special-care units. Klebsiellae are isolated fairly easily on blood agar or MacConkey's agar where, characteristically, they produce large mucoid colonies that have a tendency to coalesce. Often if the colony is touched with an inoculation loop the growth can be drawn out for a centimetre or two away from the colony.

Members of the genus are difficult to classify biochemically, although the name *Klebsiella pneumoniae* is used for the organism which causes the rare lobar pneumonia and which is pathogenic for laboratory animals, and the name *K. aerogenes* for the mainly saprophytic organism which is non-pathogenic for animals, but which is frequently found in faeces and causes urinary tract infections. The klebsiellae possess O antigens, but typing is better done using the K antigen. Seventy-two capsular types have been identified and pooled sera are employed in the typing, such as those produced by Difco Laboratories, Detroit. The antisera produce agglutination, but the Quellung reac-

tion is the one observed in the test. In this reaction the capsule is seen to become clearer and may appear enlarged when compared with the same organism treated with a negative control serum. Those members of the genus called *K. aerogenes* are MR-negative and VP-positive and grow in KCN medium, whereas those described as *K. pneumoniae* are MR-positive, VP-negative and do not grow in KCN medium. *Klebsiella* species are usually resistant to ampicillin but otherwise show large variations in their sensitivity to antimicrobial agents and sensitivity tests should always be performed.

Enterobacter

Species of the genus *Enterobacter* are found in water, soil, dairy products and as a part of the normal bowel flora of man and animals. They are sometimes isolated from urine in patients with urinary tract infections and from blood in septicaemias.

Salmonella

Salmonellae are motile, non-lactose fermenting, Gram-negative bacilli. They are found as parasites in the intestinal tracts of man and animals ranging from terrapins to birds, and they cause a spectrum of disease, from enteric fevers to mild diarrhoea.

Salmonella typhi and the three types of *S. paratyphi* (A, B and C) are only found in man for whom they are highly pathogenic and cause enteric fever, which is essentially a septicaemic illness. The other sixteen hundred or so salmonellae are derived from animal sources and usually cause acute gastroenteritis called salmonella food poisoning in man, but sometimes cause a more generalised illness which may be serious in the very young and the very old.

S. typhi causes typhoid fever, which is a severe form of enteric fever. Patients with the disease and carriers excrete typhoid bacilli in their faeces and sometimes in their urine. Water and food contaminated with excreta containing typhoid bacilli are the vehicle for its spread and the source of epidemics. After being swallowed, typhoid bacilli travel to the lymphatic system of the intestinal tract where some reach the blood stream which carries them to the reticuloendothelial cells of the liver, spleen and bone marrow where they multiply. About 10 days after ingestion at the end of the incubation period, large numbers of bacilli are liberated into the blood giving rise to fever and some of the other symptoms characteristic of the disease. *S. typhi* can often be isolated from blood cultures taken at this time. Ulceration of the Peyer's patches (part of the lymphatic system of the small intestine) may lead to diarrhoea and, sometimes, intestinal haemorrhage and perforation. The gall bladder soon becomes infected and typhoid bacilli in the bile and from the ulcerated Peyer's patches are liberated into the gut, and from this time they can be isolated from the faeces. In a proportion of cases typhoid bacilli can also be isolated from the patient's urine.

During the septicaemic phase of the illness, typhoid bacilli are carried to all parts of the body and abscesses can form as a complication, particularly in bones. After apparent recovery from typhoid fever, some patients become carriers. These patients continue to excrete small numbers of typhoid bacilli in their faeces, the source of which is usually the gall bladder, and a smaller number excrete the bacilli intermittently in their urine. These patients are called convalescent carriers, or excreters. Some patients are met with who have never had a clinical attack of typhoid fever, but who nevertheless excrete the organism. Phage typing helps with epidemiology.

S. paratyphi also causes enteric fever, but this is usually somewhat milder than that caused by *S. typhi*. *S. paratyphi* B is the most common serotype isolated in the United Kingdom. *S. typhi* and *S. paratyphi* A are category B1 pathogens according to the Howie Code of Practice.

Laboratory diagnosis of enteric fever

Laboratory diagnosis depends upon isolation of the organisms from blood, faeces or urine and upon detection of specific antibodies in the patient's serum.

Culture

It is unusual to isolate the organism during the incubation period of about 10 days. However, blood cultures are positive in about 80% of cases during the first week of illness, but this percentage decreases as the disease progresses. The *Salmonellae* may be isolated from the faeces during the first week of illness but the chances of success are greater during the second and third weeks, when up to 80% will yield positive results. Urine culture sometimes yields the organism but usually not until the third week of the illness. Faeces, rectal swabs and urine are plated on to DCA and/or XLD medium. For enrichment, about 1 g of faeces is placed in 10 ml of selenite F broth, and if *S. typhi* is suspected a

tetrathionate broth is also inoculated. All these media are incubated overnight at 37°C. First thing next morning the enrichment media are sub-cultured on to plates of DCA and XLD medium and the primary plates are examined for non-lactose-fermenting colonies. These are sub-cultured with a straight wire to urea broth which is incubated at 37°C in a water-bath. Urea broth cultures which are negative after 6 hours' incubation are then sub-cultured on to:

(a) MacConkey's agar for purity
(b) Peptone water for the indole reaction
(c) Peptone water sugars: glucose, mannite, sucrose, lactose and dulcite
(d) Agar slope for agglutination reactions.
Alternatively a commercial identification system can be used.

If the biochemical reactions are those of a *Salmonella*, slide agglutination tests using polyvalent *Salmonella* antisera are carried out, and if these are positive the appropriate monovalent antisera are used as described later in this chapter. The sub-cultures from the enrichment media are dealt with in the same way.

Blood cultures are sub-cultured in the same way as the enrichment media after incubation on to DCA and XLD in addition to the usual blood agar plates and MacConkey's medium.

Organisms giving typical biochemical and positive agglutination reactions of a *Salmonella* must be reported to the pathologist at once. A pure culture of the organism is kept either for further tests or to be sent to the *Salmonella* reference laboratory for identification. If negative, or doubtful agglutination reactions are obtained on a suspected non-lactose-fermenting organism, then an ONPG test is done and further biochemical reactions carried out to confirm the identification of the organism if necessary.

Widal reaction

About the end of the first week of the illness, anti-salmonella antibodies begin to be detectable in the patient's serum by agglutination reactions. A rising titre of antibodies in sera taken a few days apart is a valuable diagnostic test. Specific O (somatic) and H (flagella) antigens are used and if *S. typhi* infection is suspected, a Vi antigen in addition (see Fig. 14·1). Demonstration of antibodies against specific O antigens, rising to a titre of greater than 1 in 80 in the second specimen, is helpful in diagnosis and any titre against the Vi antigen indicates the persistence of the organism within the patient. Detectable Vi antibodies disappear when the *S. typhi* has been eradicated and are therefore a useful guide to treatment. Some other salmonellae, e.g. *S. paratyphi* C, also have a Vi antigen. The serum from many patients may agglutinate the test suspensions in low dilutions such as 1 in 40, and no diagnostic significance is attached to these reactions. Sometimes during the course of an illness a rise in an antibody is detected which is apparently not connected with that particular illness. This has been called an 'anamnestic' reaction, and if not remembered may lead to confusion in interpreting the results.

Patients who have been inoculated with TAB vaccine in the past may have H-agglutinating antibodies in their sera to both typhoid and the paratyphoid bacilli, but they will not generally have any appreciable O-titres unless they have had a recent infection. It is common practice to look for antibodies for other salmonellae (non-specific) and to brucellae at the same time as performing the Widal reactions. This is to save both time and effort, because if the Widal reaction is negative it is likely that the clinician will request further tests to include *Brucella* when he is investigating a pyrexia of unknown origin.

The bacterial suspensions

The full set would include:

Salmonella typhi O and H suspensions
S. paratyphi A, O and H suspensions
S. paratyphi B, O and H suspensions
S. paratyphi C, O and H suspensions
Salmonella non-specific H suspension only
(if *S. typhi* and *S. paratyphi* C give positive agglutinations a Vi test suspension is included)
Brucella abortus and *B. melitensis* suspension
(or more conveniently a suspension of a *B. abortus* with both A and M antigens).

When examining sera from residents of Great Britain who have not been abroad, it is common practice to omit the suspension of *Salmonella paratyphi* A and C since these are not endemic here. The bacterial suspension for use in these agglutination tests can be prepared in the laboratory as described in the section on Serology, but it requires both great skill and care to prepare standardised suspensions which are specific and do not present other antigens, such as fimbrial antigens for detection. Suitable bacterial suspensions may be obtained from commercial sources such as Wellcome. For the *Salmonella* non-specific H a suspension of *S. typhimurium* with the H in phase 2 is used.

The *Salmonella* O and H suspensions will keep for two years, the Vi and *Brucella* suspensions for one year at 4°C.

Reagents

　(i) Wellcome agglutinable and *Brucella abortus* suspensions
　(ii) 0·25% phenol saline
　(iii) Inactivated patient's serum (56°C for 30 min).

Method

(a) 'O' suspensions
　(i) Prepare 3 rows of eight 75 × 12 mm round-bottomed glass tubes.
　(ii) Add 1·9 ml phenol saline to the first tube in each row.
　Add 1·0 ml phenol saline to the other seven tubes.
　(iii) Add 0·1 ml patient's serum to the first tube in each row.
　(iv) Mix contents and transfer 1·0 ml to the second tube and mix. Continue this double diluting to tube seven then discard the last 1 ml. Tube eight is a saline only control.
　(v) Add 0·05 ml (one drop from calibrated pipette) of the appropriate concentrated suspension, well shaken, to all the tubes in each row, i.e. *Salmonella typhi* O—row 1; *S. paratyphi* B O—row 2; *Brucella abortus* O—row 3.
　The final dilutions are 1 : 20 in tube one to 1 : 1280 in tube seven.
　(vi) *Salmonellae*—mix and incubate for 2 hr at 37°C then leave in a refrigerator at 4°C overnight. Next morning leave on the bench for 2 hr.
　Brucella—incubate for 24 hr at 37°C.
　(vii) Examine for agglutination using a concave mirror, without disturbing the deposit.
Positive result: diffuse granular layer over the bottom of the tube.
Negative result: compact button of cells—see control.
(b) 'H' suspensions
　(i) Prepare 3 rows of eight Dreyer's tubes.
　(ii) Add 0·9 ml phenol saline to the first tube in each row.
　Add 0·5 ml phenol saline to the other seven tubes.
　(iii) Add 0·1 ml patient's serum to the first tube in each row and double dilute (0·5 ml amounts to tubes two to seven). Tube eight is a negative control.
　(iv) Add 0·5 ml of well-shaken suspension to each tube in appropriate rows. This gives the same final dilutions as the 'O' suspensions.

(v) Mix and incubate at 56°C for 2 hr.

(vi) Examine for agglutination without shaking.

Positive result: flake-like agglutination in the bottom of the tube.

Negative result: contents remain as a smooth suspension.

Salmonella food poisoning

The majority of salmonellae can cause food poisoning or gastroenteritis if eaten with the food. These organisms are commonly found in the bowels of animals and birds, so it is not surprising that they frequently contaminate animal products such as meat and eggs. Normal cooking processes will kill the salmonellae but inadequate cooking, such as may occur with spit-roasted chickens, may fail to do so. Furthermore, cooked, presumably sterile food can be easily contaminated with salmonellae from uncooked meat if strict hygiene is not observed in kitchens and shops.

If food contaminated even by a few salmonellae is not refrigerated then these organisms are likely to multiply to numbers exceeding the several millions per gram required as an infecting dose. A proportion of those eating contaminated food will develop diarrhoea and vomiting usually 12–36 hours after the meal, the diarrhoea lasting between 36 hours and a week. Others may become symptomless excretors who must be careful not to contaminate food and so must observe strict hygiene. Food may also be contaminated from the droppings of rodents, by flies and contaminated cooking utensils. Faeces, rectal swabs and ground food specimens are cultured directly on DCA and/or XLD medium, and for enrichment in either selenite F or tetrathionate broth. These cultures are dealt with in the same way as described for *S. typhi*. If organisms are grown with the appearance and biochemical reactions of a *Salmonella*, then slide agglutination tests are carried out to identify the organism. This identification is needed for epidemiological purposes.

Salmonella serotypes (Table 10.11)

The Kauffmann-White scheme for the classification, by serology, of the salmonellae divides the 1600 or more serotypes into a series of groups designated A to Z with capital letters, and sometimes into sub-groups of these using suffixes such as C_1 and C_2. There are a number of different somatic antigens which have designated numbers such as 1, 2, 3, 4 in sequence. Each serotype may

Table 10.11. The antigenic structure of a few salmonellae to illustrate the Kauffmann-White classification

Group	Type	Somatic antigens	Flagellar antigens Phase 1	Phase 2
A	*S. paratyphi* A	1, 2, 12	a	—
B	*S. paratyphi* B	1, 4, 5, 12	b	1, 2
	S. typhimurium	1, 4, 4, 12	i	1, 2
	S. saintpaul	1, 4, 5, 12	e, h	1, 2
	S. stanley	4, 5, 12	d	1, 2
	S. reading	4, 5, 12	e, h	1, 5
	S. heidelberg	4, 5, 12	r	1, 2
	S. abortus-equi	4, 12	—	e, n, x
	S. abortus-ovis	4, 12	c	1, 6
C_1	*S. paratyphi* C	6, 7, Vi	c	1, 5
	S. cholerae-suis	6, 7	c	1, 5
	S. thompson	6, 7	k	1, 5
	S. bareilly	6, 7	y	1, 5
	S. montevideo	6, 7	g, m, s	—
C_2	*S. muenchen*	6, 8	d	1, 2
	S. newport	6, 8	e, h	1, 2
	S. bovis-morbificans	6, 8	r	1, 5
D	*S. typhi*	9, 12, Vi	d	—
	S. dublin	1, 9, 12	g, p	—
	S. enteritidis	1, 9, 12	g, m	—
	S. gallinarum	1, 9, 12	(non-flagellate)	

have one or more of these antigens. The groups are so designed that each member of a particular group possesses one particular somatic antigen which is common throughout the group and not shared with any other group. For example, Group A contains antigen 2, Group B contains antigen 4, Group C contains antigen 6; the sub-group C_1 contains 6 and 7, and the sub-group C_2 contains 6 and 8. Sera can be prepared using absorption techniques to remove all antibodies except that of the determining or group-specific antigen, so that we can have a number of sera called Group A or factor 2 serum, Group B or factor 4 serum etc. The majority of the strains isolated in this country belong in Groups A to F; for example, *S. typhimurium* which is found in about 40% of cases and is in Group B. Identification of the serotype of an organism within a group depends upon the H antigen. H antigens can occur in two phases, a specific phase called phase 1 and a non-specific phase called phase 2. All cultures of a *Salmonella*, which is motile, and therefore possesses flagella, will have a proportion of organism in phase 1 and a proportion in phase 2. Most often one phase predominates. The different phase 1 flagella antigens are designated by small letters, a, b, c, and so on. The individual phase 2 H-antigens have designated numbers, 1, 2 etc., but sometimes by small letters when a particular antigen can occur in both phases.

If the organism being tested is found to be predominantly in phase 2, as it may be after sub-culture, and it is wished to test for the antigens in phase 1, then a technique using a Craigie's tube is used. A universal bottle, half-filled with sloppy (0·2%) nutrient agar and containing an open-ended glass tube, as in Fig. 10.4, is

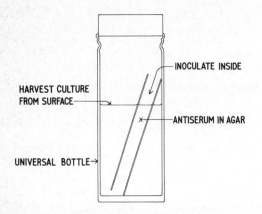

INOCULATE INSIDE

HARVEST CULTURE FROM SURFACE

ANTISERUM IN AGAR

UNIVERSAL BOTTLE→

Fig. 10.4.   Craigie's tube.

prepared. A drop of high-titre (e.g. 1:320) H phase 2 antiserum is mixed with the medium in the glass tube before this is inoculated with the culture. The phase 2 organisms are agglutinated and prevented from swimming. The organisms in phase 1 swim down the tube and up to the surface of the medium outside the tube, where they can be harvested after overnight incubation. By using an H phase 1 antiserum a culture in phase 2 can be obtained similarly.

The procedure for testing is as follows.

A loopful of a suspension of the suspect organism is placed in the centre of a microscope slide and after sterilising the loop, a loopful of polyvalent O *Salmonella* antisera is mixed with it. Nearly all salmonellae found in medical laboratories will be agglutinated by such an antiserum. This test is repeated using a polyvalent H, phase 1 and a polyvalent H, phase 2 antiserum. If these tests are positive, then it is traditional to find the O group first using each group serum in turn, then having found the O group, test with sera against all the available H antigens of both phases which might occur in this group. It is uneconomic for the average laboratory to possess all the antisera necessary for the identification of all salmonellae and many laboratories get by with the polyvalent sera, the first few O-group sera and

some of the more common H sera such as phase 1i, found in *S. typhimurium*. If these do not reveal the identity then the organism is sent to a Reference Laboratory.

Systems for serotyping, utilising combined sera called rapid salmonella diagnosic sera (RSD sera) are available (e.g. Difco), and instructions for their use are included with them.

Shigella

Shigellae cause acute bacillary dysentery. This illness can range from a few loose stools to the classical presentation which includes the sudden onset of abdominal pain, anal spasm, pyrexia and malaise, together with diarrhoea at frequent intervals. The stool may contain pus, and usually blood and mucus are present. The large volume of diarrhoea may lead to electrolyte and fluid deficiencies which may have severe consequences if untreated in the very young and the very old. Human cases and carriers are the sources of infection, which occurs by ingestion. The bacteria multiply in the large intestine producing inflammation of the mucosa which in severe cases may ulcerate so that sloughing of large areas of mucous membrane may occur. The infection is confined to the intestine and only very rarely is there spread into the blood stream, which accounts for the lack of detectable antibodies in the blood. After clinical recovery it is common for patients to continue to excrete the shigellae in their stools for a few weeks, and a small proportion do so much longer.

The shigellae are divided into four groups on the basis of their biochemical and antigenic reactions. These are *Sh. dysenteriae, Sh. flexneri, Sh. boydi* and *Sh. sonnei*. The disease caused by *Sh. sonnei* is frequently mild in character whilst that caused by *Sh. dysenteriae* is often very severe. *Sh. sonnei* is very common in Great Britain, particularly in children, and tends to occur during the winter months sometimes in epidemics. *Sh. flexneri* is less common but is isolated more frequently than *Sh. dysenteriae* or *Sh. boydi* which are comparatively rare in this country.

The shigellae grow on DCA medium where they appear as pale non-lactose-fermenting colonies. They will also grow as non-lactose-fermenting colonies on MacConkey's medium, and some strains grow quite well in selenite broth which should be sub-cultured on to DCA after overnight incubation. Suspicious colonies on solid media are picked off with a straight wire to urea broth which is incubated at 37°C in a water-bath.

Urea broth cultures which are negative after 6 hours' incubation are then sub-cultured onto:

(a) MacConkey's agar or DCA for purity.

(b) Peptone water for indole reaction.

(c) Peptone water sugars: glucose, mannite, sucrose, lactose and dulcite or a commercial kit system.

(d) An agar slope for agglutination reactions. If the biochemical reactions are those of *Shigella*, slide agglutination tests are carried out using *Sh. sonnei* phase 1 and 2 first, then *Sh. flexneri* polyvalent 1 to 6 plus x and y. If these give negative results then try *Sh. dysenteriae* 1, 2 and polyvalent serum containing 3–10. If these are negative, continue with *Sh. boydi* polyvalent 1 serum containing 1–6, then polyvalent 2 serum containing 7–11 and finally *Sh. boydi* polyvalent 3 serum containing 12–15. If negative results have been obtained in all these agglutination tests, it is very doubtful whether the organism is a *Shigella*.

Sh. dysenteriae serotype 1 is sometimes called *Sh. shigae* and is the only one to produce an exotoxin, albeit in very small amounts. *Sh. dysenteriae* serotype 2 is also called *Sh. schmitzi*. The six serotypes of *Sh. flexneri* each have a specific antigen, but the two strains x and y are strains which have lost those but retain the group antigens. *Sh. flexneri* serotype 6 includes the Newcastle and Manchester variants which, unlike other shigellae which are anerogenic, produce a small volume of gas in glucose fermentation. *Sh. sonnei* phase 1 antiserum reacts with the antigen found in the smooth phase which is different from the antigen found in the rough phase (phase 2).

If there is a strong likelihood that the patient has bacillary dysentery, slide agglutination tests for *Sh. sonnei* and *Sh. flexneri* may be carried out on likely colonies from the original DCA plate before it is sub-cultured, but it may be remembered that non-specific reactions are more likely to occur with cultures taken from selective media.

Slide agglutination test

(a) Two separate drops of saline are placed on a glass microscope slide.

(b) Parts of the same colony are emulsified in each drop to give a smooth, dense suspension.

(c) To one suspension a loopful of saline is added and mixed in (control for auto-agglutination). To the other suspension a loopful of undiluted antiserum is added and mixed in.

(d) The slide is gently rocked to and fro for one minute. A positive result is agglutination within that time.

In the case of *Sh. sonnei* a positive report may be issued if the biochemical reactions are correct and there is a clear positive slide agglutination test. For other shigellae the serum should be titred out using the tube agglutination test and the organism sent to the reference laboratory.

A preliminary report should be issued.

Tube agglutination test

(a) Suspend some of the growth from the agar slope (not from selective media) in 5 ml of 0·25% phenol saline to a density of approximately 4×10^8 organisms per ml, using a Wellcome opacity tube number 1 as a standard.

(b) In a rack place eight 75×12 mm round-bottomed glass tubes.

(c) To the first tube add 0·5 ml of phenol saline, to the second tube 0·9 ml of phenol saline and to the remainder 0·5 ml of phenol saline.

(d) Add 0·1 ml of the appropriate antiserum to the second tube and mix, then make doubling dilutions using 0·5 ml amounts discarding 0·5 ml at the end of the row.

(e) To each tube add 0·5 ml of the antigen suspension and mix.

The first tube is a negative control, and the remainder doubling dilutions of the antiserum from 1 in 20 to 1 in 640.

(f) Mix well and incubate at 56°C for 4 hr.

(g) Examine for granular agglutination indicating a positive reaction compared with the lack of change in the negative control tube. The end-point should be at or near the titre stated on the label of the tube of antiserum, usually about 1 in 320.

Wellcome agglutinating sera are suitable for this purpose.

Alkalescens-dispar (A/D) group

These organisms are mentioned here mainly because they have similar biochemical reactions to the shigellae and may, therefore, be confused with them. They can usually be differentiated using agglutination tests with a specific alkalescens-dispar serum. The suspension should be heated in a boiling water-bath for an hour before being used in the tube agglutination test.

Proteus species (Table 10.12)

Members of the genus *Proteus* are found in faeces, sewage and soil. They may cause primary infections, for example, urinary tract infections or the secondary infections of wounds and ulcers, such as bed-sores and varicose ulcers. *Pr. mirabilis* is the species most commonly isolated from human sources and is readily recognised by its spreading growth on blood agar and its characteristic fishy smell. This heavy swarming growth appears to occur in waves around the colony and may completely overgrow other organisms on the plate. To overcome this, many different culture media have been formulated such as chloral hydrate agar (1 in 500) and sodium azide agar (1 in 1000). Swarming does not occur on DCA and not very often on MacConkey's medium.

Sometimes a Gram-positive organism lying underneath a swarming *Proteus* can be recovered using the

Table 10.12.   Proteus species

	Pr. vulgaris	Pr. mirabilis	Pr. morgani	Pr. rettgeri
Urea	+	+	+	+
Mannitol	–	–	–	Acid only
Maltose	+	–	–	–
Indole	+	–	+	+
Cephaloridine	R	S	R	R

+ = acid + gas; R = resistant; S = sensitive.

ether wash or ether shake technique. These techniques must be carried out well away from naked flames. In the ether wash technique a small volume of ether is poured on to the plate, covering the surface, and 10–20 seconds later the chosen colony is sub-cultured on to a fresh medium. In the ether shake technique a suspension of the colony in a few millilitres of saline is shaken up with some ether for 30 seconds. The ether is then allowed to separate as a layer on top of the culture which is sub-cultured, using a Pasteur pipette, immediately and after a further 30 seconds. This method cannot be guaranteed to work.

Proteus species do not ferment lactose, but do split urea in 2–4 hours, except *Pr. morgani* which may take 8 hours. Two species, *Pr. mirabilis* and *Pr. vulgaris*, swarm on ordinary media at 37°C and can be distinguished by the indole reaction. *Pr. mirabilis* is indole-negative. The other two species, *Pr. rettgeri* and *Pr. morgani*, although not swarming at 37°C will do so at room temperature on soft agar. *Pr. rettgeri* ferments sugars anaerogenically, which helps to distinguish it from the others.

Pr. mirabilis can sometimes produce penicillinase, in which case it is resistant to ampicillin which otherwise can be used for treatment. *Pr. mirabilis* is sensitive to

the cephalosporins unlike the other *Proteus* species which are usually resistant to this and ampicillin. All *Proteus* species are resistant to the polymyxins, and they are usually sensitive to gentamicin and other aminoglycosides

Serratia marcescens

Organisms of this species are often found in soil, water, milk and food. They are opportunist pathogens and have been incriminated in pulmonary infections, septicaemia and middle-ear infections. They grow well on ordinary nutrient media, and about 30% of strains are chromogenic producing an orange to red pigment at room temperature, but not often at 37°C. The characteristic appearance of these chromogenic strains on nutrient agar is of a mixture of red and white colonies. The small size and characteristic appearance of this organism make it suitable for use in the biological testing of filters. The strains isolated in clinical laboratories tend to be resistant to a number of antibiotics.

SMALL GRAM-NEGATIVE BACILLI

Haemophilus (Tables 10.13, 10.14)

Organisms belonging to the genus *Haemophilus* require one or both of two accessory growth factors, namely the X factor or haematin, and V factor or nicotinamide adenine dinucleotide. Some nutrient agars are deficient in both, so a small cocco-bacillus suspected of belonging to this genus can be tested for by streaking the organism over the surface of a nutrient agar plate, then placing on the surface three filter-paper discs impregnated with X factor, V factor and a mixture of X and V factors respectively. After incubation, if the organism is an *Haemophilus*, there will be growth around discs, depending upon the species, but not on the rest of the plate. Blood agar contains haematin (X factor) and *Staphylococcus aureus* produces nicotinamide adenine dinucleotide, which diffuses into the surrounding medium. If a blood agar plate is streaked with a *Haemophilus*, and upon this streaking a point inoculum of a culture of *Staph. aureus* is made, then after incubation an organism requiring V factor or X and V factors will be found growing in the region of the *Staphylococcus* (satellitism). Chocolate agar contains sufficient X and V factors to support the growth of all *Haemophilus* species. Two species are haemolytic, and the genus can be classified as in Table 10.13 using the need for X and V factors and the production of haemolysis on horse-blood agar as criteria. Vancomycin chocolate agar can be used as a selective medium for the isolation of *Haemophilus* species from sputum.

Table 10.13.   Haemophilus *species requirements*

	X factor	V factor	Haemolysis on blood agar
Haemophilus influenzae	+	+	−
H. haemolyticus	+	+	+
H. para-influenzae	−	+	−
H. para-haemolyticus	−	+	+
H. ducreyi	+	−	−

Haemophilus influenzae

This organism is commonly carried in the normal nasopharynx of man. Of the strains carried, a small percentage possess an antigenic polysaccharide capsule. These can be divided into six serotypes (Pittman types) using specific antisera by the Quellung capsular swelling test or by agglutination reactions. Capsulate strains of type b are one of the most common causes of meningitis particularly in young children. Non-capsulate strains are frequently found in the sputum of patients with chronic bronchitis and bronchiectasis. *H. influenzae* causes other infections such as otitis media, epiglotitis, cellulitis and various other acute infections. *H. influenzae* is sensitive to chloramphenicol which is used for the treatment of haemophilus meningitis and usually to ampicillin but resistance to it is seen increasingly.

H. aegyptius (Koch-Weeks bacillus) is probably a variety of *H. influenzae* and causes acute conjunctivitis.

H. haemolyticus is usually a commensal in the throat but is sometimes associated with acute upper respiratory tract infections. Its cultural appearances are similar to those of beta-haemolytic streptococci.

Table 10.14.   *Features of some of the small aerobic Gram-negative bacilli (parvo bacteria)*

	Film	Culture	Oxidase	Catalase	Tests
Haemophilus spp.	1·5 × 0·3 µm bacilli, regular in host, pleomorphic in culture. Capsulate forms occur	No growth without X and/or V factor in medium, blood agar or chocolate agar. 1–2 mm dia cols., some haemolytic	Varies	−	Species distinguished by requirements for X and V factors, haemolysis on blood agar and capsule. Serological (Pittman) typing of *H. influenzae*
Brucella spp.	0·5–1·0 × 0·5 µm cocco-bacilli. Capsulate forms occur	Protein-enriched medium, takes 2 or 3 days. 1 mm dia cols. transparent, convex, Castaneda's method useful, *Br. abortus* requires additional CO_2	Varies	+	Biochemical and dye inhibition tests. Several biotypes and serotypes. Bacteriophage (Tbilisi) sensitivity of *Br. abortus*
Bordetella pertussis	1·5 × 0·3 µm regular bacilli. Capsulate in young culture. 'Thumb print' distribution on film	Complex enriched media, e.g. chocolate agar and Bordet-Gengou, moist atmosphere 2 or 4 days at 37°C. Tiny dome-shaped, highly refractile, pearly grey 'mercury droplets'	+	Varies	Slide agglutination with specific antiserum
Pasteurella spp.	1·5 × 0·3 µm bipolar staining. Pleomorphic, ovoid	Ordinary media. 1 mm dia cols., transparent on nutrient agar. No growth (or poor) on MacConkey's medium	+	+	Biochemical tests
Yersinia spp.	1·5 × 0·7 µm bipolar staining. Pleomorphic 'safety-pin' forms. Capsulate	Ordinary media, better on blood agar. 1 mm dia cols., semi-transparent, greyish. Grow on MacConkey's medium	−	+	Biochemical tests. *Y. pseudotuberculosis* is motile at 22°C

H. para-influenzae and *H. para-haemolyticus* are commensals of the upper respiratory tract but nevertheless sometimes cause infections.

H. ducreyi is the cause of a venereal disease, chancroid or soft sore. The organism is found in exudate from the ulcer and from pus obtained from nearby lymph nodes, but it is very difficult to cultivate although it has been grown on media containing a high proportion of rabbit blood. It has the same requirement of X factor but not V factor as *H. canis*, a commensal of the dog.

Brucella

Brucellae are primarily pathogens of animals, and man only becomes infected as a result of contact with infected animals or animal products. Brucellae have a world-wide distribution, and a number of different species have been described. Those which cause undulant fever in man, *Br. melitensis, Br. abortus* and *Br. suis* are primarily pathogens of goats, cattle and pigs respectively. Undulant fever is so called because patients with the disease have recurrent bouts of fever with a relatively normal temperature in between. Other features of the disease are tiredness, malaise, sweating, headaches, anorexia and skeletal pains. The eradication programme for *Br. abortus* in cattle should be complete in the United Kingdom by the early 1980s. The disease can be contracted by drinking unpasteurised milk or eating milk-products, and it is an occupational hazard of veterinary surgeons, farm workers and others in close contact with the animals. In cattle it causes contagious abortion; having gained access to the body the brucellae become widely distributed by the blood stream, and cause multiple tiny granulomatous nodules and abscesses in affected tissue where the brucellae are mainly intracellular.

The disease may present as an acute fever in which case the organisms can be recovered from the blood and antimicrobial treatment is likely to be effective. In the chronic form of the disease it is less likely that blood cultures will be positive, although serology will be helpful in establishing the diagnosis. Antimicrobial treatment of the chronic form is not usually effective. A clinical diagnosis of brucellosis depends upon accurate history taking and less on physical examination because the disease is so variable in its presentation. *Br. melitensis* was first described in Malta where it causes Malta fever but is found in other Mediterranean countries, Africa, the Far East and America. *Br. suis* infects pigs, mainly in the United States, South America and Denmark.

Laboratory diagnosis in man

Culture

In the acute stage, repeated blood cultures should be carried out using Castañada's method (*see* section on Blood Cultures, p. 51) which should be incubated continuously for at least 6 weeks in an atmosphere containing 5–10% carbon dioxide. Alternatively, glucose serum broth or liver digest broth can be used. *Br. melitensis* is occasionally isolated from the urine.

Serology

The following serological tests are used:

Agglutination test
Complement fixation test
Anti-human globulin (Coombs) test for non-agglutinating antibodies
Mercaptoethanol or di-thiothreitol (IgG) test

A method for detecting brucella agglutinating antibodies is described together with the Widal test for salmonellae, p. 94. The serology is fully described by W. R. Kerr *et al.*[1]

Laboratory diagnosis in animals

Culture

Uterine swabs, cervical swabs or products of conception plated on blood agar or liver infusion agar.

Cream and milk deposits injected into guinea-pigs with subsequent culture of spleen etc. after post-mortem.

Serology

Serum agglutination tests; whey agglutination tests; brucella milk ring test.

The brucellae are dangerous pathogens (Category B1) which are likely to cause laboratory infections if handled carelessly. It is doubtful whether these organisms should be handled in ordinary medical laboratories, and it is suggested that once the genus has been identified, subsequent identification into species and biotypes should be done in reference laboratories used to handling these organisms.

Br. abortus, Br. melitensis and *Br. suis* are very similar, and strains occur which have intermediate properties. *Br. abortus* is distinguished from the others by its requirement of carbon dioxide for initial isolation, its production of hydrogen sulphide, its sensitivity to the dye thionin and resistance to basic fuchsin, action in other biochemical tests, sensitivity to the Tbilisi phage and its antigenic properties. (Predominance of A antigen in some strains and M antigen in others.) There are nine biotypes, which is helpful in epidemiology.

Whey agglutination test

A 10 ml sample of milk is clotted by adding 0·5 ml of rennin and incubated at 37°C in a water-bath for 30 minutes. The milk is then centrifuged and the whey decanted. In a row of nine 75 × 12 mm glass tubes prepare doubling dilutions of the whey in 0·25% phenol saline from 1 in 10 to 1 in 2560 using 1 ml volumes. To each tube add one drop of standard concentrated *Br. abortus* suspension, mix and incubate in a water-bath at 37°C for 24 hours. Examine for agglutination using a concave mirror without disturbing the deposit. A positive result is signified by a diffuse granular layer over the bottom of the tube, a negative result by a compact button of cells. A titre of 1 in 80 or more is evidence of an udder infection.

Brucella milk ring test

The antigen is made from haematoxylin-stained *Br. abortus* organisms, and can be obtained from Wellcome. To perform the tests, 1 ml of well-mixed raw milk is placed in a test tube 75 × 12 mm and one drop of the antigen is added and mixed in. The test is then incubated at 37°C for 30–45 minutes during which time the cream rises to the surface. *Brucella* antibodies agglutinate the antigen and the stained aggregates of bacilli rise with the cream to form a blue line on the surface. If there are no antibodies, the cream line remains white. This test is both simple and effective.

Bordetella

Bordetella pertussis causes whooping cough during which it is found in the upper respiratory tract. Whooping cough is a febrile respiratory tract infection in children characterised by paroxysms of coughing which the child is unable to stop, and at the end of which there is a large and much needed intake of breath which makes a whooping noise. A similar syndrome is seen sometimes in infections with adenoviruses and myxoviruses. True whooping cough caused by *B. pertussis* was something of a rarity in Britain since the majority of children were given the triple vaccine containing antigens of *B. pertussis*, *Clostridium tetani* and *Corynebacterium diphtheriae* in early infancy, which produces active immunity. However following controversy over the safety of the vaccine fewer children are being immunised and more cases are being seen. *Bordetella pertussis* contrasts with *Haemophilus influenzae* in that it is only present in the respiratory tract during the disease and does not inhabit normal throats, neither does it require X and/or V factor for its cultivation. For culture, either per-nasal (through the nose) swabs or post-nasal (through the mouth) swabs bent tip uppermost to reach the nasopharynx are obtained. Alternatively, with less unpleasantness for the patient but less satisfactory from a diagnostic point of view, cough plates can be used. In this procedure a Petri dish containing a suitable medium, such as Bordet-Gengou, is held in front of the mouth during a coughing fit, in the hope that expectorated material landing on the plate will contain the bacilli.

Culture on enriched medium is required and chocolate agar of Bordet-Gengou agar with added penicillin may be used. It is essential that the plates are moist, and they should be incubated aerobically at 37°C in a moist atmosphere or in a polythene bag for several days before being discarded as negative. Colonies of *Bordetella pertussis* are tiny, less than 1 mm diameter after 48–72 hours incubation, and appear like mercury droplets or tiny bisected pearls. These colonies can be sub-cultured on to more ordinary media such as blood agar for further tests. *In vitro* testing of these organisms will show them to be sensitive to tetracyclines, erythromycin and ampicillin but these have little effect on the acute disease unless given very early on, although they may prevent secondary pneumonia which is a common complication. Colonies of *B. pertussis* can be distinguished from *B. parapertussis*, which is culturally rather less exacting, by a slide agglutination test performed in the usual way.

Pasteurella

Organisms formerly grouped together as pasteurellae have been divided into three separate genera, namely:

Pasteurella, containing the haemorrhagic septicaemia-producing organisms.

Yersinia, including the plague bacillus and the causative organism of pseudotuberculosis in guinea-pigs.

Francisella, containing the bacillus which causes tularemia, which is micro-aerophilic and requires special media for growth.

Pasteurella septica, often called *P. multocida*, causes haemorrhagic septicaemia in many animals. Strains causing disease in a particular animal are frequently named after that animal, for instance, the organism causing haemorrhagic septicaemia in cattle is sometimes called *P. boviseptica* or *P. bovicida*. These organisms may be transferred to man by bites and scratches which become infected and occasionally lead to septicaemia. *P. septica* is occasionally found in the sputum of patients with chronic bronchitis or bronchiectasis, but its place in the pathogenesis of this disease is doubtful. Other similar organisms occur and are usually distinguished on biochemical grounds. *P. septica* will grow on nutrient agar but not on MacConkey's medium. It is oxidase-positive, urease-negative, indole-positive, and ferments sucrose and mannitol. It is not haemolytic.

Yersinia pestis is the causative organism of plague, which was the black death of medieval times. Plague is a disease of rats and other rodents, which is endemic in parts of Asia, including India, Africa and America. Port Authorities take great care to see that rats infected with plague do not enter this country. The bacillus is transmitted from rat to rat and from rat to man by the flea *Xenopsylla cheopis*. The flea becomes infected by feeding on rat blood containing the bacilli which then multiply inside the flea. The rat dies from the infection so that the flea must seek another host, and if no rat is available the flea will bite man. Organisms are regurgitated and inoculated into the new host next time the flea feeds. There are two main forms of plague. Bubonic plague is the most common form, and follows a bite from an infected flea. The infection spreads to the regional lymph nodes which become enlarged to form bubos with subsequent invasion of the blood stream. Pneumonic plague is when a rapidly spreading haemorrhagic pneumonia occurs in the course of bubonic plague. The sputum becomes loaded with *Yersinia pestis* and the patient is highly infectious, since transmission occurs by droplets.

Diagnosis is by finding characteristic organisms in aspirates from bubos, in sputum in pneumonic plague, and blood cultures. *Y. pestis* is a Category B1 pathogen. In Gram-stained films from the lesions the organisms appear as short, thick, ovoid bacilli with areas of deeper staining at either end (bipolar staining).

They have been likened to tiny safety-pins. The appearance of organisms in culture is more variable, often with filament or chain formation and pleomorphism in old cultures. Specimens should be cultured on nutrient agar and blood agar, both aerobically and anaerobically, and on MacConkey's medium. Unlike most pathogens the optimum temperature for growth of *Y. pestis* is 27°C and not 37°C. Incubation should be at least 48 hours. *Y. pestis* grows on nutrient agar, and on MacConkey's agar, is oxidase-negative, urease-negative, indole-negative, does not ferment sucrose, but does ferment mannitol.

Inoculation of laboratory animals with clinical material or material from dead rats is done by applying the material to the nasal mucous membranes or to a shaved area of skin, since other virulent organisms which may be present in the specimen are not likely to infect this way. Cultures can be injected subcutaneously. The animal will die in a few days, and at postmortem examination there is marked inflammation at the site of inoculation with regional lymphadenopathy, a septic spleen and septicaemia, in all of which characteristic organisms can be demonstrated.

The clinical infection is treated with tetracycline, which is highly effective in a disease which is usually fatal if allowed to follow its natural course. These highly dangerous organisms are likely to cause laboratory infections unless handled with great care.

Y. pseudotuberculosis causes pseudotuberculosis in guinea-pigs and other animals including rats, where it might be confused with plague. It has been incriminated in human abdominal diseases such as mesenteric lymphadenitis from time to time, particularly in children. It can be distinguished from *Y. pestis* by its motility at room temperature, its production of urease, production of hydrogen sulphide and its inability to ferment maltose.

GRAM-NEGATIVE ANAEROBIC BACTERIA

This is a large and heterogeneous collection of strictly anaerobic, non-sporing Gram-negative bacilli. They form the major part of the flora of the intestinal tract, particularly the large bowel where the concentration may reach 10^9 per gram, and they are also found in the mouth and vagina. Anaerobic infections are very common and are frequently caused by mixtures of bacteria including both Gram-negative anaerobes and facultative bacteria such as *E. coli* and *Proteus* spp. as well as various cocci and Gram-positive bacteria. Hence the usefulness of selective media like kanamycin agar. Such infections include appendix and other deep-seated abscesses, wound infections, especially following large-bowel surgery, dental abscess, puerperal sepsis and septicaemia.

The size and shape of anaerobic Gram-negative bacilli (GNABs) is particularly variable. *Bacteroides fragilis*, which is the most numerous organism in faeces and the most important pathogen in the group, is frequently seen as thin Gram-negative bacilli 2–3 μm long but it may vary from cocco-bacillus to large, fat, possibly mis-shapen bacillus. As its name implies *Fusiformis fusiformis* appears typically as a large bacillus with pointed ends referred to as spindle-shaped but is often pleomorphic or filamentous. It is seen together with the spirochaete *Borrelia vincenti* and pus cells in Gram-stained smears from lesions of Vincent's angina.

There must be no delay in anaerobic incubation of cultures from specimens since many species are killed by a very short exposure to atmospheric oxygen. For this reason, and because of drying, it is most important that specimens are not delayed in transit between patient and laboratory. Where diagnosis is important there is much to be said for plating specimens on to pre-reduced media at the bedside and putting the cultures into an anaerobic jar at once, using a gas-generating envelope such as a Gas-Pak. Anaerobic jars should not be opened too soon since tiny colonies of the more sensitive species are killed on exposure to air and will not grow on subsequent anaerobic incubation. Isolation and manipulation of anaerobes must be done as quickly as possible and some workers have advocated the use of an anaerobic cabinet for this. However, most of the apparent medically important anaerobes can be handled in air if it is done quickly.

B. fragilis will grow on blood agar incubated anaerobically for 24 hours to form circular, semi-opaque 1 mm colonies, but many anaerobes are more fastidious and require either freshly poured or pre-reduced blood agar which in some cases needs to be supplemented with menadione (vitamin K), haemin or cysteine and incubated for a much longer period. Columbia blood agar with added cysteine is suitable for most GNABs but some workers prefer Bacto Brucella Agar (Difco) with added horse blood for fusiforms. *B. melaninogenicus*, after a few days' culture, appears as brown or black circular convex colonies about 1 mm in diameter which will fluoresce with a coral pink colour under a Wood's (UV) lamp.

Classification and identification of GNABs is difficult since their cultural characteristics and colonial appearances are so alike. One way to recognize *B. fragilis* is by its relative resistance to antibiotics compared with the others, and this is the basis of an identification system first devised by Suter and Finegold and in common use in diagnostic laboratories (*see* Table 10.15). Biochemical tests, including the gas–liquid chromatography of the products of glucose metabolism, are used to distinguish these organisms further and are fully described in the *Anaerobe Manual* of the Virginia State Polytechnic Institute. However the API 20A system which uses 21 biochemical tests in a strip of microtubes has made this task much easier for routine laboratories.

Virtually all GNABs isolated in this country are sensitive to metronidazole which is firmly established in the prophylaxis and treatment of anaerobic sepsis as well as in trichomoniasis, amoebiasis and giardiasis. They are also generally sensitive to clindamycin and chloramphenicol, whilst many are sensitive to erythromycin and tetracycline. Although most species are sensitive to the penicillins, the most numerous and important pathogen, *B. fragilis*, produces a potent β lactamase and is therefore resistant.

SPIROCHAETES

Spirochaetes are slender unicellular organisms with a flexuous structure in the form of a spiral of at least one but usually several complete turns. They are all motile and movement is effected by flexing and spinning about the long axis. Their structure is more complex than that of ordinary bacteria and may consist of a central axial

Table 10. 15. *Antibiotic disc susceptibility pattern for rapid presumptive identification of B. fragilis*

Antibiotic	Erythromycin	Rifampicin	Colistin	Penicillin	Kanamycin
Disc content	60 μg	15 μg	10 μg	1·2 μg (2 units)	1000 μg
B. fragilis	S	S	R	R	R
Other	V	V	V	S	S

S = sensitive, R = resistant, V = sensitive or resistant.

filament with the protoplasm wound round it, the whole of which is enclosed in a thin membrane. Spirochaetes cannot usually be stained by the Gram staining method, but if they do they are Gram-negative. They are best demonstrated in wet preparations by dark-ground illumination, in smears stained by Romanowsky methods, or in tissue by silver impregnation. Spirochaetes have a wide distribution, some are saprophytic and some are parasitic. Those which are pathogenic for man belong to the genera *Borrelia*, *Leptospira* and *Treponema*.

Borrelia

The genus *Borrelia* contains a large number of species, some of which are human pathogens whilst others are found on healthy mucous membranes as saprophytes. Borrelia are fairly easily stained by normal methods. They can be differentiated from the treponemes by their morphology which is relatively large and thick having a spiral wavelength of 2–3 μm. They are difficult to cultivate or keep alive on artificial culture media.

Borrelia vincenti is the species most commonly encountered in medical laboratories in Great Britain where, together with *Fusiformis fusiformis*, it is found around the gums of most people. These two, together with pus, are found in large numbers in the ulcers of Vincent's angina and occasionally in gangrenous lungs. Smears of material from the lesions of Vincent's angina can be stained with crystal violet, Giemsa or dilute carbol fuchsin which stain both organisms. The fusiform normally stains more intensely than the spirochaete. *Borrelia vincenti* is 5–10 μm long with 2–5 loose, irregular spirals.

Leptospira

Leptospira are thin, flexuous, tightly coiled spirals approximately the same size as *Treponema*, but one or both ends of the spirochaete may be bent to form a hook. They are 5–20 μm long, about 0·1 μm in width with a wavelength of about 0·5 μm. *Leptospira* can be fairly easily cultured on artificial culture media, but those which are parasitic and cause disease in man require serum-containing media.

Leptospira occur as one species, *L. interrogans*, and within this species there are two complexes called *interrogans* and *biflexa*. As it happens, nearly all the human pathogens belong to the *interrogans* complex which contains about 130 sero-types arranged in a number of sero-groups. The best known sero-groups causing disease in this country are the icterohaemorrhagiae and canicola groups. These two groups of organisms have as their hosts, rats, pigs, dogs and cattle which form the source of infection. The illness in man begins after an incubation period of a week or so when there is a leptospiraemia causing a 'flu'-like illness lasting a few days. This is followed by a phase in which there are increasing concentrations of specific antibodies in the blood, often leptospiruria and meningitis. In *L. icterohaemorrhagiae* infections (Weil's disease) jaundice may occur and in the more severe cases there is a tendency to haemorrhage.

Laboratory diagnosis

The *Leptospira* may be isolated from the blood in the acute stage if the diagnosis is suspected, but serology will be negative at this time. During the second phase, antibodies can be detected using a genus-specific antigen in a complement fixation test which is often used for screening. The sero-group can be determined using pools of antigens in slide agglutination tests. Suitable agglutinable antigens can be obtained from commercial sources, for example, Bacto-leptospira antigens from Difco.

Treponema

The genus *Treponema* contains several species, some of which produce disease in man. They are very thin, flexible and have eight to fourteen small, tight, regular spirals. They rotate quickly, but forward movement is slow. *Treponema* are extremely difficult to stain and are best examined in wet preparations by dark-ground illumination. (Disposable impervious gloves should be worn for this examination.) Some of the non-pathogenic *Treponema* found in the mouth and around the genitalia can be cultured, but this is not true of the three human pathogens, *T. pallidum*, *T. pertenue*, and *T. carateum*.

Treponema pallidum

This organism causes syphilis. Syphilis is a human disease nearly always acquired by sexual intercourse. Nine to ninety days after infection an indurated ulcer, called the primary chancre, appears usually on the genitalia. By the time this appears the spirochaetes are widely distributed through the body and there is a generalised lympadenopathy. At this time the spiro-chaetes can be demonstrated in large numbers in the exudate from the primary chancre or in fluid obtained by puncture of a lymph gland. Nine weeks later, approximately, the secondary stage develops and may include a fever, a generalised non-itchy red macular rash, snail track ulcers in the mouth and throat, and condylomata, but these lesions are extremely variable and may be severe or pass unnoticed.

The third or tertiary stage may not occur for many years (nine, plus or minus five). In this stage the spirochaetes become localised in chronic inflammatory lesions called gummata in the cardiovascular system, the central nervous system, skin, bones or other internal organs. Late manifestations of syphilis appear as degeneration of the spinal cord (tabes dorsalis), of the brain (general paralysis of the insane), and the upper part of the thoracic aorta (aortic aneurysm). Syphilis can be contracted *in utero* from an infected mother and results in a child with congenital syphilis. For this reason most pregnant women in Great Britain are subjected to a serological test for syphilis. If this is positive they are then given a course of treatment, usually with penicillin.

T. pallidum is not cultivated in the laboratory but can be propagated by intrastesticular inoculations of a rabbit with transfer to a new rabbit every three weeks or so.

Diagnosis of syphilis

(a) Primary syphilis. Demonstration of spirochaetes having the characteristic appearance of *T. pallidum* in exudate from the primary chancre or lymph node aspirates examined by dark-ground illumination. The experienced eye can distinguish these from other non-pathogenic spirochaetes which may be present.

(b) Secondary syphilis. Spirochaetes may be found in the lesions of secondary syphilis, 2–4 weeks after the appearance of the chancre and certainly by the secondary stage when the disease can be detected by serology.

(c) Latent and tertiary syphilis. Detection by serology only.

Serological tests for syphilis

In syphilis and other treponemal diseases three distinct types of antibody can be detected, these are:

(a) reagin
(b) group antitreponemal antibodies

(c) antibodies specific for *T. pallidum* and other pathogenic treponemes.

(a) The antibody here referred to as reagin has no relationship to the cell-sensitising antibodies found in allergic conditions or atopy. This reagin reacts with lipoidal material extracted from animal tissues in complement-fixation or flocculation tests. The best known of these tests is the Wassermann reaction (W.R.) which is a complement-fixation test. The Venereal Disease Reference Laboratory slide test (V.D.R.L.) and the Kahn test are flocculation tests. Tests for reagin are called the Standard Tests for syphilis or sometimes 'conventional' tests. These tests are not specific and occasionally the so-called biological false-positive reactions may occur due to other conditions not related to syphilis but where there is an increase in the reagin content of the blood. The most common of these conditions in Great Britain is pregnancy. Nevertheless, the Wassermann reaction using a cardiolipin anitigen consisting of lipid extract of bovine heart muscle with added lecithin and cholesterol is a sensitive and reliable serological test. These lipoidal antigen tests detecting reagin become positive early in the primary stage of syphilis, and in untreated cases remain positive through the secondary stage and sometimes into the late tertiary stage. In treated syphilis the tests will usually become negative after a few months.

(b) The antigen used in the Reiter protein complement-fixation test (R.P.C.F.T.) which detects group antitreponemal antibodies is an extract of Reiter's treponema. This test is more specific than the lipoidal antigen tests but is rather less sensitive.

(c) Tests for antibodies specific for *T. pallidum* are the treponemal immobilisation test (TPI), *Treponema pallidum* haemagglutination test (TPHA), and the absorbed fluorescent treponemal antibody (FTA-ABS) test. These tests are highly specific but are not able to distinguish between syphilis and the allied diseases of yaws, pinta and endemic non-venereal syphilis including bejel. These tests become positive rather later than the lipoidal antigen tests and once positive remain so much longer, often for life.

The serological diagnosis of venereal disease is described fully by A. E. Wilkinson *et al.*[3]

VIBRIOS

The genus *Vibrio* consists of Gram-negative motile, curved bacilli (comma-shaped) which are oxidase- and catalase-positive. The genus includes *V. cholerae* which

causes Asiatic cholera in man and the closely related El
Tor vibrio which also causes cholera. There are a large
number of other species which cause disease in animals,
some of which occasionally cause disease in man, and
saprophytic species found in water, soil, sewage and
sometimes in the human intestinal tract. One species,
V. para-haemolyticus, may be present in sea-foods
and if these are not prepared properly, it is a potent
cause of food poisoning, particularly in the Far East,
including Japan, but also in Britain. Cholera is an
infection of the intestinal tract resulting in the passage
of copious thin rice-water stools containing flakes of
mucus and desquamated epithelial cells. Cholera symptoms range from severe vomiting and diarrhoea with
dehydration and collapse to mild gastroenteritis. This
dehydration, collapse and toxaemia may result in death
if electrolyte replacement therapy is not given. In this
disease the vibrios are limited to the bowel and do not
invade the rest of the body.

Cholera is endemic in parts of Bangladesh, China,
India, Pakistan and other parts of the Far East.
Epidemic spread occurs from time to time. An
epidemic caused by the El Tor vibrio began in the
Celebes at the beginning of the 1960s and has subsequently spread from the Philippines and Indonesia to
India and Pakistan by the mid 1960s, reaching the
Middle East, and by the early 1970s West Africa,
Turkey, the Southern USSR, and on to Spain and Italy
(1973). Occasionally people with cholera arrive in Great
Britain usually after holidays in the affected areas. The
source of cholera is infected human faeces and it is
spread in water, food by direct contact, and indirectly
by flies. Convalescent patients frequently excrete the
organism, but long-term chronic carriers are fairly rare.
Control depends largely on hygiene and provision of
adequate sanitation.

Vibrio cholerae

V. cholerae is a curved or comma-shaped bacillus,
$1 \cdot 5$–$3 \ \mu$m $\times \ 0 \cdot 5 \ \mu$m. It is highly motile with a characteristic darting motion and in a wet preparation the
field has an appearance resembling a swarm of midges
due to the motion of the organism. In flakes of mucus
from a patient with the disease the vibrios are said to lie
parallel like fish in a stream. In liquid cultures the
organisms may be single, but particularly in older
cultures they are seen in chains with the direction of the
curve of the bacilli alternating. In culture the appearance is less typical and odd-shaped involution forms
often occur.

Culture

Cholera vibrios are aerobic and have a preference for
alkaline media with an optimum pH of $8 \cdot 2$. They will
grow on ordinary nutrient agar and blood agar producing, after overnight incubation, colonies 1–2 mm in
diameter which are regular, moist and translucent. A
number of selective media have been devised but have
largely been replaced by the TCBS (thiosulphate-
citrate-bile-salt-sucrose) agar which can be used for the
isolation of cholera-causing vibrios and those which
cause food poisoning. TCBS inhibits the enterobacter-
iacae. *V. cholerae* and the El Tor variant grow as yellow
colonies 2–3 mm in diameter whilst the food-poisoning
organism *V. para-haemolyticus* (Group 1) produces
much larger green colonies. The yellow
colour of the cholera vibrios is due to the fermentation
of sucrose causing an acid reaction in the indicator
bromothymol blue which is incorporated in the
medium. This dehydrated medium is available from
Difco, BBL and Oxoid and can be reconstituted with
boiled water (removes chlorine), and the plates poured
without further sterilisation which makes it ideal for use
in remote areas.

Isolation from specimens

On arrival in the laboratory the specimen is plated on
to TCBS medium and an alkaline peptone water is
inoculated, both are incubated at 37°C. Four to six
hours later the alkaline peptone water is sub-cultured
on to TCBS and into another alkaline peptone water.
After overnight incubation the second alkaline peptone
water is sub-cultured on to TCBS in the hope of
obtaining a pure growth of vibrios.

Most cholera vibrios are indole-positive and reduce
nitrates to nitrites. These tests can be done separately
or can be combined in the 'cholera red' nitroindole
reaction. This reaction occurs when cholera vibrios are
incubated in nitrate-containing peptone water following which a few drops of concentrated sulphuric acid
are added to the culture causing a red coloration to
appear at once.

All true cholera vibrios belong to Heidberg's Group
1, that is they produce acid from mannitol and sucrose
but not from arabinose. The El Tor vibrio can be
distinguished from the classical Asiatic vibrio in the
laboratory by its resistance to polymyxin, Mukerjee's
phages and a positive Voges-Proskauer reaction (Barritt's method).

Serological confirmation of *V. cholerae* is by slide
agglutination tests using a polyvalent 'O' antiserum and

specific Inaba type and Ogawa type antisera. (Inaba and Ogawa are two different standard strains.)

Detailed confirmatory tests are best done in a specialised laboratory, but can be found in *Identification Methods for Micriobiologists (Part B)* (1968), p. 9 (London: Academic Press).

SPIRILLA

Campylobacter

Campylobacters are tiny, non-sporing, highly mobile, spirally curved Gram-negative bacilli about $0.5 \mu m \times 0.5$–$5.0 \mu m$. They may appear as single curved rods, S-shaped pairs or spiral filaments. Superficially they look like vibrios but on further examination are quite different. Of the many species whose natural habitat is the intestinal or genital tract of animals and birds, the one which interests medical microbiologists most is *Campylobacter jejuni* because it is a common cause of enteritis involving the small intestine of man. This species is microaerophilic to anaerobic, oxidase-positive, catalase-positive and non-saccharolytic like the others, but belongs to a thermophilic group and will grow at 42–43°C as well as at 37°C.

Isolation from faeces may be accomplished on a selective lysed blood agar medium described by Dr M. B. Skirrow and containing vancomycin, polymyxin and trimethoprim to suppress common facultative bowel organisms. Incubation should be in about 6% oxygen and 10% carbon dioxide in an anaerobic jar without its catalyst at 42°C, which also aids selectivity. After 24 or sometimes 48 hours of incubation the organism appears as small semi-opaque circular or effuse colonies. It is because of its unusual growth requirements, which are not provided by traditional methods of faeces culture, that it was not recognised as a common cause of enteritis until 1977. In many laboratories, including the author's, *C. jejuni* is isolated rather more often than salmonellae and shigellae.

In some ways the infection resembles food poisoning by salmonellae in that it seems more common in summer, the source is usually animal, often chicken or meat insufficiently cooked or raw, but milk, untreated water and pet dogs have been implicated and cross-infection in man can occur. Typically the incubation period is around 5 days and contains a variable 'flu-like' prodromal phase before the onset of profuse diarrhoea. This is often accompanied by pyrexia, malaise, abdominal pain, cramps, generalised aching, vomiting and sometimes rigors. The stool is usually fluid, offensive and contains blood and pus. The diarrhoea lasts 1–3 days and may return, usually in a milder form, at intervals of a few days. In the acute phase some patients are ill enough to warrant admission to hospital, sometimes under the surgeons, because of suspected appendicitis or 'acute abdomen'. The illness lasts from a few days to 2 or 3 weeks. Occasionally the organism is invasive and it has occasionally been isolated from blood and rarely from bile and urine. The organisms are sensitive to erythromycin, which may be chosen for treatment, to aminoglycosides, tetracycline and chloramphenicol.

Spirillum minus

This organism is in the form of a spiral 2–5 μm in length. It has an active, darting motion like the vibrios but is non-flexuous, that is it does not bend like the spirochaetes do. It can be demonstrated by dark-ground illumination, or in Romanowsky-stained films. It cannot be cultured on artificial culture media, but laboratory animals, such as guinea-pigs and mice, are susceptible to infection and it can be demonstrated in their blood after one or two weeks. The organism infects the respiratory tracts of wild rats and is one of the causes of rat-bite fever, during which the organism may be found in the bite wound, in the regional lymph glands and in the blood. *S. minus* is sensitive to penicillin and tetracycline.

REFERENCES

1. Kerr, W.R., McCaughay, W.J., Coglan, J.D., Payne, D.J.H., Quaiffe, R.A., Robertson, L. and Farrells, I.D. (1968) *J. Med. Microbiol*, **1**, 181.
2. Holdeman, L.V., Cato, E.P. and Moore, W.E.C. (1977) *Anerobe Laboratory Manual.* (Fourth Edition) Blacksburg, Virginia, VPI Anerobe Laboratory, Virginia Polytechnic Institute and State University.
3. Wilkinson, A.E., Taylor, C.E.D., McSwiggan, D.A., Turner, G.C., Rycroft, J.A. and Lowe, G.H. (1972) *Laboratory Diagnosis of Venereal Disease.* Public Health Laboratory Service Monograph Series No. 1. London: HMSO.

11. Fungi

The fungi of medical importance can be divided into four groups.

1. Yeasts

These are single, round or oval bodies which reproduce by budding and grow on culture media in colonies similar to those of bacteria, for example, *Cryptococcus neoformans*.

2. Yeast-like fungi

These also reproduce by budding, but in the body they can grow in the form of chains of elongated filamentous cells called pseudohyphi giving rise to a mycelial-like mass, a pseudomycelium, for example, *Candida albicans*.

3. Filamentous fungi or moulds

These grow as branched, tubular filaments called hyphae which interweave into a tangled mass of mycelium. Part of the mycelium will grow into the culture medium and some will be raised into the air giving the mould appearance. These fungi reproduce asexually, for example, *Aspergillus* species, *Penicillium*, *Mucor*, *Microsporum* species, *Trichophyton* species and *Epidermophyton* species.

4. Dimorphic fungi

These are filamentous in the saprophytic phase such as when growing on culture medium or in the soil at ordinary temperatures, but are yeast-like in the parasitic phase when growing in the body or at 37°C, for example, *Histoplasma* species, *Blastomycetes* species, *Coccidioides immitis* and *Sporotrichum* species. These very rarely cause disease in Great Britain and are not described here.

The diseases caused by fungi are usually classified into superficial diseases of the skin, nails and hair, and the deep infections of the tissues which may be systemic.

Mycological examination of clinical material should include direct microscopic examination and culture on appropriate media.

Identification of fungi is primarily based on their growth and their microscopic appearances, particularly in culture, but it may be necessary to carry out various physiological and nutritional studies such as sugar fermentation and even animal pathogenicity tests. Serology using precipitin and agglutination reactions is often helpful with the systemic mycoses.

YEASTS (Fig. 11.1)

Cryptococcus neoformans causes a rare but often fatal form of meningitis. The yeasts are seen in the cerebrospinal fluid surrounded by a thick gelatinous capsule. For demonstration use the nigrosin or Indian ink method. Other infections such as infections of the lungs and skin occur. Torulosis is a synonym for cryptococcosis. In common with other fungi, there is a strong association between cryptococcal infections and debilitating diseases such as leukaemia, lymphoma and tuberculosis; patients on immunosuppressants are also susceptible. *C. neoformans* can be cultured on blood agar at 37°C and Sabouraud agar at room temperature.

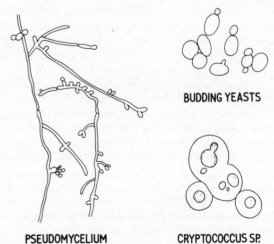

BUDDING YEASTS

CRYPTOCOCCUS SP.

PSEUDOMYCELIUM

Fig. 11.1.

After several days' incubation the organism appears as whitish, wrinkled colonies which on further incubation develop into typical very mucoid, creamy-brown colonies. Further identification is by biochemical tests, and the pathogenicity is demonstrated in mice by intraperitoneal or intracerebral injections.

YEAST-LIKE FUNGI

Candida albicans is a normal inhabitant of the mouth, intestinal tract and vagina. It is the causative organism of thrush which usually occurs in infants in whom white patches develop on the mucous membrane of the mouth. *Candida* is a common cause of vaginitis and its resultant discharge. *Candida* also sometimes infects the skin and nails and, more rarely, behaves as an opportunist pathogen causing both pulmonary and generalised infections. Whenever a patient is treated with broad-spectrum antibiotics there is general multiplication of the *Candida* and other yeasts in the body, but in the vast majority of cases this is not significant. *Candida* can often be seen in both Gram-stained and Ziehl-Neelsen stained films of specimens sent for bacteriological examination. Skin and nail scrapings should be examined directly using the potassium hydroxide method described for the dermatophyte fungi. Microscopically, *Candida* appears as small 2–4 μm oval or budding yeast-like cells, and in clinical material there may in addition be pseudomycelial fragments, all of which are strongly Gram-positive.

C. *albicans* will grow on blood agar and Sabouraud agar. In the isolation of *Candida* from clinical specimens, such as sputum or vaginal swabs on blood agar, it may be helpful to place a disc containing chloramphenicol on the secondary part of the inoculum to inhibit bacteria which may otherwise overgrow the *Candida*. Tiny colonies can be seen after overnight incubation, but after three or four days they appear as medium-sized, cream-coloured, smooth colonies which have a characteristic yeasty smell. C. *albicans* is differentiated from the other *Candida* species, some of which are pathogenic to man, by fermentation of sugars and other biochemical tests. A useful screening test is the germ tube test. In this test part of a colony suspected of being C. *albicans* is inoculated into a small quantity of horse serum in a 75 × 10 mm test tube. This is incubated at 37°C for 3 hours, after which the culture is examined microscopically in a wet preparation. Nearly all strains of C. *albicans* produce germ tubes which are tubelike extensions from the parent organism several milli-

microns long. Few, if any, of the other *Candida* species will produce germ tubes in this time.

FILAMENTOUS FUNGI

Dermatophytes

These are fungi which cause ringworm or tinea affecting the skin, hair and nails, but never deeper tissues.

There are three genera:

Epidermophyton
Microsporum
Trichophyton

Epidermophyton floccosum is the only species in this genus. It does not attack hair, and the *Microsporum* species do not attack nails. These infections are acquired in a number of ways; for example, *Trichophyton rubrum* and *T. mentagrophytes* which are common causes of tinea pedis or athlete's foot are frequently picked up from wet floors around swimming pools. *Microsporum audouini* which causes epidemic ringworm of the scalp, tinea capitis, in children can be acquired by using infected combs and brushes. *M. canis* found on dogs and cats and *Trichophyton verrucosum*, a cause of ringworm in cattle, are spread by close contact with these animals.

Diagnosis

Hairs and skin infected with some *Microsporum* species and *Trichophyton schoeleini* fluoresce under a Wood's lamp (a UV source with a special filter). Scrapings are taken from the active periphery of skin lesions with a scalpel blade into an empty Petri dish or on to a piece of black paper. Hairs which fluoresce or which look abnormal, lustreless, or broken are extracted with forceps. Full-thickness clippings of affected nails are taken together with debris from under the nails. These specimens are divided into two, one for culture, the other for microscopy.

Microscopy

Small fragments of the skin, hair or nail are placed in a drop of 20% aqueous potassium hydroxide on a microscope slide. A coverslip is carefully placed over it and the slide is gently warmed over a small flame but not allowed to boil. After cooling, the coverslip is sealed to the microscope slide in the same way as other wet

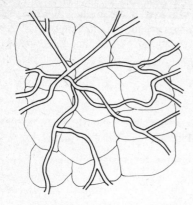

Fig. 11.2.   Appearance of mycelium in potash preparation of skin.

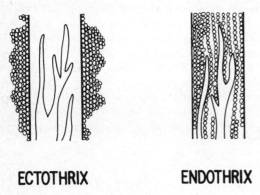

ECTOTHRIX   **ENDOTHRIX**

Fig. 11.3.   Infected hair shafts.

preparations. The slide is then examined with the ×10 and the ×40 objectives of a microscope using reduced light for the presence of the highly refractile, long, branching threads of young hyphae or older septate hyphae; occasionally arthrospores and budding yeasts are seen. The fungal elements must be differentiated from fibres of cotton, wool and other fabrics, as well as from the mosaic produced by the cells and other artefacts (Fig. 11.2). If after the initial heating the keratin has not dissolved, the preparation may be left on the bench for 24 hours or so. An organism which invades the inside of the hair is called endothrix, and one which infects the outside of the hair shaft is called an ectothrix. *Microsporum* and some *Trichophyton* species behave as an ectothrix, other *Trichophyton* species as an endothrix (Fig. 11.3).

Culture

The remainder of the specimen is inoculated both on to .the surface and into Sabouraud's agar and kept at room temperature. Species identification depends on the rate of growth, colonial appearances and microscopical appearances of the fungus and, in particular, of the type of spores (*see* Figs), namely macroconidia, micro-conidia or chlamydospores. Colonies of *Candida* species often appear overnight or in a day or so; the dermatophytes take 1–3 weeks to appear. Sporulation of dermatophytes generally occurs within 5–10 days of inoculation. Microscopic examination of the spores is accomplished by teasing out part of the colony taken from mid-way between the periphery and the centre with needles on a microscope slide in a drop of alcohol.

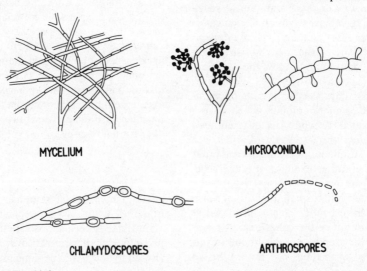

MYCELIUM   MICROCONIDIA

CHLAMYDOSPORES   ARTHROSPORES

Fig. 11.4.

Immediately before the alcohol evaporates, a drop of lactophenol blue is placed on the specimen followed by a coverslip. Penetration of the dye is aided by gentle warming over a flame but the preparation must not boil. The edges of the coverslip are sealed and the preparation is then ready for examination.

Slide culture

This technique is used for the microscopic observation of fungi in the natural state.

Method

A clean microscope slide is sterilised by dipping in alcohol using a pair of forceps and then burning off the excess alcohol in a flame. The sterilised slide is then placed on some layers of blotting paper moistened in 20% aqueous glycerol in a Petri dish. A square of Sabouraud agar 2 mm thick and about 10 mm square is cut from a plate and placed in the middle of the microscope slide. Each of the four edges of the square is inoculated with the fungus into the agar and a sterilised coverslip placed on top. The lid of the Petri dish is replaced and the culture is incubated at about 20°C. The culture is examined microscopically every two or three days for growth and spore formation. If it is necessary to stain the spores this can be done by gently lifting up the coverslip and removing the square of agar. A drop of lactophenol blue is then placed on the slide where the culture had been and the coverslip replaced. The preparation is then treated in the same way as the tease preparation before the parts of the culture adhering to the slide and coverslip are examined microscopically.

Microsporum species produce a colony which varies in colour from white to yellow, grey, buff or brown. The reverse sides of the colonies are pigmented, the colour depending to some extent upon the species, varying from yellow to orange to red and brown. The frequency of macroconidia formation depends upon the species, but when present they have a characteristic spindle shape being $8–15\,\mu m \times 35–150\,\mu m$ with thick walls and having between 4 and 15 septa. The microconidia are much smaller being $3–7\,\mu m$ across, club-shaped and borne on the hyphae (Fig. 11.5).

Trichophyton mentagrophytes produces rapidly growing colonies of two types. The granular type of colony is creamy or buff coloured on the upper surface and a browny red colour on the reverse. Numerous microconidia in grape-like clusters can often be demonstrated, and when present the macroconidia are pencil-shaped and approximately $6–20\,\mu m \times 8–50\,\mu m$ in size with 2–5 septa. The other colony type is fluffy and paler in colour with microconidia lying alongside the hyphae.

Trichophyton rubrum is slow-growing, white to reddish in colour and may have a velvety or fluffy surface. A characteristic cherry-red colour may be seen on the reverse side of the colony. Microconidia arranged alongside the hyphae occur in some strains but are rare in the more fluffy varieties. Macroconidia are rarely seen. There are several other species of *Trichophyton*.

Epidermophyton floccosum is slow-growing and produces pale, powdery, khaki-coloured colonies which are a yellow-brown colour on the reverse. Macroconidia are numerous and may be single or in groups of two or three. They are thin-walled, have 2–4 septa and are rounded at the tip. Microconidia are not seen but chlamydospores are frequent.

Pityriasis versicolor is a form of ringworm caused by *Malassezia furfur*. This organism cannot be cultured, but is seen in potash preparations of scales from the lesion as clusters of thickwalled, round budding cells $3–8\,\mu m$ in diameter and short, irregular lengths of mycelium.

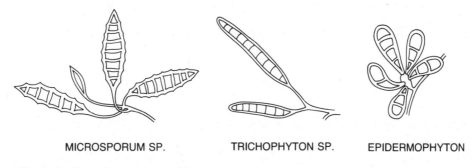

MICROSPORUM SP. TRICHOPHYTON SP. EPIDERMOPHYTON

Fig. 11.5. Examples of macroconidia.

Aspergillus

Aspergillus species are common saprophytic moulds and are frequent contaminants of laboratory cultures. *A. fumigatus* is the most important species which causes human infections, particularly in patients with pre-existing pulmonary disease such as tuberculosis and bronchiectasis. It causes pulmonary disease in three ways:

Aspergilloma, in which the fungus grows as a giant colony consisting of a mass of mycelia lying within a cavity in the lung.

A more generalised bronchopneumonia which fortunately is rare.

A hypersensitivity to the spores can develop leading to asthma-like bronchial spasms.

Aspergillus species, notably *A. niger*, but also *A. fumigatus* and *A. flavus*, can cause chronic ear infections or otomycosis affecting the external auditory meatus which becomes filled with fungal growth. Aspergilli are found so frequently in the environment that it is essential that the fungus be repeatedly demonstrated in large numbers in direct smears of fresh material and in cultures before it is considered a pathogen.

Microscopy

Mycelia and sometimes conidia can sometimes be seen in smears of sputum or other infected material. It is unusual for the fungus to be demonstrated in sputum from patients with aspergilloma or allergic aspergillosis.

Culture

Aspergillus species grow rapidly on blood agar and Sabouraud's medium with characteristic fruiting heads consisting of a conidiophore which expands into an inverted flask-shaped vesicle covered with small sterigmata in a single row. From the sterigmata parallel chains of small conidia or spores with characteristic colours extend.

Precipitins to *Aspergillus* species may be demonstrated in the serum of patients with systemic aspergillosis and this may be helpful in the absence of cultural evidence. *A. fumigatus* has smoky green conidia. *A. niger* has fruiting heads which are large enough to be seen with the naked eye and are covered with black conidia. *A. flavus* has greenish-coloured conidia, not yellow as the name suggests. The different species are also distinguished by differences of detail in morphology (Fig. 11.6).

Penicillium

This genus contains a large number of saprophytic fungi which are often grown from clinical material which they are contaminating. Penicillin was first obtained from *P. notatum*, but now it is extracted from *P. chrysogenum*.

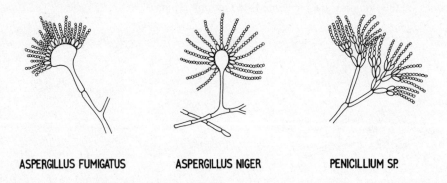

ASPERGILLUS FUMIGATUS   ASPERGILLUS NIGER   PENICILLIUM SP.

Fig. 11.6.   Examples of morphology of fruiting heads.

Mucor and Rhizopus species

Members of these species are found universally and are common contaminants of cultures and clinical material. *Mucor* is well known as pin-mould often found on old bread etc. *Mucor* mycosis occasionally occurs in diabe- tics or patients on prolonged antibiotic treatment or immunosuppression. It usually begins in the paranasal sinuses and extends to the orbit and meninges, but pulmonary disease has been recorded. On microscopy, the organisms appear as non-septate mycelial frag- ments with typical sporangia. They grow rapidly on Sabouraud's agar.

12. Parasitology

The range of parasites mentioned in this chapter is limited to those commonly found during the routine examination of faeces, urine and vaginal swabs in ordinary hospital laboratories. The diagrams are intended as a reminder of the morphology and as an aid to identification. As a general principle, the advice of an experienced person should be sought if there is any doubt about the identity of any object found during the examination of specimens. The books listed at the end of the chapter have been found useful for reference and information on the biology of parasites. Examination of blood for malaria and trypanosomes, of stools for amoebae and the vegetative forms of other intestinal protozoa is beyond the scope of this book.

Faeces

Fresh specimens of faeces are preferred and, theoretically, the whole specimen should be sent to the laboratory although this is not always a practical proposition. Ordinary rectal swabs are not satisfactory for examination for parasites. Stools produced in response to a laxative are said to have a higher yield of parasites.

Macroscopic examination

The stool is examined macroscopically for blood or mucus and the presence of worms or parts of worms such as tapeworm proglottids and scolices.

Following treatment for tapeworm if the head can be found in the faeces it is proof that the treatment was successful. If the head is not dislodged by the treatment it will produce a complete worm again. The head is found by sieving the complete post-treatment stools. This is done by carefully emulsifying the stool in 10% formol saline and leaving for 30 minutes to kill any pathogenic bacteria. The stool is then washed through a sieve sufficiently fine to hold particles of 1 mm, using a jet of tap water. A search is then made of the debris for the pin-head-sized scolex.

Microscopic examination

Using isotonic saline a wet preparation of any tissue or mucus is examined microscopically in addition to the faeces. The wet preparation of small amounts of faeces in saline is made with the help of a disposable wooden applicator stick. One drop of saline is placed on the slide and enough faeces is emulsified in it so that, when the coverslip is in place the opacity is such that ordinary newsprint can just be read through it. This preparation is suitable for examination for schistosomes such as *Sch. mansoni* and trophozoites (vegetative protozoa) in which visible movement is a distinguishing feature. When the examination is for cysts, ova and larvae only, then the addition of a loopful of Lugol's iodine to the drop of emulsion is helpful in making internal structure easier to see, but it kills trophozoites. Examine all the preparation systematically with the ×10 objective using the ×40 dry objective to examine details. Experience is required to distinguish between parasites and the many artefacts, food remnants and fungi found in faeces. For example, *Blastocystis hominis*, a saprophytic yeast, can be mistaken for *Giardia lamblia* cysts. To increase the chance of finding ova and cysts when they are few in number a concentrate is prepared.

Formol-ether concentration of faeces

1. Emulsify 1–2 g of faeces in 7 ml of 1% Teepol in formol saline in a test tube.
2. Allow to stand for 10 min to kill the bacteria.
3. Strain through a wire sieve (40 mesh to the inch) into a centrifuge tube.
4. Wash sieve for 3 min in running tap water between specimens.
5. Add 3 ml of ether to the centrifuge tube and shake vigorously for 1 min by hand or 15 sec using a whirlimix.
6. The tube is then centrifuged in a bench-size centrifuge, the speed is increased gradually over 2 min to a speed of 2000 rev/min, then the centrifuge is allowed to come to a stop.
7. Loosen the fatty debris at the interface between the two liquids with an applicator stick if necessary, and decant the supernatant into a discard jar.
8. The small deposit is shaken and poured on to a slide where it is covered with a coverslip before examination.

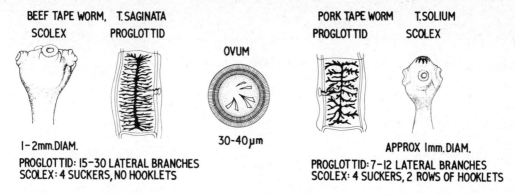

BEEF TAPE WORM,   T. SAGINATA
SCOLEX   PROGLOTTID

OVUM

PORK TAPE WORM   T. SOLIUM
PROGLOTTID   SCOLEX

30-40μm

1-2mm. DIAM.

APPROX 1mm. DIAM.

PROGLOTTID: 15-30 LATERAL BRANCHES
SCOLEX: 4 SUCKERS, NO HOOKLETS

PROGLOTTID: 7-12 LATERAL BRANCHES
SCOLEX: 4 SUCKERS, 2 ROWS OF HOOKLETS

Fig. 12.1.   Comparison of morphology of *Taenia saginata* and *T. solium*.

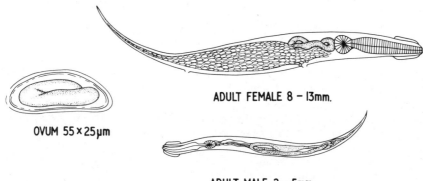

ADULT FEMALE 8 - 13mm.

OVUM 55 × 25μm

ADULT MALE 2 - 5mm.

Fig. 12.2.   Thread worm (*Enterobius vermicularis*).

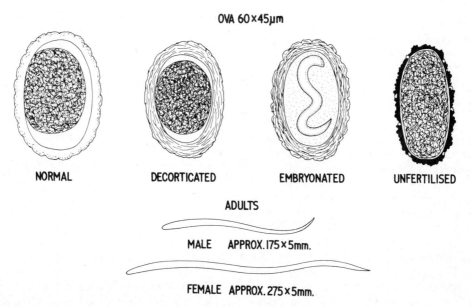

OVA 60×45μm

NORMAL   DECORTICATED   EMBRYONATED   UNFERTILISED

ADULTS

MALE   APPROX. 175 × 5mm.

FEMALE APPROX. 275 × 5mm.

Fig. 12.3.   Round worm (*Ascaris lumbricoides*).

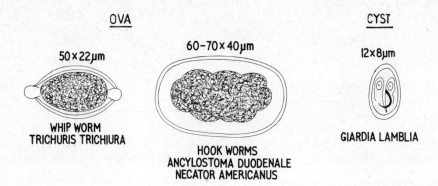

Fig. 12.4.

Ova of *Enterobius vermicularis* can be demonstrated using transparent adhesive tape such as Sellotape. The sticky side of a piece of Sellotape is applied to the anus first thing in the morning and then stuck, sticky-side down on to a microscope slide for transport to the laboratory where microscopic examination for characteristic ova is made. This method is more rewarding than examination of faeces for threadworm ova and can also be used to demonstrate tapeworm ova.

Not included with the parasites in the diagrams is a tiny worm which is the rhabditiform larva of *Strongyloides stercoralis*. These are quite often seen during microscopy of wet preparations of fresh stools from patients who have been in the tropics or subtropics. They differ morphologically from the hookworm larvae which are hardly ever seen in fresh stools.

Vaginal swabs

Trichomonas vaginalis is a major cause of vaginal discharge due to the vaginitis which infection with this flagellate produces. A pear-shaped organism, it is seen in fresh wet microscopical preparations where its jerky motility makes it easily visible. Examination of air-dried smears stained with Acridine orange by fluorescent microscopy is useful. In clinics where a microscope is available, a specimen of discharge can be collected with a Pasteur pipette and examined directly using the ×10 objective first then the ×40 objective for confirmation. When a specimen must be sent to a laboratory for examination then it should be put into a transport medium such as Stuart's or Amies.

Alternatively the swab can be broken off into a culture medium such as Feinberg's which is incubated at 35°C on arrival at the laboratory.

Microscopical preparations are made from the swab and the Feinberg's medium is examined at intervals up

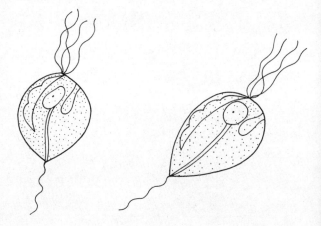

Fig. 12.5.   *Trichomonas vaginalis* (approx 15 μm diameter)

to one week for the motile flagellates which appear somewhat smaller and more round after culture. *Candida albicans*, the other major cause of vaginal discharge, also grows well in Feinberg's medium. The best results are obtained using a combination of methods. A related organism, *Trichomonas hominis*, is sometimes seen in diarrhoeal stools, but its pathogenicity is doubtful.

Urine

Trichomonas vaginalis can cause urethritis in males as well as females, and can be demonstrated in wet preparations of spun deposits of initial specimens of urine or of urethral swabs.

Schistosoma haematobium causes bilharzia or genitourinary schistosomiasis, and the ova are frequently passed in the urine of those with early disease giving rise to haematuria, cystitis and other genitourinary disturbances. This disease occurs mainly in Egypt and Africa. Ova are concentrated from a 24-hour specimen of urine by simple sedimentation, preferably in a conical urinalysis glass. The deposit is examined as a wet preparation for the typical ova. Specimens, which are treated in the same way, may be taken after prostatic massage. It is important that a number of urine specimens are examined since ova may be very scanty. It is valuable to determine whether the ova are still alive or not by examination under the ×40 objective for movement of cilia. If fresh water is introduced into the preparation at one side then sometimes mature ova are stimulated to hatch producing the motile miracidia. Alternatively, sterile water at 60°C can be added to the whole of the deposit from a 24-hour urine sample and the meniscus examined with a hand-lens in direct light for the miracidia.

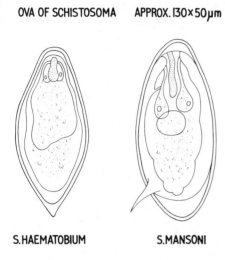

OVA OF SCHISTOSOMA   APPROX. 130×50 μm

S.HAEMATOBIUM   S.MANSONI

Fig. 12.6.

BIBLIOGRAPHY

1. Spencer, M.F. and Monroe, L.S. (1961). *The Color Atlas of Intestinal Parasites*. Springfield, Illinois: Charles C. Thomas.
2. Jeffrey, H.C. and Leach, R.M. (1966). *Atlas of Medical Helminthology and Protozoology*. Edinburgh and London: Livingstone.
3. Donaldson R.J. (Ed.) (1979). *Parasites and Western Man*. Lancaster: MTP Press Ltd.
4. Faust, E.C., Russell, P.F. and Jung, C.R. (1977) *Craig and Faust's Clinical Parasitology*. (Eighth Edition) London: Henry Kimpton.

13. Culture media and biochemical tests

CONSTITUENTS

The following are common constituents of culture media which are used to provide nutrient and other requirements of bacteria as described in the chapter on bacterial cultivation.

Agar

Agar is made from certain types of seaweed and is usually obtained in the laboratory as a highly refined powder. It is used because of its ability to form a gel. The main constituent of agar is the calcium salt of a sulphuric acid ester of a complex polysaccharide which is generally inert to bacterial metabolism. Solution occurs on heating it in water above 98°C but setting does not occur until it has cooled down below 42°C. A satisfactory gel for most purposes is produced by using a 1% concentration. Repeated melting or sterilisation of the medium will decrease its power to form a gel. Heat-sensitive materials such as blood are added to the agar solution when it is at about 50°C. Formerly it was necessary to examine all agar for its cleanliness, clarity in solution and solidifying properties, but with the refined products now available this is largely unnecessary; however, different batches do vary in their inhibitory effects on some delicate organisms.

Meat

The most commonly used meat is beef heart, muscle and liver. Meat and meat extracts form the basis for the most useful of all basic media, namely, nutrient broth. Meat extracts are readily available from commercial sources and contain soluble organic bases, protein degradation products, vitamins and minerals. They are easy to use since quality control is carried out by the manufacturers and they have largely superseded laboratory-made fresh meat infusions.

Peptone

Peptones are made by the enzymic hydrolysis of protein-containing materials of both animal and vegetable origin, such as muscle, liver, blood, milk and soya beans. The composition will depend upon the raw material and the method of manufacture, but they contain such derivatives as polypeptides, dipeptides and amino acids. Peptone provides a water-soluble source of nitrogen which is not damaged by sterilisation and is therefore suitable for use in culture media. The production of peptones is undertaken commercially, and different peptones are available with widely different properties designed for special purposes and subject to stringent quality control. In addition to all-purpose peptones with a wide range of applications, refined peptones with properties like freedom from fermentable carbohydrates are available for special purposes.

Meat extract

Specially manufactured beef extracts for use in microbiological culture media are available, such as Lab-Lemco beef extract. These are manufactured under strict control to give a product which only varies between very fine limits. Beef extracts have been widely used to replace beef infusions.

Yeast extract

Yeast extract is obtainable in the form of a paste or a powder from the water-soluble part of autolysed brewer's yeast, concentrated by a process which preserves the constituents. Yeast extract appears to contain growth-stimulatory substances and is a traditional constituent of many culture media.

Liver digest

Liver digest is a papain digest of ox liver and is used to provide growth factors and amino acids in culture media.

Fildes' extract

Fildes' peptic digest of blood is prepared by the action of pepsin on defibrinated sheep's blood; it is a source of growth factors including haematin and the coenzymes required by *Haemophilus* species. The extract is preserved with a tiny amount of chloroform in screw-cap bottles and before use it is held at 56°C for 30 minutes to remove the chloroform, but care must be taken not to exceed this temperature since some of the growth factors are thermolabile. The extract is added to the medium after it has been allowed to cool sufficiently. Fildes' extract is used in the preparation of Nagler's medium.

Blood

The blood most commonly used in culture media is horse blood although occasionally the blood from other animals, such as rabbits, is used. The blood is collected using aseptic precautions to prevent bacterial contamination and is prevented from clotting by defibrination. Sterile horse blood can be obtained commercially.

Serum

It is preferable that serum collected for use in culture media is collected with aseptic precautions, but if necessary it can be filtered to sterilise it. Sterile horse serum and other sera can be obtained from commercial sources.

Water

For many purposes it is sufficient to use tap water if it has a low mineral content. When the requirements are more exacting then glass-distilled or demineralised water may be used.

Ingredients used in the manufacture of culture media must be specified as 'bacteriological quality'. Chemicals and reagents should be of Analar quality or of the quality prescribed by the BP (British Pharmacopoeia), Eur P, USP or equivalent standard. Even small amounts of impurities, such as copper or zinc, will inhibit bacterial growth.

Many formulations of culture media are obtainable in a dehydrated form. These are generally easy to store and prepare, are quality-controlled by the makers and are constant in their performance. When making up these media it is important to follow the maker's directions which are usually supplied on the bottle label or with supplementary literature.

The pH of culture media, particularly those prepared in the laboratory, should be checked and adjusted if necessary by the addition of acid or alkali. To test the pH, aliquots of the medium are dispensed into glass tubes, previously washed with neutral distilled water. They are allowed to cool before being tested. One way is to add a few drops of phenol red to the test aliquot and a similar quantity to a standard buffer in a similar tube. The colours are compared, and if necessary N/20 caustic soda or hydrochloric acid is added to the medium until the colours match. Alternatively a Lovibond Comparator can be used. The disc appropriate for the indicator used, e.g. phenol red, is rotated until the colours seen through the apertures match, when the pH of the medium can be read off from the scale. The disc is then rotated until the required pH figure is seen on the scale and then alkali or acid added to the medium, with mixing by inversion, until the required pH is obtained. Another method using colour comparisons and an indicator involves the use of standard tubes and a set of comparator tubes of different shades covering a range of pH, each containing a liquid having the same colour and shade as would be exhibited by a named indicator at a stated pH. This sort of standard must be checked from time to time using buffers of known pH.

A more sophisticated method involves the use of a pH-meter with a glass electrode. Using a pH-meter the hydrogen ion concentration can be calculated accurately even in coloured solutions. It is essential to rinse the electrode carefully in buffer after use.

Containers

Media should be prepared in glass vessels and dispensed into sterile glass or plastic containers. Before use, glassware must be thoroughly cleaned and new glassware may require special treatment to remove excess free alkali. Media can be dispensed into test tubes, stoppered with non-absorbent cotton wool, slip-on metal caps or foil. Bottles made of flint glass and having screw-on metal caps with rubber or Neoprene washers are used. Neoprene washers are better than rubber because they can withstand autoclaving. Cotton wool plugs are inserted so that they are firm enough to pick the tube up by them, but not too tight. They allow air to pass through them excluding bacteria and fungi, but the medium tends to evaporate if stored for any great length of time. Screw-cap bottles on the other hand are air-tight. Suitable bottles for use include the 5 ml glass bijou bottles, the 28 ml (1 oz) glass universal containers, 125 ml medicine flats with screw-caps and 250 ml and 1000 ml screw-capped bottles.

Identification of media

Many media do not have a distinctive appearance when they are made up and a simple but reliable system of marking must be devised which will withstand the rigours of autoclaving. It is common practice to use a colour code for this purpose, colouring either the cotton wool of the stopper or the cap of screw-cap bottles, or by the addition of opaque coloured glass beads. The beads are boiled once or twice in distilled water and dried before use. The colour code recommended by Cruickshank in *Medical Microbiology*[1] is widely used and is noted where applicable in the description of the various culture media described later in this section. After preparation, all media should be labelled with their batch number and the date of preparation using a fibre-tip pen or adhesive labels. The hand-held price-labelling machines, as used in supermarkets, can be useful for this.

Sterilisation of media

When the ingredients of a medium are not likely to be damaged by heat, then autoclaving is the method of choice. At 121°C the usual minimum sterilising time of small bottles is 15 minutes. For universal bottles containing 10 ml of fluid, 10 minutes should be allowed; for bottles containing 100 ml of fluid, 25 minutes; for 500 ml, 30 minutes; and for 1 litre, 40 minutes. When a medium contains a heat-sensitive ingredient such as a carbohydrate, then this can be sterilised separately by filtration and added to the rest of the medium after it has been autoclaved. Alternatively the complete medium can be disinfected by steaming for 30 minutes at atmospheric pressure or by autoclaving at 5 p.s.i. for 20 minutes. Other heat-sensitive ingredients such as egg yolk, blood and serum are obtained sterile and added without further processing.

LIQUID MEDIA

Nutrient broth

This is a general-purpose beef-infusion broth for the cultivation of micro-organisms which are not exacting in their nutritional requirements.

Formula

Fat-free ox heart or lean beef	500 g
Peptone	10 g
Sodium chloride, AR grade	5 g
Distilled water	1000 ml

Preparation

Mince the meat finely, mix into the water and allow to soak or infuse overnight in a refrigerator at 4°C. Strain through a gauze, removing as much fluid as possible. Boil for 15 min and skim any fat from the surface with a filter paper. Filter through a heavy-duty filter paper such as Green's number 904 and make up to 1000 ml with distilled water. Dissolve the peptone and the sodium chloride in the fluid using gentle heat if necessary. Then adjust the pH to 8·0. Steam again for 45 min and if necessary filter to clarify by removing excess phosphates producing a clear straw-coloured fluid.

If a solid medium is required, that is nutrient agar, add 12 g of agar such as Oxoid Agar No. 3 and allow to soak for 15 min. Then dissolve the agar by bringing to the boil with frequent mixing.

Bottle, for example, in 200 ml amounts in 250 ml bottles, leaving the caps loose, autoclave at 15 p.s.i. for at least 15 min, the holding time depending upon the volumes used. Check that the final pH is 7·4. Colour code: yellow.

An equivalent medium can be prepared from commercially produced dehydrated ingredients in the form of granules or tablets, for example, Oxoid Nutrient Broth No. 2.

Formula

Lab-Lemco powder	10 g
Peptone (Oxoid L.37)	10 g
Sodium chloride	5 g
Distilled water	to 1000 ml

Preparation

(a) Granules: 25 g are dissolved in 1 litre of distilled water, the solution is distributed into its final containers and autoclaved.

(b) Tablets: one tablet and 10 ml distilled water are placed in a glass universal bottle and sterilised by autoclaving at 15 p.s.i. for 15 min.

Serum broth

This is made by adding sterile horse serum aseptically to nutrient broth in bulk after it has cooled to about 50°C. It is usually used at approximately 5% (add 50 ml to 1000 ml broth) or approximately 10%. As an alternative to serum, sterile hydrocoele fluid or ascitic fluid can be used. This enriched medium is used for growing the more exacting pathogens. Colour code: blue/white.

Glucose broth

To prepare glucose broth a nutrient broth is prepared as described above except that the volume is made to 950 ml. After the medium has been autoclaved, 50 ml of a sterile 20% solution of glucose is added to the broth to produce a 1% glucose broth. The glucose is added to the medium after autoclaving to prevent caramelisation and also to prevent the production of inhibitory substances which can be produced by reaction of the glucose with salts such as phosphates present in the medium. Glucose solutions can be sterilised by filtration, or if this is not possible, by autoclaving the solution with a pH of 7·0 or less at 115°C for 20 min. Colour code: green.

Sterile 10% solutions of glucose (dextrose) can be obtained from Oxoid.

A glucose serum broth can be prepared using nutrient broth as the basis.

Liver digest broth

This broth has a similar formula to that of nutrient broth except that the peptone is replaced weight for weight by liver digest. Liver digest broth can be used for growing fastidious organisms such as the brucellae, protozoa, including *Trichomonas vaginalis*, fungi and mycoplasmas.

Todd-Hewitt meat infusion broth

This is a 0·2% glucose broth containing sodium bicarbonate and sodium phosphate as buffers to counteract acid fermentation of the glucose which is added as a growth promoter for streptococci. This broth is useful for growing haemolytic streptococci prior to typing and grouping. It is most conveniently made from dehydrated ingredients such as those produced by Oxoid.

Selenite F broth

This is an enrichment medium for the isolation of salmonellae from faeces. Most coliforms including *Escherichia coli* do not multiply to an appreciable

extent in this medium but the salmonellae are less inhibited, and so after incubation of faeces containing both organisms the proportion of salmonellae present will be greater than that in the original sample, which increases the chance of their recognition when the selenite broth is sub-cultured on to DCA. The medium is used for the recovery of salmonellae and some shigellae from faeces or contaminated food.

Formula

Peptone	5 g
Lactose	4 g
Disodium hydrogen phosphate (anhydrous)	9·5 g
Sodium dihydrogen phosphate	0·5 g
Sodium hydrogen selenite (anhydrous)	4 g
Water	1000 ml

Preparation

The solids are dissolved in the distilled water by gentle heating. The medium is then dispensed in 10 ml amounts into glass universal bottles and sterilised by steaming at atmospheric pressure for 10 min. Excessive heating, such as would occur in autoclaving, results in precipitation of selenium as a reddish coloured deposit. Store in a refrigerator. The letter F in its name is for faeces and distinguishes this broth from Selenite S broth which is used for the enrichment of sewer swabs. In use about 0·5 g of faeces is emulsified in the medium which is then incubated at 37°C overnight and sub-cultured on to DCA and XLD medium.

Tetrathionate broth

This is another enrichment medium for salmonellae.

Formula

Base solution:	
Nutrient broth	780 ml
Calcium carbonate	25 g
Solution 1:	
Sodium thiosulphate	
Molar solution	150 ml
Solution 2: Iodine M/2 solution	40 ml
Solution 3:	
Phenol red, 0·02%	
Solution in 20% ethanol	30 ml

Preparation

Base solution:

Add the 25 g of calcium carbonate to the nutrient broth at pH 6·0 and sterilise by steaming at atmospheric pressure for 1 hr.

Solution 1:

Molar sodium thiosulphate solution is prepared by adding 248 g to 1000 ml of distilled water. This is sterilised by steaming at atmospheric pressure for 30 min.

Solution 2:

The iodine solution is made by dissolving 50 g of potassium iodide in 100 ml of distilled water, adding 31·75 g of iodine and making up the volume to 250 ml.

Solution 3:

0·05 g of phenol red is dissolved in 50 ml of ethyl alcohol and made up to 250 ml with distilled water.

Preparation for use

The four solutions are mixed together in the proportions indicated in the formula, care being taken to maintain a uniform suspension of the calcium carbonate. The medium is dispensed aseptically in 10 ml amounts into 28 ml universal bottles. This medium deteriorates rapidly and although storage at 4°C retards the deterioration, the medium should be made up freshly each week.

The medium depends for its sensitivity on the tetrathionate portion of the medium and those organisms such as *Salmonella* and *Proteus* species which are able to reduce it grow well in its presence. The *Proteus* species can be discouraged by the addition of novobiocin at the rate of 40 μg/ml to the base solution.

Recovery medium for spores (Tryptone soya broth)

This medium is recommended for the cultivation of spore strips after they have been used to test sterilisation cycles. Tryptone soya broth can also be used in blood culture and as a general-purpose highly nutrient broth. For the culture of anaerobes it is helpful to add 0·2% of agar to prevent convection currents and to use freshly prepared media. It is available in a dehydrated granular form from Oxoid.

Robertson's cooked-meat medium

This medium is used for the cultivation of anaerobic organisms and the maintenance of stock cultures.

Formula

(a)	Fresh ox heart, fat-free and finely minced	500 g
	M/20 sodium hydroxide	500 ml
(b)	Nutrient broth	2000 ml

Preparation

(a) Heat the sodium hydroxide solution to boiling and add the mince. Simmer for 20 min, stirring occasionally. Check the pH and adjust to approximately 7·5 by the addition of a further volume of N/20 sodium hydroxide. Simmer for 10 min or until the reaction of the medium remains constant at pH 7·4. Strain through muslin and express as much fluid as possible from the meat. Using large filter papers blot the meat so that the mince is dry enough to place into bottles without soiling them.

(b) Adjust the reaction of the stock nutrient broth to pH 7·4, heat in steam at 100°C for 30 min and filter through a heavy-grade filter paper.

Distribute the dry mince in approximately 2·5 g amounts into 28 ml bottles with perforated screw caps fitted with neoprene liners. Add to each bottle 10 ml of the nutrient broth. The bottles are then sterilised by autoclaving at 15 p.s.i. for 20 min. The final pH should be 7·4. If the medium is required for blood cultures, it is advisable to fit Viskaps after sterilisation.

Brewer's thioglycollate medium (modified)

This medium is used for the culture of anaerobic and microaerophilic organisms without the use of special apparatus because of the reducing action of the thioglycollate and dextrose in the medium. It is used for the sterility testing of biological fluids and may be used in blood culture.

Formula

Peptone	15 g
Yeast extract	5 g
Sodium chloride	5 g
Agar	1 g
Sodium thioglycollate	1·1 g
Distilled water	1000 ml
Glucose	5 g
0·02% aqueous methylene blue	10 ml

Preparation

The solids are dissolved in the water using gentle heat. The thioglycollate is added last and the pH adjusted to

7·3 with sodium hydroxide. Autoclave at 115°C for 10 min, then add the glucose and methylene blue solution. Mix well and distribute into universal bottles adding at least 20 ml to each, or for blood culture bottles, adding 45 ml of medium then sterilise by autoclaving.

The medium is stored in the dark with the caps tight. Oxidation of the medium is shown by blue colouring at the surface (the agar prevents convection currents making the blue colour general). If the blue colour extends more than 15 or 20 mm below the surface, the screw cap should be loosened and the bottle placed in a boiling water-bath for a few minutes until the blue colour disappears, when the cap should be tightened and the medium cooled before use. Some workers omit redox dyes from media because of possible inhibitory effects.

Fluid thioglycollate medium

This medium is useful as a basis of a blood culture medium, is recommended for use as the basal medium in place of tryptose-citrate medium in Castañeda's biphasic medium and is also suitable for the growth of anaerobes.

Bacto-fluid thioglycollate medium (Difco) is recommended for this purpose.

Preparation

29·8 g of the dehydrated medium is added to 1000 ml of cold distilled water which is brought to the boil to dissolve the medium. The medium is then distributed into bottles of a suitable size and sterilised by autoclaving at 121°C for 20 min. For use as the solid part of biphasic medium, 3% of agar is added.

This medium should be kept in tightly-closed bottles in the dark. The redox indicator in this case is resazurin, which is pink in the oxidised form and colourless in the reduced state. If more than 30% of the top part of the medium is pink, the medium is not suitable for use until it has been reheated to drive off any absorbed oxygen.

Stuart's transport medium

Stuart's and other similar transport media provide a suitable substrate in which to transport swabs of clinical material containing bacteria, fungi and parasites. It is particularly useful with delicate pathogens such as

Neisseria gonorrhoeae, *Haemophilus influenzae* and *Bordetella pertussis*, although many other organisms are kept alive for 24 hours or longer by its use.

Formula

Sodium thioglycollate	1 g
Sodium glycerophosphate	10 g
Calcium chloride	0·1 g
Methylene blue	0·002 g
Agar	2 g
Distilled water	1000 ml

It can be obtained as granules, as tablets or ready to use in bijou bottles.

A blue colouration of the methylene blue in the sterilised medium indicates oxidation and the medium should not be used unless it is resteamed with the screw cap loosened to remove any air present.

Feinberg's medium

This medium is used for the detection of *Trichomonas vaginalis* and *Candida* species in genitourinary specimens. The swab is broken off into a bijou bottle containing the medium which is incubated at 35°C and examined at intervals for up to a week.

Formula

Liver digest	25 g
Sodium chloride	6·5 g
Glucose	5 g
Agar	1 g
Sterile horse serum (inactivated at 56°C for 30 min)	80 ml
Distilled water	1000 ml

Optional: 1 mega unit of benzyl penicillin and 500,000 units of streptomycin.

This medium can conveniently be obtained in a dehydrated form (except for the serum and antibiotics) or ready made from Oxoid.

Peptone water

Peptone water is used as a growth medium in its own right and as the basis of carbohydrate fermentation media, frequently referred to as peptone water sugars. Peptone water may also be used in the performance of the indole test, although it may be better to use a medium containing a higher percentage of tryptophan, such as tryptone water. Alkaline peptone water, that is peptone water with the pH adjusted to 8·4, is suitable for the cultivation and enrichment of *Vibrio cholerae*.

Formula

Peptone	10 g
Sodium chloride	5 g
Distilled water	1000 ml

Preparation

The ingredients are dissolved in the distilled water, thoroughly mixed and distributed into the final containers such as 7 ml bijou bottles. Sterilisation is by autoclaving at 121°C. Colour code: white.

BLOOD CULTURE MEDIA

These are usually dispensed in 45 ml volumes to which are added about 5 ml of blood for culture, except for Robertson's cooked-meat medium which is commonly in 10 ml volumes to which 2 ml of blood are added. The preparation of glucose broth and Brewer's thioglycollate and Robertson's cooked meat medium has already been described.

Castañeda's medium

Castañeda originally described a tryptose-citrate medium for the isolation of brucellae from blood; this consisted of an agar slope in a bottle which also contained a broth of a similar composition.

Formula

(a) Tryptose (Difco)	20 g
Sodium chloride	5 g
Sodium citrate	5 g
Agar	30 g
Distilled water	1000 ml
(b) Tryptose (Difco)	20 g
Sodium citrate	20 g
Distilled water	1000 ml

Preparation

(a) Soak the agar in about 800 ml of the water for

15 min, then dissolve by boiling. Dissolve the other ingredients in the remaining 200 ml of water and combine with the molten agar, mixing thoroughly. Distribute in approximately 40 ml amounts into 125 ml medical flat bottles with perforated metal screw caps fitted with a suitable liner. These are sterilised by autoclaving at 115°C for 20 min. After they have been removed from the autoclave the bottles are arranged on their sides so that the agar sets in the form of a slope.

(b) Dissolve the tryptose and sodium citrate in the water and sterilise the solution at 115°C for 20 min. Aseptically add 30–40 ml amounts to the bottles containing the agar slopes.

All the bottles should be incubated at 37°C with daily tilting of the bottles so that the broth covers the agar slope each time. Examine for contamination, bacterial debris or other sediments after 3–4 days, following which the bottles are fit for use.

Using a similar biphasic method of preparation, other media can be employed for blood culture in the same way. The following are recommended.

Brain-heart infusion (Oxoid)

Formula

Calf brain infusion solids	12·5 g
Beef heart infusion solids	5 g
Proteose peptone (Oxoid)	10 g
Glucose	2 g
Sodium chloride	5 g
Disodium phosphate	2·5 g
Agar	13 g
Distilled water	1000 ml

The broth is the same except for the absence of agar and the addition of 0·5 g of Liquoid to 1000 ml.

Preparation

37 g of brain–heart infusion granules and 13 g of agar are added to the distilled water and soaked for 15 min then heated to dissolve. The remaining preparation is as for tryptose-citrate medium above.

Bacto fluid thioglycollate medium (Difco)

This can be used in the same way but will in addition support the growth of anaerobes without special anaerobic incubation.

SOLID MEDIA

Solid media generally contain approximately 1% of agar as a gelling agent. If less than 1% is used then the result is a sloppy agar which is semi-solid. If very much less is used, say 0·2%, then this is just sufficient to inhibit convection currents in the medium which can be convenient in the culture of anaerobes in, for example, Brewer's medium. If more than 1% of agar is used then this may be inhibitory for some organisms and has effects, such as inhibition of swarming of *Proteus* species, which may be useful. The media are usually dispensed as slopes in bottles and test tubes, or as plates for general use. For the isolation of individual strains of bacteria, plated media are used most commonly in amounts of 10–15 ml in a 90 mm diameter Petri dish, giving a depth of about 4 mm. Petri dishes can be made of glass to British Standards Specification 611:1952, and are approximately 95 mm diameter. Glass dishes can be fitted with aluminium tops, both parts of which have to be recycled. Disposable plastic Petri dishes, 90 mm diameter, are made from clear polystyrene. After use they are either incinerated in a suitable incinerator or autoclaved first then thrown away or incinerated. There is available a large variety of plates for holding media, some smaller, some very much larger, for instance the 140 mm diameter disposable plastic dishes; some containers have partitions, some are circular, some are square, each having its own particular use.

To prepare plates for streaking approximately 15 ml amounts of melted sterile medium are poured into sterile Petri dishes to a depth of about 4 mm taking care to avoid contamination. The outside of the tube or bottle from which the medium is dispensed should be wiped dry before pouring to avoid water droplets falling into the dish. The mouth of the flask or bottle containing medium is flamed after removal of the cotton wool plug or top and the lid of the Petri dish is raised just enough to allow easy access. When the plates have been poured the surface of the medium is flamed momentarily to remove bubbles, then the medium is allowed to solidify on a flat level surface. Next they must be dried since the presence of moisture on the surface of the medium can interfere with the production of discrete colonies. However, some organisms such as *Bordetella* prefer to be grown on a moist surface. Plates can be dried in an incubator at 37°C for 20 minutes or so; the lid of the Petri dish is first laid on the incubator shelf and the part of the dish containing the medium is inverted and placed with one edge resting on the lid so as to avoid contamination from dust. Alternatively the plates may be laid in the same manner in a drying cabinet at a higher temperature for a much shorter period.

Nutrient agar

Nutrient agar can be made by incorporating 12 g per 1000 ml of agar into nutrient broth. This is a relatively simple basal medium and is used with additions and modifications for a host of special purposes such as antibiotic assay.

Blood agar

Where extra nutrient is required for growth or to provide a more luxuriant growth, then nutrient agar can be enriched with defibrinated sterile horse blood up to about 7%, by increasing the peptone fraction of the medium or by adding extra nutrients such as liver digest and yeast extract. An example of such a medium which has an almost universal application is the Oxoid Columbia Blood Agar Base to which is added the horse blood.

Formula

Special peptone	23 g
Starch	1 g
Sodium chloride	5 g
Agar	10 g
Horse blood	70 ml
Distilled water	1000 ml

Preparation

39 g of the Oxoid Columbia Blood Agar Base are suspended in 1000 ml distilled water and dissolved by boiling. This is sterilised by autoclaving at 121°C for 15 min.

Alternatively a more nutritious base such as Oxoid Blood Agar Base No. 2 may be used, particularly where good growth of streptococci, pneumococci and *Haemophilus* species is important.

Formula

Proteose peptone	15 g
Liver digest	2·5 g
Yeast extract	5 g
Sodium chloride	5 g
Agar	12 g
Horse blood	70 ml
Distilled water	1000 ml

Preparation

40 g of the Oxoid Blood Agar Base No. 2 are added to the distilled water and allowed to soak for 15 min. It is then mixed and sterilised by autoclaving at 121°C for 15 min.

After autoclaving, some workers prefer first to pour approximately 7 ml amounts, that is, to about 2 mm depth, into Petri dishes to form a base for the subsequent addition of blood agar. The blood agar is prepared by adding the sterile defibrinated horse blood to the agar base when it has cooled to about 50°C and mixing with gentle rotation in a large flask to ensure adequate aeration of the blood without forming air bubbles. After mixing, the medium is ready for pouring into Petri dishes in 12–15 ml amounts unless a base is already laid, in which case half this quantity will be used.

Crystal-violet blood agar

This is a selective medium for haemolytic streptococci and is made as for blood agar with the addition of 10 ml of a 0·02% aqueous solution of crystal violet to each 1000 ml of medium, which inhibits a number of other organisms.

Kanamycin blood agar

A selective medium for anaerobic bacteria is made using Columbia Blood Agar Base to which is added 0·75 g kanamycin sulphate per litre. A supplement of 0·4 g per litre of cysteine hydrochloride is often added to this to aid growth. Some workers also add menadione at 5 mg per litre and haemin.

It is important that for the growth of anaerobes the medium is inoculated whilst fresh or after being 'pre-reduced'.

Chocolate agar

Fastidious organisms such as the pathogenic *Neisseria* and *Haemophilus* species can be grown on blood agar media, particularly those with a base such as Columbia agar (Oxoid, BBL); however, ordinary blood agar can be made more nutritive by disrupting the blood cells and altering the nature of the haemoglobin by heat. In practice, blood agar is prepared as described but once the blood has been added, the medium in its original container is placed in a water-bath at 75°C until it turns

brown, which takes 10–15 minutes. The medium should not be left too long in the water-bath because if it is, it will have a flakey appearance after it has been poured, and will not grow bacteria at all well. When the medium has turned brown, plates are poured in the usual way. For occasional use a plate of blood agar can be heated judiciously until the whole medium is an even brown colour.

Vancomycin chocolate agar

This is used as a selective medium for the isolation of *Haemophilus influenzae* from the upper respiratory tract. Prepare chocolate agar as above using Blood Agar Base No. 2, and when the temperature has fallen to 50°C add 0·8 ml of a 5000 μg/ml solution of vancomycin.

Thayer-Martin medium

This medium is selective for *Neisseria gonorrhoeae* and *N. meningitidis*, and is particularly useful for the isolation of *N. gonorrhoeae* from rectal swabs and vaginal swabs because of the suppression of most other bacteria and yeasts. This marked suppression of other bacteria enables a larger inoculum to be used than otherwise, resulting in a higher yield. Chocolate agar is prepared as described, using Columbia Blood Agar Base, and when it is cool, colistin-methane-sulphonate (7·5 μg/ml), vancomycin (3 units/ml) and nystatin (12·5 units/ml) are incorporated in the chocolate agar. This mixture of antibiotics, VCN, can be obtained from Difco or BBL.

Lysed blood agar

Disrupting the red cells before blood is added to the agar base is thought to make the nutrients more easily available and therefore better for the isolation of bacteria like *Corynebacterium diphtheriae* and subculture of *Neisseria*. The blood is laked by alternate freezing and thawing 4 or 5 times before use then used as in ordinary blood agar.

Skirrow's medium (Campylobacter-lysed blood agar)

Antibiotics are added to Oxoid Blood Agar Base No. 2 containing 7% lysed horse blood to suppress the growth of commensal bowel organisms like *Escherichia coli*, *Proteus* spp. and *Streptococcus faecalis* and allow the growth of *Campylobacter jejuni* when incubated at 42°C. The additives are vancomycin 10 mg per litre, polymyxin B sulphate 250 i.u. per litre and trimethoprim lactate 5 mg per litre. A combined additive is obtainable from Oxoid Ltd.

Hoyle's medium (tellurite-lysed blood agar)

This is a selective medium as an aid in the isolation of *Corynebacterium diphtheriae* and *Listeria monocytogenes*. It is a nutrient agar containing 5% lysed blood to which is added 10 ml of a sterile aqueous solution of potassium tellurite.

Cystine serum tellurite medium (CST)

This is a differential medium for the isolation and recognition of *Corynebacterium diphtheriae*.

Formula

Proteose peptone	16 g
Glucose	1 g
Sodium chloride	2·5 g
Sodium thiosulphate	0·3 g
Ammonium ferric citrate, 0·6% solution	5 ml
Citric acid, 4% solution	5 ml
L-cystine in N/10 HCl	60 ml
Potassium tellurite, 8% solution	25 ml
Calf serum	50 ml
Iso-Sensitest Agar (Oxoid)	16 g
Distilled water	500 ml

Preparation

The agar, peptone, glucose and sodium chloride are added to 500 ml distilled water, mixed and allowed to stand for 15 min before being sterilised by autoclaving for 15 min at 15 p.s.i. After cooling to 60°C the other ingredients are added, the pH adjusted to 7·6 and plates poured. *Corynebacterium diphtheriae* develops brown halos around its colonies because it produces hydrogen sulphide from the sodium thiosulphate which reacts with the ammonium ferric citrate producing a black colour whilst diphtheroids do not.

Salt mannitol agar

This is a selective medium for the isolation of *Staphylococcus aureus*. Most bacteria are inhibited by the high salt concentration in this medium but staphylococci and micrococci are able to grow. Coagulase-positive staphylococci are nearly always able to ferment mannitol, so its incorporation in the medium together with phenol red as a pH indicator results in coagulase-positive staphylococci being surrounded by a bright yellow zone, whilst *Staph. epidermidis* is surrounded by a reddish-purple zone. Slide coagulation tests should not be done directly from this medium. The medium can conveniently be obtained in dehydrated form, e.g. Oxoid.

Formula

Lab Lemco beef extract	1 g
Peptone	10 g
Mannitol	10 g
Sodium chloride	75 g
Phenol red	0·025 g
Agar	15 g

DNase agar

This medium is also for the selection of coagulase-positive staphylococci since coagulase production is paralleled by DNase production in most strains. DNase hydrolyses the deoxyribonucleic acid (DNA) to nucleotides. DNase produced by the organisms diffuses into the agar hydrolysing the DNA in a small area around the colony. After incubation, the plates are flooded with normal hydrochloric acid which precipitates the DNA in the medium but has no effect on the nucleotide fraction, so that organisms producing DNase are surrounded by a clear halo. A satisfactory DNase agar can be obtained from Oxoid.

Formula

Tryptone	20 g
Deoxyribonucleic acid	2 g
Sodium chloride	5 g
Agar	12 g
Distilled water	1000 ml

Phenolphthalein phosphate agar

This is another selective medium for *Staph. aureus* since phosphatase production parallels coagulase production and DNase production. The medium is made by adding 10 ml of a 1% solution of phenolphthalein phosphate (obtainable from Koch-Light Laboratories) to 1000 ml of nutrient agar, before pouring plates. The solution is sterilised by filtration. Organisms which produce phosphatase split the phenolphthalein phosphate, which is inactive as a pH indicator, leaving phenolphthalein which is pink in alkaline solution. Accordingly after incubation the plates are exposed to a few drops of '880' ammonia placed in the lid of a Petri dish with the medium uppermost. Colonies of phosphatase-producing organisms turn pink.

Liver infusion agar

This medium, recommended for the growth of brucellae, is prepared in the same way as liver digest broth with the addition of 12 g of agar per 1000 ml of medium at an early stage in its preparation.

Sensitivity test agar

It is important that a medium used for sensitivity testing in a routine medical laboratory should have the ability to support growth of a wide range of pathogens and not be inhibitory to the antimicrobial agents being tested. (*See* Chapter 16 on sensitivity testing.) It is recommended that commercially produced media should be used for this purpose because they are so constant and have been quality-controlled by the manufacturers. Suitable media can be obtained from Oxoid, Difco, BBL and Wellcome. The Oxoid product, DST agar base, has the following composition.

Formula

Proteose peptone	10 g
Veal infusion solids	10 g
Glucose	2 g
Sodium chloride	3 g
Disodium phosphate	2 g
Sodium acetate	1 g
Adenine sulphate	0·01 g
Guanine hydrochloride	0·01 g
Uracil	0·01 g
Xanthine	0·01 g
Aneurine	0.00002 g
Agar	12 g
Distilled water	1000 ml

MacConkey's agar

This is a differential indicator medium for the isolation of intestinal organisms from pathological material,

water and dairy products. Only organisms which will grow in the presence of bile salts can be cultivated. The medium contains lactose and neutral red as an indicator of pH so that organisms which ferment lactose appear after incubation as pink colonies, whilst those which do not ferment lactose are their own usual colour. This medium can be prepared from the double strength MacConkey broth, used in the performance of the presumptive coliform count in the bacteriological examination of water supplies, by dilution and the addition of agar. However, it is more convenient to use the following formula.

Formula

Peptone	20 g
Sodium taurocholate	5 g
Sodium chloride	5 g
Neutral red solution, 2% in 50% ethanol	3·5 ml
Lactose, sterile 10% aqueous solution	100 ml
Distilled water	1000 ml

Preparation

The agar, peptone and taurocholate are added to the distilled water and soaked for 15 min before bringing to the boil to dissolve the agar. Adjust the pH to 7·5, add the lactose and neutral red solution. Mix and steam at atmospheric pressure for 1 hour. Autoclave at 115°C for 15 min. Cool and pour plates. The medium should be a reddish-brown colour.

MacConkey-aesculin medium

This is a selective medium for *Streptococcus faecalis* which is able to grow on bile-salt-containing media and has the ability to hydrolyse aesculin. The products of this hydrolysis react with the ferric citrate to produce a black-coloured compound which is readily visible. 1 g of aesculin and 0·5 g of ferric citrate are added per litre of molten medium before it is autoclaved.

Deoxycholate citrate medium (DCA)

This medium is used for the selective isolation of *Shigellae* and food-poisoning salmonellae and *Salmonella paratyphi* B. It is less good for the isolation of *S. typhi* but is better than MacConkey's medium for this purpose. This medium is tedious to prepare from basic ingredients and different batches of sodium deoxycholate vary in quality. A medium of constant quality can be obtained in a dehydrated form, for example, Oxoid.

Formula

Lab Lemco beef extract	5 g
Peptone	5 g
Lactose	10 g
Sodium citrate	5 g
Sodium thiosulphate	5 g
Ferric citrate	1 g
Sodium deoxycholate	2·5 g
Neutral red	0·025 g
Agar	15 g
Distilled water	1000 ml

This medium is a pale pink and is semi-opaque.

Lactose-fermenting organisms produce pink colonies and may be surrounded by a zone of precipitated deoxycholic acid. The colonies of non-lactose-fermenters are colourless and may be surrounded by a clear, orange zone because of their alkaline reaction. *Shigella sonnei* grows as colourless colonies about 1 mm in diameter which become a pink colour on further incubation because of late lactose fermentation which distinguishes them from the other shigellae. *Salmonella typhi* produces colonies up to 1 mm in diameter after overnight incubation which are a very pale pink initially but later become colourless, often with a central grey dot. Other *Salmonella* species, including *S. paratyphi* B, produce colonies 1 mm or more in diameter after overnight incubation which are colourless initially but later may produce a central black dot. *Proteus* and *Pseudomonas* species also grow on DCA and may produce colonies similar to those of salmonellae and shigellae, but proteus colonies are often glossy with a large central black dot.

Xylose lysine deoxycholate agar (XLD)

This is a selective medium for enterobacteria and a differential medium for the isolation of enteric pathogens, particularly *Shigella* species.

Formula

Xylose	3·75 g
Lactose	7·5 g
Sucrose	7·5 g
L-Lysine HCl	5 g

Sodium chloride	5 g
Yeast extract	3 g
Ferric ammonium citrate	0·8 g
Sodium thiosulphate	6·8 g
Sodium desoxycholate (Difco)	2·5 g
Phenol red 1% solution	8 ml
Agar	15 g
Distilled water	1000 ml

This medium can be obtained in a dehydrated form from Difco (Bacto XLD agar). To rehydrate this medium suspend 57 g in 1000 ml of distilled water. Bring to the boil and remove from the heat as soon as the medium is dissolved, then pour plates.

The medium has a short shelf-life because of the relative instability of the thiosulphate/ammonium citrate solution which, if the medium is to be made completely in the laboratory, should be dissolved in 10 ml of water and added to the medium just before pouring the plates.

Xylose is fermented rapidly by most enterobacteria except shigellae and the related Providence group. Salmonellae (and the Arizona group) decarboxylate lysine, neutralising the acid produced by the smaller amount of xylose fermented, so that their colonies mimic shigellae. In order that lysine-positive coliforms should not also do this, the medium contains very large amounts of lactose and sucrose for their fermentation with acid production. As a further aid, sodium thiosulphate is added as a substrate for production of hydrogen sulphide which is detected by the blackening of the ferric ammonium citrate. Red colonies are produced by salmonellae and shigellae, and occasionally by some strains of pseudomonas and *Proteus rettgeri*. Salmonellae (other than *Salmonella paratyphi* A, *S. choleraesuis*, *S. pullorum* and *S. gallinarum)* produce red colonies which have black centres due to hydrogen sulphide production; other enterobacteria such as *Escherichia coli, Klebsiella* and *Proteus* species produce yellow colonies. Further differentiation depends on biochemical testing and serology.

Thiosulphate-citrate-bile-salt sucrose (TCBS) cholera medium

This medium gives a high isolation rate for vibrios and is very easy to prepare, making it ideal for use in remote areas and where cholera is endemic. The dehydrated medium is available from Difco, BBL and Oxoid.

Formula

Yeast extract powder	5 g
Peptone	10 g
Sodium thiosulphate	10 g
Sodium citrate	10 g
Ox bile	8 g
Sucrose	20 g
Sodium chloride	10 g
Ferric citrate	1 g
Bromothymol blue	0·04 g
Thymol blue	0·04 g
Agar	14 g
Boiled water	1000 ml

Preparation

88 g of the powder are suspended in 1 litre of water which is brought to the boil for complete solution. It must not be autoclaved. After being brought to the boil, plates are poured without further heating. For use, see section on vibrios. After 24 hr incubation at 37°C the cholera vibrios produce colonies which are yellow and 2–3 mm in diameter. *Vibrio parahaemolyticus* Group I grows as greenish colonies 3–4 mm in diameter. Other vibrios may produce yellow colonies which are larger than those of the cholera vibrios. The enterobacteria and *Pseudomonas* species are suppressed for the first 24 hr and produce only minute colonies that do not yellow, but *Streptococcus faecalis* grows as small colonies with yellowing of the medium.

Egg-yolk agar plus Neomycin (for Nagler's reaction)

Formula

Nutrient agar base	100 ml
Fildes' extract	5 ml
Concentrated egg-yolk emulsion (Oxoid)	10 ml
Neomycin sulphate	0·007–0·02 g

Preparation

Melt the nutrient agar, add the Fildes' extract, and steam for 20 min to remove the chloroform from the extract. Cool to 55°C and add 10 ml of egg-yolk suspension and the neomycin. Mix well, and pour in plates to at least 4 mm depth.

Organisms which produce lecithinase, such as some *Bacillus* species, clostridia and *Staphylococcus aureus*, grow as colonies surrounded by a white precipitate since the lecithinase splits the soluble lecithovitelin of the egg-yolk to produce an insoluble compound. For the Nagler reaction, *see* section on *Clostridium welchii* (p. 82).

Elek's medium

This medium is used in the identification of virulent (toxin-producing) strains of *Corynebacterium diphtheriae*.

Formula

Proteose peptone (Difco)	20 g
Maltose	3 g
Lactic acid, BP	0·7 ml
Sodium chloride	1 g
Agar	15 g
Distilled water	1000 ml
Sterile horse serum	*see* below

Preparation

The agar is added to about 500 ml of the distilled water, allowed to soak for 15 min and dissolved by boiling. The maltose, lactic acid and sodium chloride are dissolved in the remaining distilled water. The two solutions are then combined and brought to the boil. Mix thoroughly and adjust the pH to approximately 7·8. The medium is dispensed in 15 ml amounts into 28 ml universal screw-cap bottles and sterilised by steaming at atmospheric pressure for 30 min on each of 3 successive days. For use, 15 ml of the agar is melted and cooled to 55°C. 3 ml of sterile horse serum is added and mixed in before pouring into a sterile plastic Petri dish.

For use, *see* section on identification of *Corynebacterium diphtheriae* (page 78).

Bordet-Gengou medium (modified)

This enriched medium for the cultivation of *Bordetella pertussis* is tedious to prepare as orginally described and is usually prepared from a dehydrated base such as that made by Oxoid, to which is added horse blood, glycerol and penicillin.

Formula

Potato infusion	4·5 g
Proteose peptone	10 g
Sodium chloride	5·5 g

Agar	16 g
Glycerol	10 ml
Distilled water	990 ml
Benzyl penicillin	150 μg
Horse blood	200 ml

Preparation

The glycerol is mixed with the water then 36 g of the base is suspended in this 1% solution and dissolved by boiling. The mixture is sterilised by autoclaving at 121°C for 15 min and cooled to 45–50°C. 200 ml of previously warmed (37°C) sterile defibrinated horse blood is then added together with the penicillin. In many laboratories one-tenth of the above amount is prepared at one time, which is enough for four 90 mm plates of media since they are poured thicker than usual. The plates are not dried and any spare ones can be stored for a few days in a polythene bag in a refrigerator. *See* section on isolation of *Bordetella pertussis*.

Sabouraud agar (modified)

This medium is used for the isolation and differentiation of fungi.

Formula

Mycological peptone (Oxoid)	10 g
Glucose	40 g
Agar	15 g
Distilled water	1000 g
pH approximately 5·2	
Maltose may be used in place of the glucose	40 g

Preparation

The agar is soaked in the distilled water for about 15 min, the other ingredients are added, the solution brought to the boil, and the pH is adjusted to 5·5. This medium must not be overheated as acid hydrolysis of the agar will occur producing a soft unusable medium. The medium can be used with the addition of 0·5 g cycloheximide, but *Cryptococcus neoformans*, *Aspergillus fumigatus* and one or two other pathogenic fungi are sensitive to cycloheximide like the saprophytic fungi which its use inhibits. Bacteria can be inhibited by the use of 20,000 units of penicillin and 40,000 units of streptomycin or 0·4 g of chloramphenicol per litre of medium, but this combination should not be used for

the culture of *Actinomyces* and *Nocardia* which are sensitive.

Gelatin charcoal discs

These are used for the gelatin liquefaction test of proteolysis.

Gelatin charcoal discs are sterile pellets (jelly babies) prepared from denatured gelatin and contain finely powdered charcoal. For use, one of the pellets is added to a broth culture. If the organism is able to liquefy the denatured gelatin then particles of charcoal are liberated into the medium, providing a sensitive indicator of liquefaction. This method can produce results comparatively quickly, and is easy to perform. Charcoal gelatin discs are difficult to produce satisfactorily in a laboratory because of the difficulty in removing the formalin used in denaturing. Satisfactory discs can be obtained from Oxoid.

Loeffler's serum medium

This medium is used in the identification of *Corynebacterium diphtheriae*. It can also be used as an indicator of proteolysis and as a medium for the prolonged keeping of stock cultures.

Formula

Nutrient broth	250 ml
Glucose	2·5 g
Sterile serum	750 ml

Preparation

Adjust the pH of the nutrient broth to 7·6. Dissolve the glucose and autoclave at 115°C for 10 min. When cool, the medium is dispensed aseptically into previously sterilised bijou bottles in 4 ml amounts. The caps are screwed on tightly and, if possible, the bottles are laid on their sides in trays in an inspissator, and the temperature slowly raised to about 80°C maintained for 2 hr, during which time the serum coagulates to a yellowish-white solid. If no inspissator is available the serum can be coagulated by placing the slanted bottles on top of a steam steriliser.

Lowenstein-Jensen medium

This medium is used for the cultivation of mycobacteria.

Formula

Potassium dihydrogen phosphate	2·4 g
Magnesium sulphate	0·24 g
Magnesium citrate	0·6 g
Asparagine	3·6 g
Glycerol	12 ml
Distilled water	600 ml
Potato starch (optional)	30 g
Fresh whole egg	1000 ml
Malachite green, 1% aqueous solution	40 ml

Preparation

The salts and glycerol are added to the distilled water and steamed at atmospheric pressure for 2 hr and allowed to cool overnight. The glycerol can be replaced by 2·4 ml of pyruvic acid neutralised with sodium hydroxide if desired. Add the potato starch and slowly raise the temperature to 70°C using the water-bath. Shake frequently to produce a smooth mixture, then cool.

About 20 standard-sized eggs are washed in soap and water using a nail brush, rinsed in running water and placed in methylated spirits for 5 min, then placed on a sterile towel to dry. Using a pair of sterile sharp-pointed forceps puncture each egg in turn at both ends and place it, air sac uppermost, over the mouth of a sterile screw-capped 2-litre bottle which should contain glass beads and be calibrated at 1000 ml. The contents of each egg are blown into the bottle until 1000 ml is reached. The bottle is then capped and shaken vigorously. The egg mixture is then filtered through a sterile gauze into the salt solution. The malachite green is added and mixed in thoroughly. It is at this point that the various amounts of anti-mycobacterial agents such as streptomycin, para-aminosalicylic acid and isonicotinic acid hydrazide are added to the medium when sensitivity tests are to be undertaken. Dispense the mixture aseptically in 10 ml amounts into previously sterilised universal bottles. Slope in an inspissator and heat at 75–80°C until solid. This medium may be obtained ready made.

BIOCHEMICAL TESTS

Biochemical tests can for convenience be divided into primary tests and secondary tests. The primary tests include the catalase test and the oxidase test. Many workers also include the oxidation-fermentation test (Hugh and Leifson), but this test is not carried out with any great frequency in routine diagnostic bacteriology.

The secondary or second-stage tests when of general application are described together with the preparation of the culture or biochemical test medium, whereas those with a more limited or particular application are described together with the group of organisms for which they are used.

The catalase test

Catalase is an enzyme which catalyses the release of oxygen from hydrogen peroxide.

Method

Approximately 1 ml of hydrogen peroxide (10 vol.) is poured over a 24-hr culture on a nutrient agar slope. If the organism is catalase-positive, bubbles of oxygen immediately appear, and if it is catalase-negative no gases evolve. Using a Pasteur pipette as a dropper, this test can often be performed on individual colonies on culture plates. However, it should not be performed on colonies on blood agar because catalase contained in the medium can give a false-positive result. Another way is to take a platinum loop or a loop made from the melted end of a Pasteur pipette to remove part of a colony and dip it into 10 vol. hydrogen peroxide in a small, clean test tube. Slide methods must not be used.

The oxidase test

This test uses a redox dye such as tetramethyl-para-phenylenediamine to detect oxidases in the bacteria which catalyse the transport of electrons between electron donors. When oxidised, these dyes have a deep purple colour.

1. Plate method

A fresh 1% solution of dimethyl-paraphenylene-diamine dihydrochloride is prepared each day. A few millilitres are poured on to the surface of the agar plate so as to cover it, then decanted. Oxidase-positive colonies turn purple within 10 sec. Sub-cultures should be done immediately. The dimethyl derivative is less toxic than the tetramethyl derivative, and is therefore preferred in this test.

2. Filter paper method

A Whatman No. 1 filter paper in a Petri dish is wetted with a millilitre or so of a freshly prepared 1% solution of tetramethyl-para-phenylenediamine dihydrochloride. Using a platinum loop or a suitably shaped piece of glass made by melting the end of a Pasteur pipette, a portion of the growth to be tested is rubbed into the surface of the dampened filter paper. The appearance of an intense purple colour within 10 sec is a positive result. Nicrome wire loops must not be used as traces of iron may catalyse the reaction and give a false positive result. Traces of some media, such as MacConkey's media, carried over on to the blotting paper may give a violet colour which is not a positive reaction.

If strips of Whatman No. 1 filter paper are soaked in a 1% solution of dimethyl-para-phenylenediamine oxalate, which keeps better than the dihydrochloride, they can be dried and stored in a dark bottle tightly sealed with a screw cap. Before use they should be dampened slightly with distilled water, otherwise the test is the same.

This test is useful in distinguishing *Neisseria*, *Pseudomonas*, *Vibrio* and a few other genera from those which give negative reactions such as Gram-positive organisms and the enterobacteria.

Peptone water sugars

These are simple media serving as an indicator of the fermentative properties of bacteria, and can be used for all those which are not fastidious in their growth requirements.

Formula

Peptone	10 g
Sodium chloride	5 g
Andrade's indicator	10 ml
Appropriate carbohydrate	10 g
Distilled water	900 ml
Distilled water (to dissolve carbohydrate)	90 ml

Andrade's indicator is made by adding normal sodium hydroxide to a 9·5% solution of acid fuchsin until the colour becomes yellow. Its concentration for use is 1%. This indicator is colourless in neutral solutions at room temperature, but is pink in acid solution or when a neutral solution is heated. Andrade's indicator has a shelf-life limited to a few months.

Preparation

900 ml of peptone water is prepared and the pH adjusted to approximately 7·2 before addition of the Andrade's indicator. The indicator is added and the mixture sterilised at 115°C for 20 min. 10 g of the appropriate carbohydrate are dissolved in the 90 ml of water and sterilised either by steaming for 30 min or by filtration. When the peptone water–Andrade's indicator mixture has cooled to 50°C, the 90 ml of the carbohydrate solution is added aseptically. The medium is mixed and distributed into previously sterilised bijou bottles in 4 ml amounts. The bijou bottles should contain inverted Durham's tubes when gas production is to be tested; these are like tiny test tubes about 15 mm long. Before use it is important to see that the Durham's tube becomes completely filled with medium by inversion of the bijou bottle. If fermentation of the carbohydrate is achieved with the production of both acid and gas, a small bubble of gas can be seen in the Durham's tube after incubation.

Commonly used carbohydrate media include the following:

Lactose: red top
Glucose: green top
Mannitol: mauve top
Dulcitol: pink top
Sucrose: blue top
Maltose: blue and white top
Starch: yellow and mauve top.

The indole reaction

Some bacteria such as *Escherichia coli* are able to metabolise the amino acid tryptophan with the formation of indole. Indole reacts with Ehrlich's reagent para-dimethylamino-benzaldehyde in acid alcoholic solution. A modification of this reagent using amyl alcohol is called Kovac's reagent.

Formula

Para-dimethylaminobenzaldehyde	5 g
Concentrated hydrochloric acid (SG 1·19)	25 ml
Amyl alcohol	75 ml

Preparation

Dissolve the aldehyde in the alcohol by incubating the mixture in a water-bath at 56°C. Allow to cool, and add the acid slowly.

Procedure for test

5 ml of peptone water or tryptone water are inoculated with the organism being tested and the culture is

incubated for 24–48 hr at 37°C. A few drops of Kovac's reagent (about 0·2 ml) are added to the culture and shaken gently. Allow the two liquid phases to settle out. A red colour developing in the reagent layer at the surface of the medium denotes the presence of indole.

Note: Kovac's reagent has poor keeping qualities and should be prepared in small amounts and kept in a refrigerator.

Serum water carbohydrate medium

This is more enriched than the peptone water sugars and is also buffered. It is used to determine the fermentative properties of fastidious organisms such as Corynebacteria.

Formula

(a) Base:

Peptone	7 g
Sodium phosphate	1·4 g
Andrade's indicator	11 ml
Distilled water	1400 ml
Sterile ox serum	250 ml

(b) Sterile carbohydrate in a 20% solution.

Preparation

The peptone and sodium phosphate are dissolved in warm distilled water and steamed for 15 min. Filter. Adjust the pH to 7·4 and add the serum. Mix well and steam for a further 20 min. Adjust the pH to approximately 7·7 if necessary. Distribute in 200 ml amounts into screw-cap bottles. Sterilise at 115°C for 10 min. Aseptically add 10 ml of the 20% carbohydrate to each bottle containing 200 ml (final dilution 1%). Dispense aseptically in 4 ml amounts into previously sterilised bijou bottles. This medium has a cloudy appearance because of the coagulation of the serum during sterilisation. Steam the media for a further 20 min.

Serum water starch medium is unstable in storage, so for this medium the serum water is dispensed into the bijou bottles without its addition for storage. A 2·5% solution of soluble starch in distilled water is prepared and sterilised by autoclaving at 115°C for 10 min. 0·8 ml of this solution is added to 4 ml of the sterile base solution in the bijou to give a final concentration of starch of 0·4 per cent.

Serum agar carbohydrate medium

This enriched medium is used usually as slopes in bijou bottles for determining the fermentative properties of fastidious bacteria such as Neisseria.

Formula

Nutrient broth	100 ml
Peptone	20 g
Sodium chloride	5 g
Agar	25 g
Phenol red 0·2% solution	20 ml
Distilled water	880 ml
Sterile serum	50 ml

Required carbohydrates in 10% solutions each of 20 ml.

Preparation

25 g of agar are added to the water and allowed to soak for 15 min. The peptone and sodium chloride are then dissolved in the water and the pH adjusted to 7·6. The pH of the nutrient broth is adjusted to 7·6 and it is combined with the peptone solution. Steam at atmospheric pressure for 45 min. Add the phenol red solution, mix and distribute in 200 ml amounts. Sterilise at 115°C for 20 min.

After the medium has cooled to 55°C, aseptically add 10 ml of the sterile serum and 20 ml of the required carbohydrate to each 200 ml aliquot. These bottles can be maintained at 50°C or so in a water-bath. Mix and dispense 3 ml amounts into previously sterilised bijou bottles. After the appropriate coloured caps have been put on the bottles, they are laid on their sides with the cap resting on a piece of dowel so that the agar sets in the form of a slope reaching to the neck of the bottle. Colour code as for peptone water agars. Phenol red is deep red when alkaline, orange when neutral and yellow when acid.

Urea agar slopes

This medium is a modification of Christensen's medium for the detection of urea hydrolysis by organisms such as *Proteus* species and *Klebsiella* species.

Formula

Peptone	1 g
Glucose	1 g
Sodium chloride	5 g
Disodium hydrogen phosphate	1·2 g
Potassium dihydrogen phosphate	0·8 g

Phenol red, 0·5% solution	2·5 ml
Agar	15 g
Urea (AR grade), 40% aqueous solution	50 ml

This medium is available from Oxoid as granules or tablets with a separate sterile 40% urea solution.

Inoculate with a pure culture of the organism to be tested. Urease-producing organisms hydrolyse the urea to form ammonia and the medium changes to red. With *Proteus* species the reaction is usually complete after 4 hr at 37°C, but other species may require 24 hr incubation or more.

Oxidation–fermentation medium (Hugh and Leifson)

Formula

Peptone	2 g
Sodium chloride	5 g
Dipotassium hydrogen phosphate	0·3 g
Bromothymol blue, 0·2% aqueous solution	15 ml
Carbohydrate (usually glucose), sterile 20% solution	50 ml
Agar	3 g
Distilled water	950 ml

Preparation

The agar, peptone and salts are added to the distilled water. Allow to soak for 15 min and then dissolve by heating. The pH is adjusted to 7·1 and the indicator added. Autoclave at 115°C for 20 min. When the solution has cooled to 55°C add the carbohydrate solution aseptically. Mix and dispense in 10 ml amounts into previously sterilised 150 × 12 mm test tubes fitted with slip-on metal caps or cotton wool plugs.

Procedure for test

Use two tubes of medium and make a stab culture in each using a pure culture of the organism to be tested. One is incubated at 37°C aerobically for 24 hr, the other is incubated anaerobically at 37°C or, alternatively, liquid paraffin to a depth of several centimetres is run on the surface of the medium, and the medium incubated aerobically with the other tube. It may be helpful, particularly if the medium has been stored for any length of time, to remove the air dissolved in the medium just before use by placing in a boiling water-bath for a few minutes and then rapidly cooling.

Results	Aerobic tube	Anaerobic tube
Oxidation	yellow	green
Fermentation	yellow	yellow
No action	blue or green	green

Since the medium contains only 0·2% peptone and a buffer, those organisms which are oxidative in their carbohydrate metabolism, producing only a very small amount of acid, do not have this action masked by any possible splitting of the amino acids in the small amount of peptone producing ammonia. If larger amounts of peptone were used, the ammonia formed might be sufficient to neutralise the very small amount of acid produced in oxidative metabolism. Baird-Parker's medium is used in a similar way except that the colour change indicating acidity is from purple to yellow.

Oxidation–fermentation medium for staphylococci and micrococci (Baird-Parker)

Formula

Tryptone	10 g
Yeast extract	1 g
Bromocresol purple, 0·2% solution	20 ml
Glucose, 20% solution	50 ml
Agar	2 g
Distilled water	950 ml

Preparation and procedure

As for Hugh and Leifson's medium.

Glucose phosphate medium for MR and V-P tests

Formula

Peptone	5 g
Dipotassium hydrogen phosphate	5 g
Distilled water	1000 ml
Glucose	5 g

Preparation

Add the peptone and phosphate to the distilled water and steam until dissolved. Filter and adjust the pH to 7·5. Add the glucose, mix and dispense in 10 ml volumes into universal bottles. Sterilise at 115°C for 10 min.

The methyl red (MR) test and the Voges-Proskauer (V-P) test

These tests are carried out on the same culture in glucose phosphate medium and are used to distinguish between various coliform organisms. All coliform organisms ferment glucose with the production of acid, and if the medium is tested 24 hr after inoculation with one of these organisms, they will all have a pH of about 4·6, that is, they are MR-positive. However, further incubation with *Escherichia coli* results in the production of more acid and after 48 hr the MR test remains positive. Other organisms which can decarboxylate and condense the pyruvic acid formed to acetyl methyl carbinol, like *Klebsiella aerogenes*, allow the pH to rise and when methyl red indicator is added, the colour is yellow or MR-negative. This test must be incubated for at least 48 hr at 37°C before the test is done.

The Voges-Proskauer test detects acetyl methyl carbinol which condenses with guanidine derivatives to form red compounds. The original test described a red fluorescent colour which appeared after the addition of potassium hydroxide to some cultures in glucose-containing media.

Methyl red test (MR)

Inoculate 10 ml of the glucose phosphate broth with a pure culture of the organism to be tested. Incubate at 37°C for at least 48 hr or at 30°C for at least 72 hr. Add a few drops of 0·04% methyl red solution. A magenta-red colour is a positive result. A yellow colour is a negative result. Pink or pale red are equivocal.

The methyl red solution is made up as follows:

0·4 g of methyl red is dissolved in 40 ml of absolute ethanol and diluted with 60 ml of distilled water.

Voges-Proskauer test (V-P)

This test can be carried out on the same culture as the MR test. Some workers divide the culture into two parts after incubation, one for the MR, one for the V-P, others use the same culture and perform the MR first.

Reagents

5% alpha-naphthol in absolute ethanol
40% aqueous potassium hydroxide.

Method

To the 10 ml culture in glucose phosphate broth add 4 ml of alpha-naphthol solution and 1·5 ml of the 40% potassium hydroxide solution and shake. Leave the cap on the bottle loose and examine after 15 min and 1 hr. A positive reaction is indicated by a cherry-red colour. This modification of Barritt's method is suitable for the differentiation of enterobacteria and vibrios but not of *Bacillus* species where a modified medium is required.

ONPG (orthonitrophenyl-beta-D-galactopyranoside)

This medium is expensive and has a short shelf-life, so it is recommended that only a small volume is made up at one time.

Formula

ONPG	0·6 g
Disodium hydrogen phosphate	0·142 g
Distilled water	100 ml

Preparation

The two chemicals are dissolved in the water and the resultant solution is sterilised by filtration. This solution can be stored in a refrigerator in the dark. When required for use, the ONPG solution is aseptically diluted 1 part plus 3 parts with peptone water and distributed in 4 ml amounts into previously sterilised bijou bottles. In this form the medium is stable for about a month at 4°C.

Procedure for test

The ONPG peptone water is inoculated with a pure culture of the organism to be tested and incubated for 24 hr, although sometimes a positive result can be seen in a very much shorter time. Beta-galactosidase activity is shown by the appearance of a yellow colour due to the orthonitrophenol produced.

The fermentation of lactose by bacteria requires two enzymes, a permease which allows entry of the lactose to the cell and a beta-galactosidase which is induced in the presence of lactose. Bacteria which are late lactose fermenters either lack the permease or require a large amount of lactose for the induction of the beta-galactosidase.

Hydrogen sulphide tests

1. Test papers

These can be prepared by impregnating strips of filter paper with a 10% solution of lead acetate and drying them. A strip of paper is placed in the top of a nutrient broth culture using the lid to hold it so that it does not touch the side of the bottle. Blackening of the paper after incubation indicates hydrogen sulphide production. This test is simple but perhaps too sensitive.

2. Iron agar

This is nutrient agar to which has been added 0·03 g of ferric citrate and 0·03 g of sodium thiosulphate to each 100 ml. The medium is dispensed in 4 ml amounts in bijou bottles and allowed to set as a slope. The method of use is to smear the surface and make a stab with a pure growth of the test organism. If the organism produces hydrogen sulphide from the sodium thiosulphate this reacts with the ferric citrate to produce a black colour which can be seen after incubation.

Potassium cyanide test medium

This medium tests the ability of an organism to grow in the presence of potassium cyanide.

Formula

Peptone	3 g
Sodium chloride	5 g
Potassium dihydrogen phosphate	0·23 g
Disodium hydrogen phosphate	5·64 g
Distilled water	1000 ml
Potassium cyanide, 0·5% solution	15 ml

Preparation

Add all the ingredients except the cyanide to the distilled water. Adjust the pH to 7·6 and sterilise by autoclaving at 121°C for 15 min. Cool to 4°C. To the cold medium add the 15 ml of the 0·5% solution of potassium cyanide. Mix and dispense aseptically in 4 ml amounts into previously sterilised bijou bottles. Seal tightly and store at 4°C. The medium keeps for about 4 weeks in the refrigerator.

Procedure for test

The medium is inoculated from a pure 20 hr-culture of the organism being investigated in nutrient broth and incubated at 37°C with the cap screwed on tightly. The medium is examined for turbidity produced by growth after 24 hr and 48 hr.

Potassium cyanide is extremely poisonous and great care must be taken when making up the 0·5% solution.

X and V factors

One or both of these factors is required for the growth of *Haemophilus* species. X factor is haematin and V factor is diphosphophyridine nucleotide and can be replaced by co-enzymes I or II; it is synthetised by *Staphylococcus aureus*. Discs impregnated with X and V factors can be obtained commercially, for example, from Oxoid.

Alternatively an X factor nutrient agar can be made by preparing a 1% solution of haematin hydrochloride in a 1% solution of sodium carbonate which is filter-sterilised. For use, 1 ml of the X-factor solution is added to 15 ml of liquid nutrient agar cooled to 50°C. Mix and pour into a Petri dish to set. The suspected *Haemophilus* is inoculated on to the surface of the plate which is then spotted, in the *Haemophilus* inoculum, with a culture of *Staphylococcus aureus* which provides the V factor. Organisms requiring both X and V factors will grow in satellite colonies around the *Staphylococcus*. Organisms which require V factor only grow on a nutrient agar plate without X factor but are spotted with *Staphylococcus aureus* around which they satellite.

DILUENTS

Saline

0·85% sodium chloride in water is isotonic for micro-organisms, and is described as physiological saline.

Ringer solution

This solution which is used at one-quarter strength is less toxic to bacteria than saline. It can be used as a diluent for both micro-organisms and specimens.

Formula: full strength

Sodium chloride, AR	9·0 g
Potassium chloride, AR	0·42 g
Calcium chloride, anhydrous, AR	0·48 g
Sodium bicarbonate	0·2 g
Distilled water	1000 ml

Preparation

The salts are dissolved in the water which is sterilised by autoclaving at 121°C for 15 min. Alternatively it can be made up directly as quarter-strength in the same way.

Calgon Ringer solution

This is quarter-strength Ringer's solution containing 1% Calgon, which is sodium hexametaphosphate, and is used for dissolving alginate wool such as from swabs.

The ingredients of saline, Ringer solution and Calgon Ringer solution can be obtained in pre-weighed tablets which obviate the tedious weighing otherwise required. They are obtainable from Oxoid.

CONTROL OF CULTURE MEDIA

Some bacteria are fastidious and will only grow when the conditions are right. Once a medium has been found which will support the growth of these organisms it is important that subsequent batches have the same qualities. In addition it has been shown that inhibitory or selective media can vary widely in their properties because of variation in the nature of their contents such as bile salts. For these reasons it is important to use known or pure ingredients and to prepare media in a standard way which is known to be satisfactory. With commercially produced media the quality control of the ingredients has been carried out by the manufacturer, and it is only necessary to follow their instructions for final preparation.

The most satisfactory method of checking solid media for the ability to grow fastidious organisms is to do surface viable counts by the method of Miles and Misra on a sample of the new batch of media and to compare the results with an identical test, performed at the same time on a sample from the previous batch. For example, *Bordetella pertussis* can be used to test chocolate agar. Liquid media are tested for their ability to support the growth of an appropriate organism using a very small inoculum obtained by dilution of a broth culture and containing only a few organisms.

Sterility testing of media is not a practicable proposition because of the large size of the sample of each batch which would be required to give statistically significant results and the time taken in such testing. Media should be used as soon as possible after preparation.

The media described in this chapter do not comprise a comprehensive list and a number of well-known special media have not been described, such as Wilson and Blair's bismuth sulphite medium for the isolation of Salmonellae which is used in some laboratories, especially where lactose-fermenting strains are likely to occur, for example, *Salmonella ferlac* in animal feeds or *S. indiana* from turkeys.

REFERENCE

1. Cruickshank, R. (1975) *Medical Microbiology* (13th Edition). Edinburgh, London and New York; Churchill Livingstone.

BIBLIOGRAPHY

1. *The Oxoid Manual* (1976) 3rd edn. London: Oxoid Ltd.
2. *Difco Manual* (1953) 9th edn. Detroit: Difco Laboratories.
3. *BBL Manual of Products and Laboratory Procedures* (1968) 5th edn. Cockeysville: BBL Division of Becton, Dickenson and Company.

14. Serology

Serology in microbiology is concerned with the examination of blood serum for antibodies using known antigens and, conversely, the examination of microorganisms for known detectable antigens using specific antisera containing antibodies known to react with particular antigens. The serum is examined for antibodies as evidence of infection whilst the microorganisms are examined serologically as a means of identification or typing. Specimens such as cerebrospinal fluid and sputum can be examined for traces of bacterial antigens from, say, pneumococci or meningococci by counter-current immunoelectrophoresis (CCIE) even after antibiotic treatment has rendered culture useless. Serological techniques like CCIE, enzyme-linked immunosorbent assay (ELISA), radioimmunoassay (RIA) and immune electron microscopy are not described because of their complexity

Antibodies which react with surface antigens of particles and cause agglutination of the particles are called agglutinins. Agglutination reactions are used frequently in the identification of bacteria such as in the serotyping of *Salmonella* species. In this example the surface antigens belong to the *Salmonella*, and are part of it. It is often possible to extend the technique to identify antigens which are not normally agglutinable such as thyroglobulin, rheumatoid factor or human chorionic gonadotrophin. In these tests the antigen is adsorbed on to the surface of inert particles such as tanned red cells, dead staphylococci, polystyrene and latex particles. Reaction of the coated particles with an agglutinin containing antiserum of the right specificity will produce visible agglutination.

Some antibodies when reacting with a suitable antigen, form a visible precipitate. These are called precipitins. Lancefield's original grouping test for haemolytic streptococci is an example of a precipitin reaction where the specific antibody reacts with the appropriate carbohydrate extracted from the surface of the streptococcus. In this test, the precipitation is seen at the interface between the antiserum and the carbohydrate extract which are contained in a narrow-bore tube. Precipitin reactions can also be carried out in gels, in which case the antigen and the antibody are allowed to diffuse towards one another in a gel, and where they meet in the correct concentration they react to form a precipitate which is visible as a line in the gel. This technique is called immunodiffusion and is used widely in diagnostic microbiology. Developments of this technique include immunoelectrophoresis and CCIE.

Some antibodies will only react together in the presence of complement. These antibodies are called complement-fixing antibodies, but their reaction is not visible to the naked eye and requires an indicator system, usually employing sensitised sheep cells. Complement fixation tests, although of wide application in microbiology, are beyond the scope of this book. Another method of detecting antibodies, immunofluorescence, involves labelling the molecules of antibody with a fluorescent dye or fluorochrome such as fluorescein isothiocyanate. In these tests the labelled antibody is reacted with the antigen such as the specific surface antigen of *Neisseria gonorrheae* then, after washing away excess antibody from the preparation, the presence of the antibody is detected by fluorescent microscopy. In this example where the antibody (globulin) sticks to the surface of the gonococci, these organisms will be seen to fluoresce whilst other organisms do not. This is the direct method. An indirect method using a fluorochrome-labelled antiglobulin, which is more sensitive than a direct method, has been developed.

Individual antigen-antibody tests when used in this book are described in the relevant section; for example, the Widal test is described in the section on Salmonellae. Likewise, when a special antigen is required such as in Lancefield's grouping test, its preparation is described in the method or the test. The following descriptions of antigens and antisera preparation are of general application.

Bacterial antigens (Fig. 14.1)

Cell wall

The cell wall of Gram-negative bacteria consists of a layer of glycopeptide covered by a lipopolysaccharide and protein. It is the polysaccharide part of this outer layer which comprises the O antigen and the specificity of the different O antigens is related to the arrangement and type of the sugar residues in their make-up.

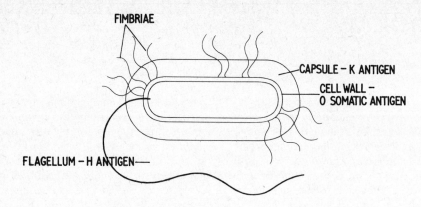

Fig. 14.1.   Diagram of sites of bacterial antigens.

Capsule

Surrounding the cell wall is a capsule of polysaccharide which is thermolabile and can be detected immunologically. It is referred to variously as the K or Vi, or sometimes as B antigen, depending upon the nature of the organism.

Flagella

These are long, thin appendages attached to the cell membrane and are responsible for the motility of the organism. They are composed of the protein flagellin and are demonstrated as the H antigen, for example, in salmonellae.

Bacterial suspensions for agglutination tests

Bacteria can be prepared so that either the K antigen, O antigen or H antigen is available for testing.

H agglutinable suspensions

These are prepared by adding 1 part per 1000 of formalin to a 24-hour broth culture or saline suspension of the organism. The suspension is then standardised using an opacity method to give a suspension of approximately 750×10^6 organisms per ml. Often the simplest way is a direct comparison with a commercially produced H suspension such as is used in the Widal test. Only motile bacteria have H antigens.

O agglutinable suspensions

The O or somatic antigen may be covered by the capsular or K antigen. The K antigen is thermolabile

and can be inactivated by heating a suspension of the organism in saline at 100°C for 30 minutes in a water-bath. Alternatively the organism can be grown on nutrient agar containing 1 part in 800 of phenol which inactivates the K antigen. If the organism has flagella, then the antigenic effects of these are removed by heating the suspension for $2\frac{1}{2}$ hours at 100°C.

To prepare the antigen, a smooth colony is selected and sub-cultured on to nutrient agar. After 24 hours incubation the growth is scraped off and emulsified in a small amount of saline which is heat-treated if necessary to remove the K antigen. The suspension is then diluted 1:20 with absolute alcohol and heated at 56°C for 30 minutes. The suspension is then centrifuged hard for 10 minutes and the deposit suspended in 0·25% phenol saline and standardised in the same way as H antigens.

These suspensions are tested by the method described for the Widal test on p. 93.

Some agglutination tests can be carried out by making a thick suspension of the colony in question in a drop of saline on a microscope slide. To this suspension is added an inoculation loopful of antiserum which is mixed into the suspension. The slide is then gently rocked to and fro for a few seconds and observed for visible agglutination. This method is used for example in the screening of *Escherichia coli* isolated from children under two years of age for enteropathogenic strains. In this case it is usually the K antigen which reacts. However, this reaction is not quantitative and may give misleading results. To make the test reliable it must be made quantitative and preferably be carried out in tubes.

To make a serological test quantitative we require to know how many antibody units there are in a given volume of serum. This is done by making serial dilutions of the serum and reacting it with a suitable amount of known antigen. The last dilution to give a reaction is called the titre of the serum and is a measure of the antibody it contains. When the titre of an antiserum is known, it can be used for the identification of unknown bacteria, because if the test organism possesses the correct antigen, it will be agglutinated by dilutions of the serum up to about that of the known titre of the serum.

Bacterial antigens for the routine testing for antibodies in serum such as in the Widal test, are best obtained from commercial sources, e.g. Wellcome, or from Reference Laboratories.

Antisera

Most antisera required by routine diagnostic bacteriology laboratories are available from commercial sources. Antisera to O antigens are prepared by the injection of heated suspensions of selected strains of the organism into rabbits using the system of repeated challenge. For example, 5 ml inoculations into the marginal vein of the ear of a 3 kg rabbit at 5-day intervals. The suspension is prepared by suspending the growth from a 24-hour slope culture in saline and heating at 60°C for 1 hour. It is usual to begin with a 1 in 20 dilution, except when the organism is highly toxic, when 1 in 100 is used. The strength is increased with each injection to a final strength of 1 in 2.

A week after the last injection serum is obtained from the rabbit by removing about 40 ml of blood from the marginal ear vein; this is repeated about a week later, and after a further week the rabbit is exsanguinated. A preservative such as 0·01% Merthiolate is added to the serum which should be stored at −20°C or better still at −70°C. Before use the serum is usually diluted, e.g. 1 in 50 in 0·5% sterile saline, the diluted sera being stored in an ordinary refrigerator. Each serum produced is tested against its own antigen and for cross-reactivity against other antigens of the same bacterial genus. A useful antiserum will have a titre of more than 1 in 200 against its homologous antigen and a titre of less than 1 in 100 against other antigens. Unwanted cross-reactivity is removed by absorption of the unwanted agglutinin by a known antigen. This is done by reacting the serum, which is diluted to about 64 times its known titre, with an equal volume of a dense suspension of the organism possessing the offending antigen.

For example, if the known titre is 1:4000 then the dilution used is 64:4000, which is 1:62·5. The dense suspension is prepared from a saline-washed growth on nutrient agar and is heated at 100°C for 30 minutes before use. The reaction is carried out by incubation at 37°C for 4 hours followed by high-speed centrifugation to separate the bacteria from the serum. The supernatant is the absorbed serum which should be tested for specificity (remembering that it has been diluted during the process). H antisera are prepared in the same way as O antisera, except that the suspensions of organisms used for injection should be predominantly motile.

BIBLIOGRAPHY

1. Wellcome (1976) *Laboratory Diagnostic Reagents*, 4th edn. Beckenham: Wellcome Reagents Limited.

15. Counting bacteria

TOTAL COUNTS

Counting chambers

The total number of bacteria in suspension or in a liquid culture can be determined by microscopical examination of the suspension contained in a calibrated counting chamber of known volume, such as a Helber chamber. This counting chamber is 0·02 mm deep and has a ruled area of 1 mm² divided into 25 large squares, 0·2 mm × 0·2 mm each containing 16 small squares whose sides are 0·05 mm × 0·05 mm. To avoid counting the same organism twice if it glides across the ruling between small squares, all the cells on the top and left-hand margin of each square are ignored when counting that square, although these cells are included in the count for the appropriate neighbouring squares.

A sample giving 5–15 organisms per small square is convenient to count, and a hand tally counter may be helpful. The whole of a large square (0·04 mm²) enclosing 16 small squares of this chamber can be seen at once using the ×10 objective and a high magnification eyepiece on the microscope. If ordinary transmitted light is to be used then the organism should be stained with methylene blue, but it may be simpler to use phase contrast. At least 500 organisms should be counted or between 50 and 100 small squares selected at random. The count per ml is $2n \times 10^7 \times$ dilution factor if any, where n is the mean number counted per small square.

Method

A scrupulously clean chamber and cover-glass are used. A few drops of formalin are added to the suspension to be counted prior to a thorough mixing, such as on a 'whirlimix'. If the suspension requires dilution, this is done using previously filtered 0·1% peptone water containing 0·1% Teepol and 1% methylene blue. Fill the chamber by capillarity and allow 5 min for the bacteria to settle before counting. Take the average of 3 counts as the result.

Counts of stained films

The Breed count uses a microscope slide upon which an area of 100 mm² is etched. Into each square is placed 0·01 ml of fluid from a microsyringe, and the fluid spread over the area. This is allowed to dry and the film is stained with methylene blue. Count the number of organisms in several fields in different parts of the ruled area using an oil-immersion lens giving a known field diameter. The count per ml is then $(n \times 4 \times 10^4) \div (\pi d^2)$ where n is the number per field and d is the diameter of the field. The organisms are more numerous at the centre than at the edges, and counts must therefore be made across the complete width of the drop to obtain an average.

Electronic counters

A number of models are now available but they are not yet in general use in routine medical laboratories. One such model uses the principle of the alteration of electric resistance across a small hole in a glass tube each time an organism passes through this hole.

Precision of total count

The precision of any total count is limited by sampling error arising from the limited number of organisms counted, and technical errors such as the errors in the volume of the chamber or counting the same organism twice, or detachment of a fraction of the organisms during fixation and staining in the Breed count.

VIABLE COUNTS

In a total bacterial count many of the organisms counted may be dead or indistinguishable from other particles. An estimate of the number of living organisms in a sample is called the viable count. In making a viable count we must assume that each living bacterium is capable of producing a colony when subsequently cultured. A second assumption is that each colony subsequently counted has arisen from one bacterium. This is often not the case, particularly with organisms such as streptococci which commonly form chains or with mycobacteria which cling together in groups. These multiples of bacteria can often be separated by shaking with glass beads or light ultrasonification. A viable count is then an estimate of the number of particles in a suspension capable of producing a colony. Dilutions should be done in 0·1% peptone water or quarter-strength Ringer's solution.

Dilution counts

Serial dilutions, such as tenfold, of the culture are made and known volumes of these dilutions are added to tubes of culture medium. After incubation the tubes are examined for growth, and the probable number of viable organisms in the original suspension is calculated with reference to the highest dilution showing growth.

Presumptive coliform count

The presumptive coliform count is an estimation of the number of coliform bacilli in water in which various quantities of MacConkey broth are inoculated with given quantities of the water being examined. After incubation, cultures showing acid and gas are counted and the probable number of coliform organisms in 100 ml of water is calculated using McCrady's tables. The method is described in the section on examination of waters of Cruickshank's *Medical Microbiology*.[1]

Pour plates

A known volume of the suspension is mixed with molten agar culture medium in a Petri dish. After setting and incubation the number of colonies is counted.

Method

(a) Make serial tenfold dilutions of the well-mixed bacterial suspension such that one of the dilutions will contain between 50 and 500 viable bacteria per ml. First pipette 9 ml amounts of diluent into each of 9 sterile test tubes.

(b) Mix well. If individual bacteria rather than bacterial cell groups are to be counted, then this mixing must be vigorous, such as on a 'whirlimix'. Alternatively the cultures may be subjected to light ultrasonifica-

tion to disrupt the cell groups, which increases the viable count.

(c) Using a sterile 1 ml 'to deliver' pipette, transfer 1 ml of the suspension into the first tube of diluent. It is important to fill and empty the pipette with the suspension several times before withdrawing from the original container, to remove any excess drop from the outside of the pipette and to delivery the contents into the tube of diluent slowly, touching the wall of the tube but not dipping into the diluent.

(d) With a fresh sterile 1 ml pipette, mix the first dilution by filling and emptying several times and then transfer 1 ml into the next tube of diluent. Make the remaining dilutions in the same way using a fresh pipette for each.

Note: The pipettes must be operated by a mechanical means such as a rubber teat; mouth pipetting is forbidden in microbiology laboratories.

(e) Beginning with the highest dilution, pipette 1 ml amounts of each dilution into each of three 90 mm Petri dishes, then pour into each dish about 10 ml of clear nutrient agar which has been melted and then cooled to between 45 and 50°C.

(f) Mix immediately by moving the plate on the surface of the bench from side to side 6 times, then to and fro 6 times, followed by making circular movements causing swirling of the medium alternately in a clockwise direction for about 10 sec and then anticlockwise for about 10 sec taking care not to spill any of the contents.

(g) Allow the medium to set, then incubate in an inverted position for 1 or 2 days.

(h) Count the colonies in the 3 plates that were inoculated with the dilution giving between 50 and 500 colonies per plate. Multiply the average number per plate by the dilution factor to obtain the viable count per ml in the original suspension.

It is convenient to use 12×100 mm rimless test tubes with loose-fitting metal caps which are previously sterilised and held in a metal rack to make the dilutions. Both tubes and Petri dishes should be labelled with the dilution, etc., using a fibre-tipped pen, before use. Experience will show that it may only be necessary to sample the higher dilutions, for example, if counting the number of organisms in a fast-growing overnight culture, then it might be quite satisfactory to begin sample at 10^5 (1 in 100,000) and omit the lower dilutions which will contain too many colonies to count. If a fresh pipette is not used for each step when diluting the bacteria the count may be as much as one hundred times too high because of the organisms retained on the wall of the pipette.

Surface colony counts

Spread plates

A known volume of the suspension to be counted, usually between 0·1 ml and 0·4 ml, is pipetted on to the surface of a nutrient agar plate and spread out evenly with a sterile spreader. L-shaped glass rods may be used for this purpose which can be sterilised in tins by dry heat and discarded after use, or can be disinfected repeatedly by immersion in a beaker of boiling distilled water. Two further methods, one using a standardised inoculation loop and one using blotting paper, which are suitable for the routine screening for bacteriuria are described in the section dealing with urine examination.

Drop method

This useful method is named after Miles and Misra who first described it. If the number of bacteria in the suspension to be counted is completely unknown, up to 10 ten-fold dilutions are made in 0·1% peptone water as previously described. If the numerical range of the count is known then only suitable dilutions are prepared.

(a) Petri dishes containing a suitable nutrient solid medium are prepared and the medium is dried more than is usually necessary, for 2 hr in an incubator.

(b) Divide the area of the medium into 6 segments by ruling lines on the bottom of the plate with a fibre-tip pen. Label one segment on each of 6 plates for each dilution to be tested.

(c) Using a sterile '50 dropper' pipette (drops of 0·02 ml at 30 drops per minute), beginning with the highest dilution and holding the pipette in a vertical position 10 mm above the plate, allow one drop of this dilution to fall on to the surface of the medium of the segment labelled for this dilution on each of 6 plates. This operation must be done confidently and without hesitation, or there will be splashing or bouncing and running of the drops on the surfaces of the media making them difficult or impossible to read.

(d) This operation is carried out for the next lowest dilution, filling and emptying the pipette three times before dispensing the drops. Repeat until all the dilutions have been sampled.

(e) Leave the plates with the medium lowermost on the bench for the liquid in the drops to be absorbed before the plates are incubated in the usual way.

(f) After incubation, count the number of colonies in the drops having 10–20 colonies; these should all be for the same dilution.

(g) Divide the total count for this dilution by the number of drops to be counted (6) and multiply this by 50 (because of the drop size), and by the dilution factor of the suspension sampled, e.g. 20 (average count) $\times$ 50 $\times 10^6$ giving organisms per ml of original.

Membrane filter counts

Sterilisable filter apparatus using thin, porous cellulose discs capable of retaining bacteria are used. The filters, wrapped in Kraft paper, are autoclaved either pre-assembled with the screw-parts loose or as individual parts. The membranes are autoclaved whilst interleaved between absorbent pads in a container, or can be bought ready for use. The sterilised filter is fitted to a filter flask, which is connected to a trap, and then to a pump giving a suction of 250–500 mm of mercury. It is usually convenient to use a filter of 50 or 66 mm diameter and a pore size of 0·45 μm. Discs with a grid marked on the surface can be obtained, and make counting easier. Both smaller and larger filters are available and can be adapted for this purpose. Obviously this method can be used only where very small numbers of bacteria are expected in the sample since each bacterium appears as a colony on the filter disc; the number of bacteria in the sample must not exceed the number of colonies, say about 100, which it is possible to count on any disc. This method is useful for the examination of drinking water, pharmaceutical products, etc., in which the bacterial count is expected to be low or non-existent.

Method

(a) Assemble all the apparatus and check that the filter is seating properly.

(b) Pour a measured volume of the fluid to be examined into the upper funnel and apply suction.

(c) When filtration is complete, slowly restore the pressure so as to avoid sucking back.

(d) Remove the filter disc from the apparatus aseptically on to a nutrient medium. This can either be a solid nutrient medium in a Petri dish, such as blood agar, or 2 or 3 ml of a suitable liquid medium can be pipetted on to a sterile Whatman 50 mm No. 17 absorbent pad in a Petri dish. In both these methods the culture medium can easily rise to the organisms on the other surface of the filter disc by capillarity.

(e) The disc may be incubated aerobically or anaerobically as required at a suitable temperature, depending on the type of organisms being looked for.

(f) The result is obtained by simply counting the number of colonies observed on the disc after incubation and referring this to the volume of liquid sampled. The result is usually expressed in organisms per ml or organisms per 100 ml as in the case of water.

Membrane filters are discussed further in chapter 17.

Opacity

The Beer–Lambert law does not hold at high bacterial concentrations which are underestimated because of secondary scattering of light by reflection from the bacterial surfaces. However, standard opacity tubes like Brown's tubes containing barium sulphate are sometimes useful where a rough estimate of bacterial concentration is required. These are best obtained commercially. A number of glass tubes containing a different concentration of barium are used; these tubes are given a number and, using a similar tube, the comparison is made by holding the unknown suspension and the standard side by side against a white card ruled with a black line. The line is set at right-angles to the tubes which are viewed by daylight whilst standing with back to a window. With practice the opacity of the unknown tube can be brought to within 10% of that of the standard. In any given set of conditions of growth of a particular bacterial species, once the concentrations of organisms which produce an opacity equivalent to each of the standards are known, they can be used repeatedly without further bacterial counts being done.

Scattered light

Within limits the amount of light scattered by a bacterial suspension is proportional to the concentration of bacteria in that suspension. This is measured by a nephelometer such as the EEL nephelometer (Evans Electroselenium Limited). The sample is contained in a round-bottomed test tube placed in the machine over an electric bulb. Light scattered from the suspension reaches a ring of photoelectric cells surrounding the base of the tube. These are connected to a galvanometer with an arithmetic scale. The reading is compared with an arbitrary standard consisting of a rod of Perspex with a ground surface which is inserted into a test tube of water. Calibration curves are prepared using dilutions of a known suspension against the standard.

REFERENCE

1. Cruickshank, R. (1975) *Medical Microbiology* (13th edn). Edinburgh, London and New York: Churchill Livingstone.

16. Laboratory tests of therapeutic antimicrobial agents

SENSITIVITY

Antimicrobial chemotherapy is the treatment of infectious diseases with drugs which either kill or inhibit the causative organisms. For such treatment to be effective, an antimicrobial agent to which the infecting organisms are sensitive must be chosen. In the case of a number of organisms such as *Streptococcus pyogenes,* the pattern of sensitivity to antimicrobial agents is pretty constant and therefore predictable, but in the case of other organisms such as *Escherichia coli*, it is not possible to predict with certainty to which antimicrobial agent a particular organism will be sensitive. In this case, it is helpful when selecting treatment to have had sensitivity tests performed on the causative organism. Where an organism is sensitive to a number of drugs, the clinician takes into account the pharmacological properties of the drug such as route of administration, distribution within the body, toxicity, and side effects. For further information on the principles of antibiotic treatment, which is outside the scope of this book, the reader is referred to *Antibiotic and Chemotherapy* by Garrod *et al.*[1] and *Antibiotics in Clinical Practice* by Hillas Smith.[2]

Antimicrobial agents may be divided into two categories, the synthetic or chemical chemotherapeutic agents which include the sulphonamides, nitrofurantoin, nalidixic acid, trimethoprim, metronidazole, and so on, and the antibiotics which are antimicrobial substances produced by living organisms. The majority of those used in clinical practice were originally produced from moulds and fungi, but bacitracin which is sometimes used as a topical spray is produced by a bacterium. Many antibiotics, such as the semi-synthetic penicillins, have had the original molecule manipulated chemically to alter both the range of antimicrobial activity and the pharmacological properties of the drug to improve them.

Antimicrobial agents, including both the synthetic chemicals and the antibiotics, can have two types of action. Bactericidal drugs are rapidly lethal, for example, penicillins, cephalosporins, aminoglycosides and polymyxins. Bacteriostatic drugs merely inhibit the growth of organisms, for example, sulphonamides,

tetracyclines and chloramphenicol. However, the difference in action may be merely one of concentration, for example, erythromycin may be bactericidal in high concentrations or bacteristatic in low concentrations. The least amount of antimicrobial agent which will inhibit the reproduction of the organism is called the minimum inhibitory concentration (MIC). The least amount of drug required to kill the population is called the minimum bactericidal concentration (MBC). Ways of measuring these concentrations will be mentioned later. Antimicrobial agents can also be divided into three main groups depending upon the range of their antimicrobial effect.

1. Active against Gram-positive organisms and Gram-negative cocci, e.g. penicillin, erythromycin.
2. Active against Gram-negative bacilli, e.g. polymyxins and gentamicin.
3. Broad-spectrum antimicrobials active against both Gram-positive and Gram-negative organisms, e.g. tetracyclines, chloramphenicol and the mixture co-trimoxazole (sulphamethoxazole-trimethoprim mixture).

Mycobacteria are a special case, but *M. tuberculosis* is generally sensitive to rifampicin and streptomycin; also to ethambutol, isoniazid and para-aminosalicylic acid which have little effect on other bacteria.

Diffusion or plate tests. In these methods, a plate of a suitable nutrient agar medium-sensitivity test agar has its surface uniformly seeded with the culture and the antimicrobial agent is allowed to diffuse into the medium from a focal source such as a disc, or is incorporated within the medium as in methicillin mannitol salt agar, a selective medium for the isolation of methicillin-resistant *Staphylococcus aureus*. These methods are also used for antibiotic assays.

Tube methods. These employ a series of dilutions of the drug in broth to which a standard inoculum of the test organism is added. After incubation the lowest concentration of the drug which visibly inhibits the growth is recorded as the minimum inhibitory concentration (MIC), whilst tubes showing no growth are sub-cultured on to drug-free medium, and the lowest concentration producing no growth is the minimum bactericidal concentration (MBC). The amount of work involved and the time taken in the performance of these tests prevent their use for routine clinical work, but they are used for special purposes such as in subacute bacterial endocarditis.

SENSITIVITY TESTS

Plate diffusion tests

Disc method

A known amount of antimicrobial agent is incorporated in a small disc of blotting paper. For the test a suitable medium is uniformly seeded with the test organism to produce a lawn after incubation. As soon as the plate has been inoculated, the piece of blotting paper is placed gently but firmly on the surface of the medium. The drug diffuses from the disc into the medium. Where it reaches a sufficient concentration it inhibits the growth of the organism, producing a zone of inhibition, which can be seen after incubation. This method is used generally in the United Kingdom for routine sensitivity testing because of its simplicity and cheapness.

Plate method

A Petri dish of sensitivity-test agar has a strip of approximately one-third of its area removed aseptically and replaced with medium containing the antimicrobial agent. A similar effect can be had by laying a strip of antibiotic impregnated paper across the plate. This method is used for testing a number of strains against a single drug, e.g. staphylococci against methicillin by streaking the organism across the plate at right angles to the strip. Each plate should be controlled using a known or standard organism.

Hole or cup method

Following inoculation, either a small hole is punched out of the sensitivity agar on a plate using a cork borer, or a small cylinder such as a 'fish spine' (porcelain electrical wire insulator) is placed on the surface of the medium. The cavity is filled with the drug solution. As with the disc method a number of different strengths of a single antibiotic may be used; alternatively a number of different drugs can be tested in this way. The drug diffuses away from the hole into the medium in the same way as in the disc test.

Factors affecting plate diffusion sensitivity tests

1. Medium

Only flat-bottom plates can be used and the medium must be of uniform depth, approximately 4 mm (pour on a level surface). The medium must support the growth of the organism to be tested and must not inhibit the action of the drug or drugs to be used, e.g. the pH of the medium is important and can affect the activity of antibiotics, notably streptomycin which is five-hundred times more active at pH 8·5 than pH 5·5, whilst tetracycline is more effective in acid solution. Some agars are inhibitory to the aminoglycosides and polymyxins. Highly protein-bound antibiotics such as fucidic acid will appear less effective on blood-containing media than on media of a lower protein content. Other contents of media which may affect the drugs being tested include electrolytes, peptones, fractions of which may inhibit sulphonamides, and reducing agents. Sugars should not be incorporated in sensitivity test agar because their fermentation will change the pH of the medium; so will incubation in an atmosphere of carbon dioxide, which should also be avoided. Anaerobic incubation may also produce uncertain results. Sulphonamide inhibitors can be neutralised by the addition of 5% lysed horse blood.

2. Inoculum

In general, the size of the zone of inhibition in a plate test is reduced as the number of bacteria present increases. With most drugs this effect is quite small but with the cephalosporins and sulphonamides, it can be appreciable.

3. Discs

The amount of drug in a disc must be such that the results of the test can be related to amounts of the drug which may be expected at the site of the infection in a patient on normal therapeutic doses. For this reason, a number of drugs are used at two strengths, the lower one for general use and the higher one for use in urinary tract infections where the drug can be expected to be excreted and concentrated in the urine or when, in special circumstances, the blood or tissue levels are expected to be higher than usual. Since there is no general agreement as to the amount of drug in each disc, it is likely that the pathologist in charge of the laboratory will prescribe the amount to be used. For most purposes it is convenient to buy the drug-containing discs from a commercial source such as Mast or Oxoid. To reduce the tedium of using a number of separate discs, there are various devices such as the Oxoid Multodisks, where satellite discs of filter paper incorporating the drugs are joined centrally for ease of handling. These are placed on pre-seeded agar plates in the same way as the discs. The discs must be stored in airtight waterproof containers in a refrigerator, and expiry dates adhered to.

Pre-diffusion, where the inoculated plate with added discs is left for about 3 hours on the bench before incubation, allowing the drug time to diffuse, has been recommended but satisfactory results can be obtained without this additional complication.

Incubation at 37°C will usually be overnight. Sometimes for special purposes, with heavy inocula and a fast-growing organism, the results can be read after only a few hours incubation. Tests should not be incubated longer than necessary to be able to read the results, because of deterioration in the drug with time.

4. Controls

Every test is an experiment and, accordingly, should be controlled. Each disc is controlled in the method described by Dr E.J. Stokes in *Clinical Bacteriology*.[3] If multiple discs are used, then control tests should be set up every day for each type of multiple disc using standard strains of *Staphylococcus aureus*, e.g. NCTC 6571, Oxford strain, for most purposes because it is sensitive to normal amounts of commonly used antibiotics. *Escherichia coli*, e.g. NCTC 10418, is used to control the polymyxins (including colistin and thiosporin) and for tests of organisms isolated from the urinary tract when larger amounts of drugs are used in the test. The choice of control organism depends more upon the site from which the organism has been isolated than upon the species. This is because the effectiveness of therapy depends upon the concentration of antibiotic at the site of infection. Whether a particular organism is relatively resistant or not for that species can be determined by using a typical member of the same species as control, other conditions being equal. For example, *Pseudomonas aeruginosa* NCTC 10662, a sensitive strain, is used to control tests of sensitivity of isolated strains of *Pseudomonas* sp. which may be relatively resistant to, say, gentamicin, using a Stokes' plate.

Interpretation of results

The size of the zone produced with the unknown organism is compared directly with that given by the control organism. Sensitivity is signified by a zone of inhibition the same size as, or larger than, that of the control. Resistance is signified by absence of a zone of inhibition or one that is less than 2 mm radius.

The term 'moderate resistance' is used when the radius of inhibition is more than 2 mm, but smaller than the radius of the control, if the inocula and other conditions are similar. Moderate resistance may be an increase in the resistance to particular antibiotics in a normally sensitive species which is not enough to justify the term 'resistant', or it may refer to the usual sensitivity of the species which happens to be more resistant than the control organism, but which may still respond to treatment with normal or high doses of the drug.

The activity of different drugs cannot be compared by comparison of the zone sizes since some diffuse readily into the agar and therefore have large zones, e.g. chloramphenicol, while others diffuse poorly, e.g. polymyxin, and produce small zones of inhibition.

Staphylococci and penicillins

A high proportion of the strains of *Staphylococcus aureus* which are isolated in hospitals produce a penicillinase (beta lactamase) which destroys the drug. However, these strains may have quite large inhibition zones around the penicillin discs in the test. At the edge of the zone of inhibition the growth is heaped up into a ridge, and this appearance distinguishes the strains from the non-penicillinase-producers which have a gradual, smooth transition from no growth to full growth. The penicillinase-producing staphylococci should be reported as being resistant to benzyl penicillin.

Methicillin, cloxacillin, flucloxacillin and, to some extent, cephaloridine, are cross-resistant. Cloxacillin and flucloxacillin should not be used in sensitivity testing because of unreliable results. Methicillin is used, but if methicillin discs are employed on ordinary sensitivity agar at 37°C only a small proportion of any bacteria capable of being resistant to methicillin will appear resistant. To overcome this, the medium can be incubated at 30°C for 18 hours using a 10 μg methicillin disc or, alternatively, 5% sodium chloride can be incorporated in the sensitivity agar and the plate incubated at 37°C for 18 hours.

Sulphonamides and trimethoprim

Many laboratory media contain substances which inhibit the reaction of sulphonamides, but in practice these can usually be neutralised by the addition of lysed horse blood; the same problem occurs with trimethoprim. Oxoid Diagnostic Sensitivity Test Agar is satisfactory for testing these drugs.

A sulphonamide (sulphamethoxazole) and trimethoprim are often used compounded together as cotrimoxazole (Septrin or Bactrim) because of the frequent synergy between the two drugs. This synergy can be demonstrated by placing two discs, each containing one of the drugs, approximately 15 mm apart on a suitably inoculated plate. When synergy is present, the zones of inhibition round each of the discs are deformed so that they coalesce. A test producing a zone of inhibition round a single disc containing both drugs merely indicates sensitivity to either the sulphonamide or the trimethoprim, and does not demonstrate possible synergy. Ideally both drugs should be tested by using separate discs. Treatment with a mixture is likely to be effective, even when the organism is apparently resistant to the sulphonamide, if it is sensitive to the trimethoprim or if there is moderate resistance to both drugs.

Sensitivity tests on primary cultures

Since different species of bacteria have different sensitivity patterns to antimicrobial agents, discs containing these agents can be used for the purpose of their selective isolation and as an aid to identification. For example, specimens from the respiratory tract plated on to blood agar may have the following discs: penicillin (10 units), neomycin (30 mg), and bacitracin (10 units). Streptococci, including pneumococci and enterococci, are resistant to neomycin and grow quite happily in the zone around the neomycin disc where other sensitive organisms are inhibited. *Haemophilus influenzae* and the haemolytic *Haemophilus* species grow with ease within the zone surrounding the bacitracin disc which inhibits Lancefield Group A beta-haemolytic streptococci. *Candida albicans*, *Pseudomonas* species and enterobacteria will grow in the zone around the penicillin disc.

It is often useful to incorporate relevant antibiotic discs in the primary culture of material from the site of an infection, particularly when future antibiotic therapy is known. If this is to be done the best method is that described by Dr E.J. Stokes in her book, *Clinical Bacteriology*,[3] mentioned earlier in this chapter.

Range of drugs to be tested

The aim of the laboratory should be to test a range of drugs which are likely to be clinically useful for the infection concerned. Usually this will be decided by the pathologist or microbiologist in charge of the laboratory in consultation with the clinicians. However, it is worth bearing in mind that the range of antibiotics used in the hospital is to a large extent influenced by those which are reported by the laboratory, and it is unwise to report the results of tests on potentially toxic drugs when they are not necessary or are pharmacologically inappropriate.

Cross-resistance may occur between a number of related antimicrobial agents, and in these cases only one of the group need be tested as follows:

Tetracyclines: tetracycline
Sulphonamides: sulphafurazole
Polymyxins: colistin-methane sulphonate
(or polymyxin B sulphate)
Penicillinase-resistant penicillins: methicillin

Preparation of discs containing antimicrobial agents

It is recommended that commercially produced sensitivity discs should be used as far as possible. However, if no such disc is available they can be prepared as follows.

Discs about 5 mm in diameter are punched from a good quality blotting paper. They are then spread out individually at 2 mm intervals in a 150 mm glass Petri dish. The Petri dish is covered with its top and sterilised in a hot-air oven at 160°C for 1 hr. After cooling, using a standard dropping pipette delivering 0·02 ml, a drop of a sterile solution of the antimicrobial agent is dropped on to each disc. The strength of the antimicrobial solution must be such that 0·02 ml contains the appropriate amount of antimicrobial agent. For example, if discs containing $10 \mu g$ of tetracycline are required then the solution must contain $50 \times 10 = 500 \mu g$ of the tetracycline per ml. The discs are then dried by placing the Petri dish with its lid tilted to one side in a desiccator which is then placed in a refrigerator for a few days, after which the discs are transferred to an air-tight container and stored at 4°C. It is important that they are kept dry. Before use, a performance test should be carried out comparing the new disc's activity with that of another known disc containing the same amount of antimicrobial agent using a susceptible organism.

Inoculation of plates for sensitivity tests

The plates must be seeded so that a dense, nearly

confluent, growth is evenly distributed over the plate to produce a lawn. This is achieved using a standardised inoculum of a pure culture of the organism to be tested.

Broth method

Five to ten identical colonies, hopefully selecting both susceptible and resistant organisms of the population, are emulsified in 2 ml of broth or peptone water. One drop of this suspension is then added to 5 ml of broth for most organisms although for slow-growing organisms, such as pneumococci and streptococci, the original suspension may be used but for very rapidly growing bacteria, such as the enteric bacteria, a further dilution may be necessary. Variations of this procedure using a turbidity standard, some of which involve incubation of the broth, have been described.

Method of inoculating plates

(a) The method obtaining the best results is to pour 5 ml of the standard inoculum broth over the surface of the plate. Tip the plate to one side and remove the surplus fluid by suction or carefully pour it in to a discard jar. The potential hazards of this procedure prevent it from being a routine method in most microbiology laboratories.

(b) A sterile cotton swab is saturated with the inoculum, excess fluid is removed by pressing it against the inside of the inoculum-containing tube or bottle, and the swab is streaked over the plate in several different planes.

(c) 0·5 ml of the inoculum broth is transferred to the surface of the agar and spread with a sterile cotton swab, or a flamed L-shaped glass rod for an inoculation in several planes. With these methods it may be necessary to dry the surface of the agar for about 30 min before applying the sensitivity testing discs.

Direct method

At least three isolated colonies of the organism to be tested are selected and an inoculum from each is transferred on to the test plate with a wire inoculation loop. The bacteria from these inocula are spread evenly all over the plate by streaking across the plate in several different directions with the inoculation loop. This method is both quick and reliable in experienced hands.

ASSAY TECHNIQUES

Several different techniques are available including plate, vertical diffusion, urease, transferase, fluoro-immunoassay, radioimmunoassay and high performance liquid chromatography. In laboratories where these estimations are done frequently, a plate method may be used to advantage, but when they are only carried out infrequently on a 'one off' basis, it is probably better to choose a broth dilution technique. These assays are performed to check whether adequate concentrations of the antimicrobial agent are being obtained in the blood; for example, in subacute bacterial endocarditis, or other body fluid such as cerebrospinal fluid in patients with meningitis. These assays are also performed when toxic antimicrobials such as streptomycin, gentamicin and kanamycin are used to ensure that the drugs do not reach a toxic level, especially in patients with impaired renal function. Overdosage with streptomycin leads to tinnitus and dizziness which is usually reversible, but overdosage with gentamicin can cause irreversible deafness. Gentamicin assays are included in the national microbiology quality control scheme run by the P.H.L.S.

It is useful to know the lowest level achieved so a specimen of the fluid, for example blood, should be taken immediately before the next dose is due. The highest level achieved depends upon the dose, the size of the patient, the route of administration and the pharmacological properties of the drug. The highest levels will be achieved within a few minutes of an intravenous injection, but after intramuscular injection it may take 30 minutes or more. The time of the sample in relation to the times of administration of the drug must be recorded on the request form. It is also essential to know whether any other antimicrobial agent is being given at the same time since this will materially affect the result of the assay unless steps are taken to destroy the second drug, for example with penicillinase, or to nullify its effect by using a resistant test organism.

In the following tests it is imperative that the antimicrobial solutions used are made up from pure chemicals with known activity and not from tablets or other pharmaceutical mixtures.

Plate diffusion methods

The size of the zone of inhibition produced by the unknown fluid, or known dilutions of it, is compared with the sizes of zones of inhibition produced by known concentrations of the antibiotics. This is done graphically with a standard curve constructed on it of zone diameter against the concentration of the standards or by using an electronic calculator. For most antibiotics the zone diameter plotted against the log of the concentration will give a straight line. At least three standards should be used in the preparation of the curve. Dilutions of the unknown are prepared so that one of them will be close to the MIC for the organism to be used during the test, for example, for blood in a 1 in 10 dilution is often the nearest, but if high levels are expected, then higher dilutions, for example 1 in 100, must be prepared. It is helpful, but not essential, that the fluid to be assayed is sterile.

Gentamicin assay: plate method

Principle

A sensitivity test agar plate is inoculated with a stock *Klebsiella* which is sensitive to gentamicin but resistant to other antibiotics like cefuroxime and carbenicillin. These may be given together with gentamicin in severe infections. Wells are bored into the agar and standard antibiotic solutions in serum are put into the wells. The serum to be assayed is placed in other similar wells. The plates are incubated for 18 hr at 37°C. Zone sizes obtained with the standards are measured and the graph plotted.

Test serum zone sizes are measured and the concentration of antibacterial substance in that test serum can be read from the graph.

Standard solutions

A concentrated stock solution of gentamicin sulphate, paediatric injectable (20 mg base in 2 ml) is prepared in distilled water, and from this the following final concentrations are prepared in sterile pooled human serum:

20 μg/ml, 5 μg/ml, 2·5 μg/ml, 1·25 μg/ml.

The concentrated stock solution is stored in the deep freeze, the final concentrations in serum are stored at 4°C. A check is kept on the potency of these solutions by measuring absolute zone sizes weekly with a standard inoculum of the organism to give a semi-confluent growth, and a record is kept. If these same sizes vary by 2 mm or more, new standard sera are prepared.

Stock organism

Klebsiella species with multiple resistance to other antibiotics such as *K. edwardsii* (NCTC 10896). This organism is stored on nutrient agar slopes and is sub-cultured weekly.

Method

(a) Inoculate 5 ml of nutrient broth with a little of the culture and incubate until cloudy (about 4–5 hr).

(b) With a Pasteur pipette transfer just sufficient culture into fresh nutrient broth to give a slightly turbid appearance.

(c) Dilute this further 1:100 (0·1 ml in 9·9 ml of sterile broth) to produce the final dilution of culture.

(d) Take a 250 mm² assay dish containing 100 ml of sensitivity agar and dry for 5–10 min. (Oxoid D.S.T. at pH 7·3.)

(e) Flood the surface of the plate with a final dilution of the culture, and after 15 sec remove the excess with a pipette.

(f) Dry the plate again for 3–5 min.

(g) Using a No. 5 cork borer (diameter of hole 9 mm) cut holes 25 mm apart. Up to 25 holes can be cut in 250 mm² plate. Place equal volumes of the standard solutions and the test sera, all in triplicate, in individual wells in sufficient amount to fill the wells, but not to overflow (70μl) using a Finnpipette.

(h) Incubate the plates, media lowermost, at 37°C for 18 hr, then read the zone diameters with the aid of callipers or a zone-measuring device. Record the zone diameters and draw a graph on semi-log paper of control zone diameters against log concentrations of controls. Read off test concentrations.

Note. Assay dishes are disinfected before use by u.v. light. A ready-poured inoculated plate can be kept for up to a week at 4°C before use.

Antibiotic assay: tube dilution method

Principle

In this method the antibiotics are assayed by titration in liquid culture using a standard sensitive organism. For this method the fluid to be assayed must be sterile; a syringe-fitting membrane filter may be used to achieve this, although small amounts of the antibiotic will remain on the membrane. Serum to be assayed should be inactivated at 56°C for 30 min before the test. The fluid to be assayed should be tested in parallel with solutions containing known amounts of antibiotic in a similar fluid.

Apparatus

Sterile 75 × 10 mm test tubes with either aluminium tops or cotton wool plugs.

Sterile graduated pipettes.

Standard solutions

A 1:1000 dilution of the pure antibiotic of the same kind as that to be assayed is made in buffer solution at pH 7·0–7·6. From this a working dilution is prepared equal to 16 times the usual MIC of the test organism to that antibiotic. The working dilution should be made in a fluid as nearly as possible the same as that which is to be assayed; for serum use sterile human serum, for urine use sterile urine at the same pH, and for cerebro-spinal fluid use buffered distilled water.

Stock organism

For most antibiotics the Oxford staphylococcus (NCTC 6751) will be suitable, but for chloramphenicol the polymyxins and carbenicillin, *Escherichia coli* (NCTC 10418), is suitable. If a mixture of antibiotics is being given to the patient, then it is sometimes possible to find an organism that is sensitive to the antibiotic it is wished to assay and resistant to the other, such as the *Klebsiella* recommended for use in the plate gentamicin assay which is resistant to carbenicillin but sensitive to gentamicin. Sometimes it is possible to neutralise the other antimicrobial agent; for instance, sulphonamides can be neutralised with para-aminobenzoic acid and many cephalosporins and penicillins by beta-lactamases obtainable commercially.

Medium

Peptone water with 10% added serum which can be increased to 50% if the drug is known to be heavily protein-bound.

Inoculum

If the inoculum is too heavy, a lower end-point may be obtained owing to the presence of resistant mutants or to the inoculum effect.

Method

(a) Inoculate the indicator organism into 5 ml of peptone water containing 10% serum and incubate overnight.

(b) Prepare two rows of 10 sterile test tubes, one marked 'Test' the other marked 'Control'.

(c) Add 1 ml of the peptone water containing 10% serum to each of the tubes, except the first in each row, aseptically.

(d) Add 1 ml of the fluid to be assayed to both the first and second tubes of the row marked 'Test', then make serial doubling dilutions in the remainder of the tubes in that row by transferring 1 ml to each tube in turn with a fresh pipette, with adequate mixing each time.

(e) Add 1 ml of the working dilution of the antibiotic to the first and second tubes of the row marked 'Control' and make doubling dilutions from the second tube to the end of the row.

(f) Take an overnight culture of the indicator organism in peptone water. Dilute until the suspension is just cloudy, approximately 10^8 organisms per ml. Dilute 1:100 (0·1 ml to 9·9 ml distilled water) and mix thoroughly. Inoculate each tube with one drop from a 50 dropper pipette of this dilution.

(g) Incubate overnight.

Result

The bacteriostatic minimal inhibitory concentration (MIC) is the concentration of antibiotic in the first tube of the control row where there is no visible growth. The concentration of the antibiotic in the test fluid is the first dilution at which there is no growth in the test row, multiplied by the MIC of the indicator organism.

Minimal inhibitory concentration (MIC)

This is a test of the sensitivity of an organism to a known antibiotic, and the method is similar in many ways to the tube dilution antibiotic assay just described.

Method

(a) Inoculate the unknown test organism into 5 ml of peptone water containing 10% of serum and incubate overnight. At the same time prepare a similar culture of a standard organism such as the Oxford staphylococcus.

(b) Prepare two rows of 10 sterile 75×10 mm test tubes with caps or plugs.

(c) Add 1 ml of the peptone water serum mixture to the first, third and subsequent tubes in each row. The first tube in each row being a control for the broth and inoculum.

(d) Add 1 ml of the fluid to be assayed to the second and third tubes in each row. Mix the contents of the third tube and transfer 1 ml to the fourth tube. Continue this double diluting to the end of each row.

(e) Dilute the test organism until the broth is just cloudy (approx. 10^8 organisms per ml). Add 0·1 ml to

9·9 ml of distilled water (1:100 dilution). Mix thoroughly and add one drop from a 50 dropper pipette (0·02 ml) to each tube (final inoculum approximately 20,000 organisms per ml).

(f) Inoculate each of the tubes in the control row with a similar inoculum of the control organism (Oxford staphylococcus).

(g) Mix all the tubes and incubate overnight.

Results

The bacteriostatic minimum inhibitory concentration (MIC) is the concentration of antibiotic in the first tube where there is no visible growth.

To determine whether there is a bactericidal endpoint, sub-culture 0·1 ml from the last tube with visible growth and all the tubes without growth on to one-quarter of a well-dried blood agar plate. Spread over the surface of the quarter with an inoculation loop and incubate overnight. The minimum bactericidal concentration (MBC) is the concentration of antibiotic in the first tube where no growth occurs.

Combinations of antibiotics

In serious infections with relatively resistant organisms, e.g. subacute bacterial endocarditis caused by a resistant streptococcus, when no single drug can be given in doses sufficient to kill the organism, then combinations of antibiotics must be tested for their bactericidal effect. Experience has shown that treatment of bacterial endocarditis with bacteristatic drugs ends in failure and that a drug with bactericidal effects must be used. When two antibiotics are used together there are three possible effects:

1. Addition or indifference, where each drug exerts only its own usual effect.
2. Antagonism, where the effect is less than would be expected.
3. Synergy, where the effect is more than expected, e.g. when each drug by itself is not completely effective but the two together are bactericidal.

The bactericidal penicillins are always antagonised by bacteriostatic antibiotics such as tetracycline or chloramphenicol. Penicillins or cephalosporins frequently act synergistically with the aminoglycosides such as streptomycin or gentamicin.

Tests of synergy or antagonism of two combined antibiotics can be carried out in broth or the technically more exacting method known as the Cellophane transfer method which employs a Cellophane tambour which is fully described by Garrod and Waterworth (1962).[4]

Such a test cannot be carried out merely by placing the two antibiotic discs near to one another on a seeded agar plate since this only demonstrates the bacteriostatic action, not the necessary bactericidal action.

Tube test of combined action

Principle

Where two antibiotics are to be tested, each antibiotic is added to broth in an amount giving a concentration which is similar to a concentration likely to be obtained in the blood during therapy, such as $10 \mu g$ per ml. A standard inoculum is added to each of 4 tubes containing, respectively, neat broth (control), each of the two antibiotics, and a 50–50 mixture of the two. The neat broth is cultured in a standard way immediately. After incubation, the antibiotic-containing broths are sub-cultured in the same standard way on to a solid medium and the results are compared with the results of the control sub-culture. A number of these tests can be conveniently carried out together, in which case the tubes are arranged in the form of a half chess-board as in Fig. 16.1.

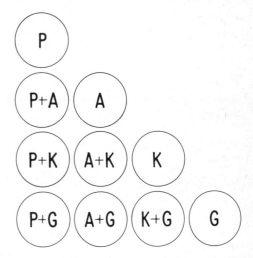

Fig. 16.1. Arrangement of tubes and contents in an example of the 'half chessboard' test of combined antibiotic action to discover a bactericidal combination P = penicillin; A = ampicillin; K = amikacin; G = gentamicin.

Method

(a) Inoculate a pure culture of the test organism (from the patient) into nutrient broth and incubate overnight. Prepare the inoculum broth by diluting the overnight culture until it is just cloudy (approximately 10^8 organisms per ml), then dilute a suitable portion of this 1 in 100 with broth.

(b) Prepare rows of sterile 72×12 mm test tubes with caps as in Fig. 16.1.

(c) Make up solutions of each antibiotic containing $100 \mu g$ per ml.

(d) Add 0·5 ml of each solution to the appropriate tubes in the rows.

(e) Add 4 ml of broth, pre-inoculated to contain 10^6 organisms per ml, to each tube containing two antibiotics and 4·5 ml to those containing only one.

(f) Mix well.

(g) Using a standard loop inoculate a quarter of blood agar plate with the inoculum broth, then incubate the plate and tubes overnight.

(h) Using the same standard loop, inoculate a quarter of an agar plate with medium from any tubes showing no growth and incubate the plates for at least 24 hr.

Results of sub-cultures

(a) No growth, indicating total bactericidal action.

(b) A growth similar in amount to that from the control tube, indicating bacteriostatic action only.

(c) A reduction in growth compared with the control tube, indicating incomplete bactericidal action.

Test of the bactericidal action of patient's serum on the infecting organism

A simple but reassuring tube test can be carried out to see whether the patient's serum contains enough antibiotic to kill the infecting organism if it has been isolated.

Using sterile capped 75×12 mm test tubes, doubling dilutions of the patient's serum in broth are made from 1 in 2 to 1 in 64. Each tube is inoculated with approximately 20,000 organisms per ml as described in the method for the estimation of the MIC using tubes. After overnight incubation the tubes are inspected for growth, and those showing no growth are sub-cultured on to blood agar which is incubated for 24 hours. The bactericidal concentration is the concentration of serum in the first tube where no growth occurs.

A 1 in 2 dilution should inhibit the organism, but it is recommended that there should be enough antimicrobial agent in the serum to inhibit the organism at a dilution of 1 in 4 or 1 in 8 to provide an adequate margin of safety.

REFERENCES

1. Garrod, L.P., Lambert, P.H., O'Grady, F. (1981) *Antibiotic and Chemotherapy* (Fifth Edition). Edinburgh & London: Churchill Livingstone.
2. Smith, Hillas. (1977) *Antibiotics in Clinical Practice* (Third Edition). London: Pitman Books Ltd.
3. Stokes, E.J. and Ridgway G.L. (1980) *Clinical Bacteriology* (Fifth Edition). London: Edward Arnold (Publishers) Ltd.
4.. Garrod, L.P. and Waterworth, P.M. (1962) *J. Clin. Path.* **15**, 328.

BIBLIOGRAPHY

Reeves, D.S., Phillips, I., Williams, J. D. and Wise, R. (1978) *Laboratory Methods in Antimicrobial Chemotherapy*. Edinburgh, London and New York: Churchill Livingstone.

17. Laboratory aspects of sterilisation and disinfection

Sterility is absolute freedom from living micro-organisms. Sterilisation is the achievement of sterility by killing or removal of all micro-organisms. Disinfection is the removal or killing of harmful or infectious micro-organisms, usually from a surface or an object which then becomes safe to handle. This is not an absolute like sterilisation since the disinfected article may not be free from spores. A chemical or chemical solution which can kill vegetative bacteria may be a disinfectant. Disinfectants are applied to inanimate objects; an antiseptic is a chemical or chemical solution which usually has a milder effect than a disinfectant and is used to disinfect skin or mucous membranes which should not be damaged by it and are sensitive to the stronger solutions.

Table 17.1 sets out the methods employed in sterilising laboratory equipment.

PHYSICAL METHODS

Dry heat

Dry heat kills by oxidation and incineration, and may be applied as a flame such as when flaming an inocula-

tion loop or the neck of a bottle, or in a specially constructed incinerator. Many hospitals have an electrically heated or gas-fired incinerator which can be used for disposing of infected articles such as dressings, pathological material and animal carcasses, in addition to the burning of a lot of inflammable rubbish. If disposable polystyrene culture plates, etc., are to be destroyed in this way, then it is necessary to use an incinerator designed with this in mind to prevent the clouds of black smoke, which are produced when polystyrene burns, escaping into the atmosphere.

Sterilisation can be achieved using hot-air ovens, and this method is commonly used in hospital laboratories. These ovens should comply with a BS 3421. Sterilising ovens must be fitted with a fan to ensure an even temperature throughout the oven. Hot-air ovens can be used for sterilising such articles as all-glass syringes, some heat-resistant glass and metal syringes, surgical instruments and glass-ware, such as pipettes. Some oils and powders are sterilised this way. Care must be taken when selecting articles since the high temperatures achieved will damage many things such as ordinary rubber. Capped bottles, such as universal bottles, when sterilised this way must be fitted with silicone-rubber

Table 17.1   Methods of sterilising

Physical	Heat	dry	flaming, incineration, hot-air ovens
		moist	water: Pasteurisation, boiling
			steam: steamers, autoclaves
	Radiation	non-ionising	ultra-violet light, infra-red rays
		ionising	gamma-rays (cobalt 60), beta-particles (linear accelerator)
	Filtration	earthenware candles	Berkefeld, Mandler and Chamberland filters
		asbestos pads	Seitz filters
		sintered glass	Buchner funnel or Gooch crucible
		cellulose membranes	cellulose nitrate: Gradocol
			cellulose acetate: Millipore
Chemical	Gaseous	formaldehyde	low-temperature steam/formaldehyde autoclave
		ethylene oxide	neat in special cabinet, 10% in CO_2 in special steriliser
	Liquid	aldehydes	formalin, glutaraldehyde

washers. Articles to be sterilised are usually placed in glass containers such as large Pyrex boiling tubes stoppered with a plug of cotton wool or in tin boxes. The cotton wool plugs are slightly charred during this operation. Ensure that there is plenty of space between articles being sterilised in the oven. Air is a poor conductor of heat and it takes some time for articles being sterilised to reach the sterilising temperature; this is the heat penetration time. The holding time depends upon the temperature selected; the following have been found satisfactory:

160°C for 45 min
170°C for 18 min
180°C for 7½ min
190°C for 1½ min

The cycle or sterilising time includes the heat penetration time, the holding time and an added extra time as a safety factor—often half the calculated holding time. Thus a sterilising time of 1 hour at 160°C is commonly used for glass-ware. An allowance of extra time must be made where there is any doubt about the penetration time, for instance, when a large object is being sterilised. In general there is less damage to the object being sterilised if a longer sterilising time at a lower temperature is used rather than a shorter time at a higher temperature.

It is better to test the sterilising process rather than to test the product which is subject to cultural, technical and statistical snags. Temperature can be measured accurately and the temperature gauge of ovens should be checked, using a thermocouple, from time to time. Thermocouples can also be used to check the penetration time by inserting the leads into the centre of packs. Chemical indicators, such as Browne's tubes (Albert Brown Ltd, Leicester), are available for testing a number of sterilising processes involving heat. They consist of glass phials which contain a heat-sensitive liquid which is initially a red colour and which changes through orange to a green colour (like traffic lights) when the desired temperature has been achieved for the correct length of time. The Browne's tube designed for hot-air ovens has a green spot and the green colour change occurs after 60 minutes at 160°C. A Browne's tube can conveniently be included in each batch and serves as a check. A biological test of the process which is much more trouble and less certain is to use the spores of a non-toxigenic strain of *Clostridium tetani* as a test piece. Paper strips inoculated with approximately 10^6 viable spores are placed in envelopes which in turn are placed inside a typical pack or item being sterilised, such as a glass syringe. At the end of the sterilising process the envelope is opened and the spore strip transferred aseptically to either Robertson's cooked-meat medium or thioglycollate broth, which is incubated at 37°C for 5 days, then sub-cultured using a large inoculum on to freshly prepared blood agar plates which are incubated anaerobically for 2 days at 37°C before inspection.

Moist heat

Moist heat kills by denaturation of protein. A variety of methods are employed ranging from the relatively low temperatures of Pasteurisation to the high temperatures achieved using high-pressure steam.

Hot water can be used for disinfection; for instance 10 minutes exposure to a temperature of 65°C (Pasteurisation) will kill most vegetative organisms, but will not kill spores or thermophilic species. Two methods are used in practice, one in which the liquid, usually milk, is held at 63°C for 30 minutes, the other where it is held at 72°C for only 15–20 seconds. Both the holder process and the flash process are able to kill brucellae, salmonellae and tubercle bacilli which can contaminate milk. Serum and other protein-containing fluids can be disinfected by heating in a water-bath at 56°C for 1 hour on each of several successive days. Many other methods on these lines have been described, none of which can be relied upon to sterilise; they only disinfect. Boiling water (100°C) kills vegetative bacteria very quickly, but some spores are able to last as long as 30 hours at this temperature. However, boiling can be used where an absolute guarantee of sterility is not necessary, such as in the sterilisation/disinfection of instruments used at autopsy. The instruments should be thoroughly cleaned before being put in the bath to which washing soda can be added (2%), which is said to aid the killing of bacterial spores and to reduce rusting and consequent blunting of sharp instruments. Addition of washing soda reduces the time of immersion in the boiling water from 10 minutes to 5 minutes. This method is not recommended for general use.

Steam

Steam at atmospheric pressure (approximately 100°C) can be used either in a specially constructed steamer, such as those of Koch or Arnold, or in a laboratory autoclave with the lid loosened. Carbohydrate-containing media which might well caramelise at higher temperatures and gelatin-containing media can be sterilised in this way, but sterility is not guaranteed. In Tyndallisation, the material to be treated is allowed a heating-up period of about 10 minutes and a holding time of 20 minutes after which it is cooled and allowed to remain at room temperature for 24 hours; after this it is again heated in the same way. A third heating is given after another period of 24 hours. The principle is that the vegetative bacteria should be killed during the first heating. Spores are given a chance to germinate during the next 24 hours and any vegetative bacteria so formed are killed by the second heating. Similarly the third heating; however, thermophilic organisms may not be killed and anaerobic spores, if present, will not have germinated unless the medium was incubated anaerobically between heatings.

Autoclaves (Table 17.2)

Saturated steam is a most efficient sterilising agent when used under pressure in a specially constructed vessel called an autoclave. In nearly all cases where the

Table 17.2.   Types of autoclave

1. Pressure cooker type
2. Downward displacement:
   (*a*) Laboratory autoclaves
   (*b*) Bowl and instrument sterilisers
   (*c*) Bottled-fluid autoclaves
3. High vacuum, high pressure: for dressings and wrapped instruments
4. High vacuum, sub-atmospheric pressure: for low-temperature steam disinfection of heat-sensitive instruments and fabrics. (Sterilisation with addition of formaldehyde during cycle.)

object to be sterilised can withstand the temperature of an autoclave without damage this is the method of choice, since the process can be controlled absolutely and the conditions required are known. Autoclaving as a means of sterilisation is suitable for many culture media, aqueous solutions, surgical bowls and instruments, surgical dressings and contaminated articles, such as used Petri dishes, bottled media, anaesthetic tubing and infected articles from patients. In the future, pressure will be measured in newtons per square metre or pascals, but for the time being in Great Britain pressure in autoclaves is measured in pounds per square inch, so these units have been retained in this section.

Boiling occurs when the temperature of a liquid is such that its saturation vapour pressure is equal to the external atmospheric pressure. If the atmospheric pressure decreases, the liquid boils at a lower temperature; similarly, increased pressure raises the boiling point. When water is boiled in a closed vessel at an increased pressure the temperature at which it boils, and therefore of the steam which is formed, rises. It takes a relatively large amount of heat to make liquid water into steam; conversely when steam is condensed back to water it liberates heat, the latent heat. A direct consequence of this is that articles put into an autoclave become heated very quickly as the hot steam condenses on their surfaces liberating the latent heat. Ideally, the steam used in an autoclave should be on the phase boundary so that it is still dry, but is about to condense back to water. Dalton's law states that in a mixture of gases each gas exerts a pressure which is the same as if it were alone and occupying the volume of a mixture. It follows that if an autoclave contains air as well as steam the partial pressure of the steam will be less than the total pressure in the autoclave by an amount depending upon the proportion of air present. Therefore the temperature, which depends upon the pressure, will be less than expected with regard to the total pressure in the autoclave. For example, if the gauge pressure of an autoclave is 15 p.s.i. and the autoclave contains hot, dry, saturated steam only, then the temperature will be 121°C. If however, at the same gauge pressure there is an equal mixture of steam and air (half air discharge), then the temperature reached will only be 112°C. If at the same pressure none of the original air in the autoclave has been discharged the temperature will be 100°C. Furthermore, air hinders the penetration of the steam into porous materials such as surgical dressings, and of containers such as glass vessels and syringes, and the air, being denser than steam, tends to form a separate cooler layer in the lower part of the vessel, pack or autoclave itself. It is therefore important that as much air as possible should be removed from the autoclave chamber and the articles of the load before sterilisation, and it is for these reasons that a vacuum is produced before the sterilisation cycle in many autoclaves.

1. Pressure-cooker autoclaves

The familiar domestic pressure cooker can be used quite well for this purpose, but there are available a number of larger vessels which work on the same principle. These consists of a vertical metal chamber fitted with a lid which can be fastened down usually by a number of thumb screws and which is sealed by a rubber gasket. They all have a discharge valve which may be quite separate or may be combined with the pressure regulator which is usually adjusted by means of small weights. Many have a pressure gauge, all must have a safety valve to prevent an explosion in the event of failure of the pressure regulator which may become blocked and a device for preventing the top from being opened whilst the chamber is under pressure or a thermal lock.

Water is placed in the bottom of the chamber and the objects to be sterilised are stood on a trivet. Heat is supplied either electrically or by gas at the bottom. The maker's directions must always be followed. First check that there is enough water, replace the trivet and stand the objects to be autoclaved on it. Apply the heat and close the lid. Leave the discharge tap open and adjust the pressure regulator. Internal turbulence when the water boils causes a mixture of steam and air to come from the discharge tap, and this should be allowed to continue until air ceases to come from the inside of the chamber. This point is detected in various ways from the rocking of the weights on the valve on some models to a change of note of the sound of the escaping steam. On some models it is possible to run a piece of rubber tubing from the discharge valve into cold water in a bucket, the steam condenses in the water and the air rises in bubbles to the surface; when the bubbling ceases there is no more air escaping from the chamber. At this point the discharge tap is closed. The pressure in the chamber now increases until it reaches the level at which the pressure regulator opens and emits excess steam. This pressure is commonly 15 p.s.i., and an appropriate holding time at this pressure is usually 15 minutes unless large articles are being autoclaved when a longer time is allowed.

At the end of the holding time the heater is turned off and the whole autoclave is allowed to cool down until the pressure gauge reads zero. The discharge tap is then opened very gently and any slight excess of pressure allowed to subside. If the discharge valve is opened too soon, liquid in the chamber will boil explosively causing a mess inside the autoclave and sometimes bursting its containing bottle. The autoclave should be allowed to cool for a further few minutes before the top is opened and the contents removed. The tops of screw-cap bottles must be loosened slightly before being sterilised in an autoclave to prevent the bottles bursting. The tops can be tightened up again when the sterilisation process is finished. These simple autoclaves can be very useful, but their air discharge is not very efficient and the load is distinctly wet at the end of the cycle. They are therefore not satisfactory for the sterilisation of apparatus and dressings which are wrapped in either paper or cloth, since bacteria travel quite easily through these materials when they are wet. This can often be avoided in the laboratory by placing the articles in wire baskets and making sure that they are dry before they come into contact with unsterile objects. The efficiency of a cycle can be tested using a spore strip (*Bacillus stearothermophilus*) or a Browne's Tube No. 1: Black spot.

2. Downward-displacement autoclaves

Air is heavier than steam and tends to gravitate to the bottom of the sterilising chamber where the discharge valve is situated. The steam is led in near the top of the chamber. This is a more efficient method than that used by the pressure-cooker type autoclave and is all right for autoclaves intended to sterilise solid articles, such as surgical instruments and bowls, which must be either upside down or on their sides to avoid trapping air in them. It is less satisfactory for porous loads such as dressings. Fitting a vacuum pump or steam ejector to the discharge makes the operation much more efficient. Autoclaves used for sterilising dressings, but not bottled liquids, can have a vacuum cycle after sterilising, following which the chamber is filled with dry filtered air. In larger autoclaves drying is further facilitated by the autoclave chamber being kept hot by means of a steam-filled jacket. In the bottom of these autoclaves is an outlet for condensed water which incorporates a strainer, a steam trap and non-return valve. The thermometer should be situated in or near this outlet. These autoclaves are operated from the mains steam supply of the hospital and are usually horizontal in position; they may be either rectangular or round in section.

To operate, follow the manufacturer's instructions. If present, the jacket is first brought up to operating temperature. The chamber is then loaded and the door closed. The load must be distributed in such a way that there is a free circulation of steam between the articles and these must be arranged so that there will be no air pockets left; for example, bowls should be upside down. The steam-to-chamber valve is then opened allowing steam into the top of the chamber, and air and condensate are forced out through the drain at the bottom. When the air and condensate have been eliminated and pure steam goes through the trap the temperature, as recorded by the temperature gauge or thermometer, rises and the steam trap closes, e.g. it will be expected to close at 121°C when a pressure of 15 p.s.i. is being used. This is the air displacement period which coincides with, but is not the same as, the heat generation time which is the time taken for the heat to penetrate completely each item of the load. The holding period starts when the thermometer in the discharge pipe first shows that the proper temperature has been reached. The exact period of the holding time depends upon the nature of the load since the heat generation time extends into it (*see* Table 17.3).

Table 17.3. Holding times for autoclaves

Pressure (p.s.i.)	Temperature (°C)	Holding time (min)
10	115	30
15	121	15
20	126	10
30	134	3

These conditions will kill gas gangrene and tetanus spores, but not necessarily a thermophile.

Timing of the cycle according to the temperature gauge is much better than by using the pressure gauge because of the air mixture problem and the notorious inaccuracy of pressure gauges. A safety time, often half of the theoretical holding time, is added to the holding time. At the end of this period the supply of steam to the chamber is stopped and that to the jacket, if fitted, is maintained. The steam in the chamber cools and the pressure falls to atmospheric pressure. The air inlet valve is then opened, after which the door can be opened and the contents removed. The design of the autoclave must be such that it is impossible to open it whilst the chamber pressure is above atmospheric pressure. On the more sophisticated machines a drying cycle can be included after the holding cycle when sterilising things other than liquids in bottles. The steam is removed from the chamber by vacuum and replaced by filtered air.

Controls. The temperature at the chamber drain should be checked during the cycle, this is most conveniently done using an automatic recorder.

(i) Browne's tubes
   Type 1 (Black spot for temperatures below 126°C)
   Type 2 (Yellow spot for temperatures above 126°C) i.e. over 20 p.s.i.
(ii) Browne's T.S.T.
   This is a colour change indicator which senses time, steam and temperature and changes from yellow to blue/purple when adequate conditions have been present in the sterilisation process (ref. Table 17.3).
(iii) Spore strips of *Bacillus stearothermophilus* are sometimes used.

Bottled-fluid autoclaves are downward-displacement type autoclaves. The bottles should have metal screw-caps and be fitted with Neoprene-flanged stoppers for pharmaceutical products. Other stoppers may be all right for laboratory use. The bottles are placed in suitable crates or wire baskets which are then put into the autoclave. The heat generation time may be prolonged and is best arrived at using a dummy bottle of the same kind as those in the load, filled with liquid and containing a thermocouple so that the temperature within the bottle or simulator can be read and recorded. The holding time is the same as for other loads. At the end of the holding time the steam supply is cut off and the autoclave is allowed to cool and come down to atmospheric pressure by itself. This process may take as long as 3 or 4 hours and can be followed by looking at the temperature in the dummy bottle. If the pressure in the autoclave is brought down quickly then the bottles are likely to explode, so it is very dangerous to open the door of the autoclave before the bottles have cooled sufficiently. Some modern bottle autoclaves are fitted with a rapid-cooling device which sprays the bottles with water at the end of the holding time; this may not be satisfactory if unsterile water is used for cooling since it has been shown that the cooling water can get into the bottles, thereby introducing micro-organisms. Special bottle caps are being designed for use in these autoclaves.

3. High pre-vacuum, high-pressure steam sterilisers

Discussion of these as used for dressings is beyond the scope of this book, and they are not found in microbiology laboratories.

4. Subatmospheric steam sterilisers

Steam at less than atmospheric pressure at a temperature of 80°C can be used for the disinfection of heat-sensitive instruments such as cystoscopes, fabrics and bedding materials. The holding time is usually about 10 minutes. The bactericidal power of the process can be increased by the addition of formaldehyde. This is usually done in a specially constructed high pre-vacuum autoclave, similar to a dressings autoclave, but fitted with a formaldehyde generator which uses bottled formalin as its source. A sterilising cycle using the subatmospheric steam and formaldehyde has a holding time of 2 hours at 73°C. At the end of the holding time a vacuum removes virtually all the formaldehyde. Spore-strip tests are not really a satisfactory control of this process but Browne's market a chemical indicator which changes from purple to green during an adequate cycle.

Spore strips

Autoclaves can be subjected to a biological test as a back-up to the physical tests using the highly resistant spores of a thermophile called *Bacillus stearother-mophilus*. They are simple to use but the results are difficult to interpret. The results depend upon the type of spores, the method of preparation, the number and concentration of the spores in the test and the conditions for the recovery. In any population of spores, some will be more resistant than others, and occasionally spores will survive an otherwise satisfactory autoclave cycle. To overcome this, standardised test strips must be made with an LD.50 closely related to the time and temperature to be used and using the spore strips in groups, such as five, remembering that a small proportion will give false positives. Spore strips are probably best obtained from commercial sources such as Oxoid or Mast, but they can be prepared in the laboratory. A culture is incubated aerobically at 56°C on nutrient agar for 5 days, a suspension of growth is made in sterile water to contain at least 10^6 spores per ml. Strips of filter paper soaked in the suspension and dried at room temperature aseptically are then placed in sterile paper envelopes, which are then sealed. One, or preferably a group of envelopes, can then be included in packs to be autoclaved. After autoclaving the strips are transferred aseptically to bottles of recovery medium. These are then incubated at 56°C for at least 7 days with another bottle of the same medium containing a control strip from the same batch which has not been autoclaved. The spores of *B. stearothermophilus* are generally killed by an exposure at 121°C for 12 minutes.

Safety

All autoclaves must be submitted to hydraulic tests by an engineer, and the laboratory must hold a test certificate showing the conditions of safe operation. All autoclaves must be insured against the risk of explosion and be examined by the insurer's engineer/surveyor at regular intervals, and recorded in the engineer's log. The maximum working pressure of the autoclaves should be clearly displayed on them at all times. Pressure gauges must be tested regularly. Insulated gauntlet gloves and a visor should be worn when unloading an autoclave.

Filtration

In bacteriology laboratories, filtration has three purposes, namely: clarification of solutions, i.e. removal of unwanted suspended particles as in the preparation of broth, sterilisation, and bacterial counting. In coarse filtration the filter acts as a sieve, but in sterilisation where the particles are smaller, much of the filter's action is due to adsorption or impaction on to the walls of the filter pores. The mean size of particles retained is often smaller than the average pore diameter of the filter. Earthenware and Seitz filters have been widely used in the past, but they are not as quick as membrane filters and absorb small amounts of filtrate which can be important when only small volumes are being used.

Sintered-glass filters

These are made of glass fragments which have been fused into a disc. There are five grades varying from Grade 1 which is a coarse filter used for clarifying, to Grade 5 for bacteria. Grade 5 filters are rather delicate and are usually made of a layer of Grade 5 laid on top of a layer of Grade 3; this is physically stronger and is sold as Grade 5/3. In the Buchner-funnel type the disc is fused into a complete funnel. Gooch crucibles, the bottom of which is the filter, are fitted to a funnel by means of a rubber gasket which encircles the crucible. Sintered-glass and sintered-steel filters are also used to support a membrane filter. After use as clarifying filters, sintered-glass filters are cleaned by passing distilled water through them in the reverse direction. This is followed by cleaning in warm concentrated sulphuric acid containing a little potassium nitrate and potassium chlorate by immersion overnight followed next day by repeated washing with distilled water. Do not wash by attaching to the mains water supply to a tap and running water through in the reverse direction because the high pressure can damage the union between the disc and the funnel. If the filter has been used for filtering bacteria, it should be washed free of protein-containing material by passing water through in the normal direction and then treated with 70% methylated spirit or isopropyl alcohol to kill vegetative bacteria, after which the filter is cleaned as above. The filters are sterilised by wrapping in Kraft paper and autoclaving at 15 p.s.i. for 15 minutes.

Membrane filters

Thin porous membranes of cellulose esters can be manufactured with remarkably even pore sizes from 14 micrometres (μm) down to 7·5 nanometres (nm) capable of retaining small viruses and high-molecular-weight proteins. These and membranes made from other materials have a wide range of applications in both industry and science which are described, together with suitable apparatus, in the manufacturers' catalogues such as those of the Millipore Corporation and Gelman Hawksley. It is recommended that these catalogues be consulted so that the range of filters and types of filter holder for different purposes can be appreciated. Membrane filters have replaced other types in many microbiology laboratories.

The main uses of membrane filters by microbiologists are the sterilisation of liquids and the viable counting of bacteria in liquid or air using known volumes. Membrane filters may also be used in the cytological examination of body fluids, since the membranes can be made transparent after filtering by filling the pores of the membrane with a substance having a similar refractive index, such as immersion oil (obtainable from the filter manufacturers), and cell stains also are not readily taken up by the membrane. The principal advantage of membrane filters is the high flow rates which can be achieved through them which may be forty or more times those of other filters. Coupled with this is the ease with which nutrients required for growth of bacteria are able to pass through in the reverse direction so that bacteria retained on the membrane can be cultured *in situ*. One way of doing this is to place the filter disc on the surface of a suitable solid medium such as nutrient agar in a Petri dish. After incubation, typical colonies from the filtered bacteria can be seen growing on the surface of the membrane. Enumerating bacteria this way is described in the chapter on counting bacteria.

For most purposes in bacteriology, membranes with a pore diameter of $0.45\,\mu$m are used. Discs of membrane in a holder are supported on a grid or similar structure in use. Filter discs can be obtained presterilised or can be sterilised by autoclaving at 15 p.s.i. for 15 minutes by themselves but separated by nonporous paper discs or absorbent pads, or alternatively they are autoclaved pre-assembled in filter holders wrapped in Kraft or other lint-free paper. The most generally useful filter apparatus is a filter funnel holding about 300 ml of fluid and having a disc diameter of 47 mm. Swinney-type 13 mm filter holders for use with a syringe are useful for small volumes. Also for small volumes a centrifugal filter holder is available in place of the older Hemmings filter which utilised an asbestos pad held in a double screw-cap holder for two 5 ml bijou bottles. For sterilising large volumes of fluids such as culture media, stainless-steel filter holders are available.

Vacuum equipment

The flasks for collection of filtrate should be thick-walled and round bottomed or specially designed Buchner flasks, which are conical side-arm flasks, because of the risk of implosion. Sudden changes of pressure must be avoided. Glass-ware under a vacuum must be held in a suitable protective cage or covered with a heavy cloth. Scratched, cracked or etched glass-ware should not be used, and it is advisable to wear goggles or spectacles with safety glass when handling vacuum equipment.

Ultra-violet irradiation

Ultra-violet light is that part of the spectrum with a wavelength of less than 400 nm. In small doses UV light behaves as a mutagen for bacteria; in larger doses it kills them, the optimum wavelength for this being 260 nm. Some light contains UV light with a wavelength of 290 nm, but this is less efficient.

Ultra-violet light can be used as a means of disinfecting the inside of exhaust protective cabinets and sterile rooms, such as media preparation rooms but is no longer recommended. A germicidal tube consists of an electric arc operating in low-pressure mercury vapour. This is mounted between electric contacts and run off the mains with a choke. About 80% of the total UV emission is at a wavelength of 253.7 nm which is slightly less effective than the optimum at 260 nm. The glass of the tube is such that it absorbs all radiation shorter than about 200 nm because such rays react with atmospheric oxygen to produce ozone which is toxic to man in very small concentrations. The system must be designed so that no UV light reaches the eyes either directly or by reflection, since it produces severe corneal irritation which is very unpleasant and can last 36 hours. Reflection occurs from polished metals and even white paper. It takes of the order of 5 minutes to kill 99.9 per cent of *Escherichia coli*, or 4 hours to kill resistant fungal spores at a disance of 3 feet from a new 15 watt tube. The intensity of the irradiation received depends upon the age of the tube, e.g. after about 3000 hours use, the intensity is down to about 80 per cent and will fall still further with time, although the lamp may still be emitting visible blue light. Distance from the light source is important, and the inverse square law holds except when very close to the lamp. Ultra-violet light is heavily absorbed by protein, nucleic acids, free bases and plastics, so penetration into culture media is very limited. In general, UV light irradiation in cabinets and sterile rooms should be regarded as an extra precaution, following cleaning and chemical disinfection.

Table 17.4.   Some disinfectants suitable for laboratory use

Disinfectant	Lab. uses	Concn.	Spectrum	Not affected	Comments
Alcohols industrial methylated spirits ethyl alcohol isopropyl alcohol	Skin prior to injection or vene-puncture: clean surfaces	70% in water	Wide, vegetative bacteria	Spores, many viruses	Rapid action, lack penetrating power; isopropyl alcohol is better than ethyl alcohol, both improved by addition of 0·4% chlorhexidine (Hibitane)
Aldehydes Formalin (40% v/u formaldehyde gas in water)	High-risk situations	10%	All microbes		Too irritant for regular use, good ventilation essential. Causes skin reactions in some people. Can be used in presence of organic matter
	P.M. room, discard containers, bench tops	5%		—	
	Preservative of bacterial suspensions	up to 2·5%			
	Fumigation, e.g. safety cabinets	Neat			
Glutaraldehyde e.g. Cidex	Discard containers, bench tops etc.	2% at pH 7·5– 8·5	Wide	—	Less irritant and damaging. Can be used to 'sterilise' utensils and instruments, e.g. cystoscopes and anaesthetic face masks. Deteriorates in working strength solutions. Poor penetration. Expensive.
Halogens hypochlorite e.g. Chloros (10% solution) Domestos	Utensils, e.g. pipettes. Clean surfaces, after blood spillage, discard jars, contaminated lab. coats and gowns	1% 10,000 p.p.m. of available chlorine (i.e. 1 in 10 Chloros)	Wide, includes viruses and spores	Mycobacteria, cysts of *Entamoeba histolytica*	Rapid action. Easily inactivated by organic material. Corrode metals, so do not use in centrifuges etc. Potassium permanganate used as redox indicator. Colourless = reduced = inactive. Starch/iodide papers turn blue at 50 p.p.m. available chlorine and deep blue at 200 p.p.m. Inactivate with thiosulphate before autoclaving to prevent release of gaseous chlorine
Povidone iodine Betadine	Hands, e.g. after contamination	Neat	Wide	—	A surgical scrub: organic iodine in detergent mixture
Phenolics Lysol	P.M. room, after spillage, discard containers, faeces, sputa, etc.	1%	Wide	Spores, hepatitis virus	Highly toxic and irritant to skin. Retains much activity in presence of organic matter, but not in presence of gross soiling. Allow to act for at least 30 min, then wash off with running water. 24 hr for tubercle bacilli
Clear, soluble phenolics, e.g., Hycolin Clearsol, Stericol, Printol	As Lysol, wiping down work benches	0·5–1·5% 1·0–2·5%			See makers' instructions for exact concentrations to use in different circumstances. Add liquid to water to prevent gel formation. Form clear solutions in soft water. These are more refined and less corrosive than Lysol. Do not autoclave, the fumes produced are dangerous to the operator

Table 17.4. *Some disinfectants suitable for laboratory use (cont.)*

Disinfectant	Lab. uses	Concn.	Spectrum	Not affected	Comments
Quaternary ammonium compounds Cetrimide (Cetavlon)	Selective medium for *Pseudomonas* spp.	0·1%	Gram-positive	Gram-negative organisms less affected	A cationic detergent
Aniline dyes Crystal violet	Selective medium for streptococci	1–2 p.p.m.	Gram-positive, especially staphylo-cocci	Gram-negative organisms, less affected, also strepto-cocci and *Erysipelothrix*	Use 0·2 ml of a 1 in 1000 solution to 100 ml medium
Malachite green	In Lowenstein-Jensen medium	1 in 2000	Most organisms at this concn.	Mycobacteria	A selective medium for mycobacteria, which grow slowly; needs an agent to suppress other faster growing microbes and prevent them from overgrowing the medium
Organic solvents Chloroform	Preservative for serum. Fildes' peptic digest, urine etc.	0·25–1·5%	Vegetative organisms	—	Easily removed by incubation at 56°C when the chloroform vaporises. Not easily inflammable
Metallic compounds thiomersal (Merthiolate)	Serum, antigen and urine preservative, also agar gels used for immuno-diffusion	0·005–0·1%	Vegetative, bacteria, fungi	—	—
Sodium azide	buffer preservative	0·01%	—	—	—

CHEMICAL METHODS

Chemicals can be used to disinfect and occasionally to sterilise. Both liquids and gases are used. Chemicals are generally less effective than physical agents.

Antibacterial spectrum. The antibacterial spectrum should be wide, but some disinfectants are more active against Gram-positive than against Gram-negative organisms; only a few will kill myobacteria, spores and viruses within a few hours.

Concentration. To be effective the exact concentrations of disinfectants must be used, and this involves the measurement of the chemical itself and its diluent.

Deterioration. A number of disinfectants such as glutaraldehyde solutions deteriorate after dilution, and these should be used freshly prepared.

Inactivation. A number of things inactivate disinfectants, notably hard water, soap, incompatible detergents, organic material like pus and faeces, cork, wood and some fabrics and plastics; prior cleaning of surfaces to be disinfected may reduce inactivation.

Sufficient time must be given for disinfectants to act. On a clean surface their action may be quite rapid and complete within a minute or two, but where there is dirt or organic material, or particularly resistant organisms, such as tubercle bacilli and the spores of *Bacillus* species and *Clostridia*, as long as 24 hours may be required even when using the optimum solution for the purpose. Some disinfectants will fail to kill all organisms and merely inhibit growth (Bacteriostatic action), e.g. *Pseudomonas* species are particularly resistant to quaternary ammonium compounds. Viruses are more resistant than bacteria to some germicides. The fat-soluble lipophilic viruses such as herpes, vaccinia, influenzae, and adenoviruses are more easily killed by the quaternary ammonium compounds and phenolic compounds than are the fat-insoluble hydrophilic viruses such as polio virus, coxsackie and echo groups. Halogen compounds such as hypochlorite are effective against all groups of viruses except in the presence of organic matter, but the susceptibility of some viruses, e.g. the viruses of hepatitis, is not sufficiently known.

Laboratory testing of disinfectants using traditional tests such as the Rideal-Walker and Chick-Martin tests (developed for testing the efficiency of phenolic disinfectants) are not usually performed in medical laboratories. In general, the testing of disinfectants is complicated and should be left to specialist laboratories; however, 'in use' tests are the responsibility of the user and should be done in every hospital where disinfectants are used. The method is described by Kelsey and Maurer,[1] and the object is to determine whether disinfectants taken from such sources as laboratory discard jars, mop buckets, stock solutions, etc., contain living bacteria, and if so, how many. No single substance is likely to be suitable for all purposes, and Table 17.4 gives a brief description of the properties of some of those which are useful in the laboratory.

Topping-up of partially empty bottles should always be avoided. Stock bottles should be cleaned and disinfected, preferably by heat, before they are refilled. Cork stoppers must never be used since they harbour bacteria, especially *Pseudomonas* spp. Many disinfectants become firmly fixed to the surfaces of materials which they contact, and this inhibits their use in the laboratory but makes them suitable for the disinfection of discarded objects such as plastic centrifuge tubes. Objects being disinfected in reservoirs of disinfectant solution must be totally immersed and contain no air bubbles.

Biological tests of sterilising systems are set out in Table 17.5.

Table 17.5. *Biological tests of sterilising systems*

Hot-air ovens	Non-toxigenic *Clostridium tetani* spore strip
Autoclaves (+ low-temperature steam and formaldehyde)	*Bacillus stearothermophilus* spore strips
Irradiation	*Bacillus pumulis* spore strips *Streptococcus faecium*
Filtration	retain *Serratia marcescens*
Low-temperature steam	*Streptococcus faecalis* (dried in serum)
Ethylene oxide	*Bacillus subtilis* var. *niger* spore strips

REFERENCE

1. Kelsey, J.C. and Maurer, I.M. (1966). *Mon. Bull. Minist. Hlth. Lab. Serv.*, **25,** 180.

BIBLIOGRAPHY

1. Maurer, I.M. (1978) *Hospital Hygiene* (Second Edition). London: Edward Arnold.

18. Introduction to experimental animals

INTRODUCTION

Laboratory animals are protected by a number of Acts of Parliament of which the most important is that known as the 'Cruelty to Animals Act 1876' and the following remarks are based on that piece of legislation. It is probable that new legislation will come into being in the near future and undoubtedly any changes will be brought to the attention of prospective users of experimental animals. Before anyone in Great Britain can perform experiments on living animals they must obtain a licence from the Home Secretary which authorises the licensee to carry out experiments in a particular stated place. All such places must be registered, but approval by the Home Office is required before a registration is granted. The premises will be visited by a Home Office Inspector from time to time without notice, to ensure that no unnecessary suffering is imposed upon the animals and that their conditions are satisfactory. The licence authorises the experimenter to carry out an experiment only on anaesthetised animals, and the animal must be killed before recovery from the anaesthetic.

If no anaesthetic is to be used, then a special certificate (Certificate A) must be obtained with the licence which will authorise the experimenter to carry out simple procedures such as subcutaneous, intramuscular, intravenous or intraperitoneal injections and scarifications. Other certificates must be obtained if it is necessary for an animal to recover from an anaesthetic for the purpose of the experiment or if it is wished to carry out experiments on cats, dogs or *equidae*. The holder of the licence is required to keep a record of all experiments and to make a return of experiments carried out at the end of each year. Tests carried out by a bacteriologist to aid in the identification of organisms and in virulence testing or in the raising of antibodies are all regarded as experiments. The licence and any accompanying certificate comprise a legal document giving authority only to the holder of the licence, and under no circumstances is delegation of that authority allowed even in his presence.

Further information can be obtained from *Notes on the Law Relating to Experiments on Animals in Great Britain*, issued by the Research Defence Society and obtainable from the Secretary, 11 Chandos Street, London, W.1.

The Animal Unit

The best animal houses are purpose-built. They incorporate a room for the quarantine of newly arrived animals, a breeding room, a room for stock animals, an entirely separate room for inoculated animals, a vermin-proof store for foodstuffs and bedding, an equipment store, a utility room for cleaning and sterilising, a room where the experiments are carried out and a room for the animal house attendant. The parts containing the animals should be maintained at a temperature of 17–19°C. Air conditioning giving 14–16 air changes per hour and maintaining the relative humidity at 45–50% is recommended. The entire animal house must be kept scrupulously clean and must be vermin-proof.

The animals are absolutely reliant on the staff of the animal house for their well-being.

Feeding

Each animal must have a plentiful supply of fresh, clean drinking water and a balanced diet which must meet the requirements of the species concerned. Cubed or pelleted diets containing proteins, carbohydrates, fats, vitamins, and minerals in adequate and balanced amounts to meet the needs of most laboratory animals are available commercially, and can be supplemented with natural foodstuffs such as fresh vegetables. The commercial diets should be stored in dry, well-ventilated, vermin-proof rooms in food bins, but should not be kept for long periods. The food bins should not be topped-up, but should be allowed to fall empty and be cleaned before being refilled. Care must be taken to avoid damp, beetles and flour mites.

Hygiene

The animals and their surroundings must be kept clean

to avoid the risk of epidemics. The animals should be provided with a fresh clean cage once a week. The dirty cages are scraped, scrubbed and then sterilised in an autoclave. Before being used again, the cage is dried and a layer of litter about 2 cm deep of an absorbent material such as sawdust, is placed in the bottom of the cage and a fresh food hopper and water bottle provided.

The rooms where the animals are kept should have their floors hosed down daily and the walls washed weekly. Each animal must be inspected daily and its general condition, behaviour, consumption of food and water, and nature of faeces observed. New animals should only be purchased from accredited breeders, and must be kept in quarantine for two weeks to prevent introduction of disease such as pasteurellosis or lice into the general stock. Any disease which occurs during the quarantine period must be fully investigated. All the animals inoculated with material containing or likely to contain micro-organisms must be kept in an isolation area and regarded as infectious. These animals should be kept in cages designed to prevent cross-contamination between the cage units. Uneaten food and litter from these animals must be handled carefully and incinerated. After handling inoculated animals, overalls should be changed and the hands washed thoroughly.

Cages

Cages are commonly made of stainless steel, but more recently autoclavable plastic cages have been introduced which are relatively cheap, durable, easy to clean and quiet. Cages are designed for each species so that each has sufficient room for rest and exercise. They must also be strong, corrosion-resistant, capable of being sterilised, and easy to clean, store and handle. Many cages have wire-mesh floors through which the excreta fall on to a tray which is removable for cleaning.

Food hoppers are preferred to dishes for species commonly found in hospital animal houses. Water is usually provided in inverted polypropylene bottles with stainless steel canullae. Each cage must have permanently attached to it a holder for a label on which is recorded the name of the experimenter, the identifying marks of the animal or animals, the date, the nature of the experiment, and the name of the patient or identifying number. This label must be placed in such a position that it cannot be reached, or excreted upon, by the animal and should be transferred to the new cage with the animal when required.

TECHNIQUES

Marking animals for identification

Staining. A small area, e.g. on the back of an animal, is deeply stained with an alcoholic solution of a dye which is applied by means of a cotton wool swab. The following stains are suitable:

Colour	Stain
Red	Carbol fuchsin
Violet	Methyl violet
Green	Malachite green
Blue	Trypan blue
Yellow	Saturated picric acid

This method is not permanent and reapplication of the dye will be necessary from time to time.

More permanent methods include tattooing, suitable for rabbits' ears; ear punching, either holes cut right through the ear or notches round the edge of the ear; ear-marking studs; rings; tags or discs on collars and neckbands. Whichever method is chosen it is essential that a suitable coding system should be drawn up and adhered to.

Euthanasia

Methods of killing animals can be divided into two types: chemical methods and physical methods.

Chemical methods

Chloroform. An overdose of chloroform is suitable for killing most animals. Mice can be killed conveniently by placing them in the top half of a glass desiccator which contains a pad soaked in chloroform in the bottom part. This method can be adapted for larger animals such as guinea-pigs, but the chloroform-soaked cotton wool must not be allowed to come into contact with the animal because it causes burning of the mucous membranes. The interior of the container should have light excluded from it because this reduces the amount of struggling that the animal will do in order to get out of the container. Ether is much less lethal and unreliable as a killing agent, but on the other hand it is a safer anaesthetic for animals.

Intravenous injection. Rabbits and other large animals can be killed by giving intravenous injections of suitable agents such as pentabarbitone sodium (Nembutal). The dose required is about three times that which produces anaesthesia.

Physical methods

Methods requiring rupture of the spinal cord require some manual dexterity and should only be learnt from a person skilled in these procedures, since they must be effective on the first attempt. The preferred method of killing guinea-pigs is dislocation of the neck. This can be accomplished by holding the animal with one hand over the top of the animal's head with a finger on either side of its neck, swinging it so that the body is vertical and then dropping the arm swiftly downwards. The weight of the animal's body swinging in this way will be sufficient to dislocate the neck. Before the carcass is disposed of it is essential to ensure that the animal is actually dead. Death is certain in the following circumstances:

if a post-mortem examination has been performed,
if the animal has been completely exsanguinated as when guinea-pig blood is collected for use as complement in CFTs,
if the heart has been removed,
if the animal has been decapitated, or
when the carcass is still and cold and has rigor mortis.

Materials for inoculation

Body fluids, such as blood, serous fluids or cerebrospinal fluid and ground tissue suspensions may require no further preparation if they are thought to contain only the suspected organism. Other fluids such as sputum and urine deposits from early morning urines, e.g. for examination for mycobacteria which probably contain other contaminating organisms, will have to be treated before inoculation, using a method such as those described in the section on mycobacteria.

Pus does not usually require any previous preparation.

Bacteria may be suspended in broth or saline for inoculation.

Tissue for inoculation, for example endometrial curettings for examination for mycobacteria and biopsy specimens, must be ground up so finely in a sterile Griffith's tube that they will go through a hypodermic needle, adding a little peptone water if necessary.

Post-mortem examination of animals

A post-mortem examination is carried out on all experimental animals. Since the animal is likely to be infected with a virulent organism, great care must be taken at all times.

Equipment

(a) Gown, rubber apron, surgical gloves and protective spectacles or goggles.

(b) A dissecting board generally made of cork (bathmat type).

(c) Cellophane sheet or other impervious disposable sheet to cover the board and four pins for attaching the legs. Alternatively a specially designed table can be used for larger animals.

(d) Instruments—these must be sterile and can conveniently be made up into sets containing the following:

3 scalpels
4 pairs dissecting scissors
4 pairs toothed forceps

(e) Assorted Petri dishes, bacteriological swabs, sterile containers and culture media.

(f) A phenolic disinfectant in strong aqueous solution such as 1% Clearsol.

Procedure

(a) Identify the animal with its cage label and any markings and record the date of death in the record book.

(b) Immerse the animal in the phenolic disinfectant for about 5 sec to prevent loose fur flying about later.

(c) Pin the animal on to a covered dissecting board so that it is lying on its back with its legs stretched outwards towards the corners of the board.

If the animal has died of an infectious disease it is recommended that the next part of the procedure should be carried out in an exhaust protective cabinet, but in any case an aseptic technique must be used, since only in this way can pure cultures of the infecting organism be obtained.

(d) Lay out the sterile instruments on a sterile plane such as their wrapping paper or the lid of the box in which they were sterilised.

(e) Make a median incision of the skin over the chest and abdomen and reflect the skin over the chest, abdomen and limbs. The instruments used (a pair of forceps and a pair of scissors or/and a scalpel, depending upon the choice of the operator) are discarded.

(f) Examine:

(i) the site of injection, for example, the right-hand thigh (left facing), and sample bacteriologically if an abscess has formed.

(ii) the regional lymphatics, for example, to see if there is involvement of the lymph nodes in the femoral triangle.

(g) Open peritoneal cavity with a fresh set of instruments and reflect the abdominal walls to each side. The presence of fluid or exudate is noted.

(h) Examine the spleen, lymphatics, liver and kidneys macroscopically and remove aseptically to sterile containers if culture is required.

(i) Open the chest by holding the sternum firmly with a pair of forceps held in one hand and, using scissors with the other, cut the ribs on each side and reflect the anterior chest wall upwards to demonstrate the heart and lungs.

(j) If the animal died from a septicaemic illness the heart blood can be sampled using a Pasteur pipette passed through the heart wall. The lungs can now be removed for culture, if necessary, using a fresh set of instruments.

(k) Discard the carcass, operator's gloves and cellophane board cover into an opaque waterproof bag and incinerate. The instruments are autoclaved, the cork board is disinfected using the phenolic disinfectant. Do not autoclave this or it will disintegrate.

(l) Record the findings.

GUINEA-PIGS

Cage. $750 \times 750 \times 230$ mm high with a wire-grid floor and a portable metal dirt tray under each cage

Diet. Commercially prepared cubes, e.g. diet SGI, and drinking water

Temperature of room. 17–19°C

Room humidity. 55%

Weight of adult. 450–700g

Rectal temperature. 37·6–38·9

Normal respiration rate. Approximately 90–120 per minute

Mating age. 15–20 weeks

Gestation period. 60–72 days, usually about 63–65 days

Weaning age. 7–14 days

Weaning weight. 120–170 g

Breeding season. Continuous

Oestrus cycle. Every 13–20 days with a duration approximately 50 hr.

Handling. To pick the animal up, place a hand over its back with the thumb behind the front leg and the finger on the other side under its chest. Place the other hand under its hind quarters and lift using both hands. For intramuscular injection of the thigh, the assistant should hold the guinea-pig with his right hand so that the thumb is below the shoulder on the left-hand side and the right front leg is between the index and middle finger, with the middle, ring, and little fingers reaching round on to the front of the chest. The left hind leg is held with the left hand. The person doing the injection holds the right hind leg out straight whilst giving the injection. It is important that the animal is approached with confidence, that no sudden movements are made to frighten the animal, and that the handling is gentle so that the animal is not hurt.

Experimental procedures

Subcutaneous inoculation

The animal is held so that the neck or flank is presented to the inoculator. Up to 5 ml of fluid can be introduced into a skin fold.

Intracutaneous inoculation

The hair is removed from the flanks of the animal with hair clippers followed, if necessary, by depilation using any commercial depilating cream. The depilator is allowed to act for at least 2 minutes and is then washed off. This operation should be carried out some time before the injection is due. A 1 ml tuberculin syringe with a fine, short needle is used. The syringe is held with the bevel of the needle uppermost and the needle is introduced into the dermis just below the surface. 0·1 ml (not more than 0·2 ml) is injected into the dermis raising a bleb. If several injections are to be made, the skin of the flanks can be divided into 25 mm squares using a ball-point pen, and the injections are made into the middle of each square carefully noting the position of each. The results are usually read 24–48 hours later.

Intramuscular injection

The animal is held as described above, and the injection is usually made into the thigh.

Intraperitoneal inoculation

The guinea-pig is held upside down and the inoculation is made in the-line in the lower abdomen. Up to 5 ml of fluid can be inoculated.

Bleeding

If only a few drops of blood are required these can be obtained by nicking an ear vein with a sterile lancet. Large volumes are obtained by cardiac puncture or the animal can be exsanguinated after death.

Anaesthesia

For a light anaesthesia of short duration halothane is suitable, for example, when carrying out cardiac puncture. For a long-acting anaesthetic, pentabarbitone sodium is given intraperitoneally, 30 mg per kg of body weight. This is given about a quarter of an hour before the experiment and will last up to 2 hours. The effects wear off after 12 hours. It would only be in very unusual circumstances that such an anaesthetic was required in an ordinary medical laboratory.

Common diseases

These include pseudotuberculosis caused by *Yersinia pseudotuberculosis*, respiratory tract infections, for example, with pneumococcus and *Pasteurella multocida*. Intestinal infections such as salmonellosis and abscesses of the lymphatic glands due to group C haemolytic streptococci.

MICE

Cage. Up to five mice of the same sex can be kept in a metal box cage 150 mm × 300 mm × 150 mm deep. The lid is made of wire and incorporates a food hopper and a place for a water bottle. Sawdust or woodchip litter is placed in the bottom of the box and the mice are cleaned out once or twice a week.

Diet. Commercially compressed food cubes such as Diet 41B and water
Room temperature. 19–21°C
Humidity. 45–55%
Weight of adult. 25–28 g
Rectal temperature. Average 37·4°C
Pulse rate. Approximately 180 per minute

Mating age. 6–8 weeks
Gestation period. 19–21 days
Sex determination. At birth the males have a larger genital papilla which is further from the anus than in the females
Weaning age. 19–21 days
Weaning weight. 7 g
Breeding season. Continuous
Oestrus. 5-day cycle
Handling. With the finger and thumb of the left hand gently take hold of the base of the tail. Using the thumb and forefinger of the right hand the mouse can then be picked up by the scruff of the neck and inverted so that its back lies in the palm of the hand. The tail and right back leg can then be restrained between the little and ring fingers.

Experimental procedures

Subcutaneous inoculation

Up to 1 ml may be injected under the skin near the root of the tail with an assistant steadying the mouse by holding the tail with one hand and the loose skin behind the head with the other.

Intraperitoneal inoculation

Up to 2 ml can be injected just to one side of the mid-line in the lower half of the abdomen.

Intravenous inoculation

The mouse is placed in a perforated cylinder just large enough to hold it. A cork is used to close the cylinder behind the mouse whose tail is allowed to protrude through a nick in the edge of the cork. The cylinder may then be held in a retort stand. The tail veins are made to dilate by warming with a lamp. Up to 0·5 ml can be injected in this way using a tuberculin syringe and a fine needle. A vein is selected as near the tip as possible where they are more firmly fixed than the slightly larger veins near the base of the tail.

Intracerebral inoculation

The mouse is lightly anaesthetised with halothane and the skin over the head is cleaned with 70% alcohol. A tuberculin syringe with a fine needle is used to inject up to 0·02 ml of fluid about 2–3 mm into the skull half-way between the eye and the ear, 3 mm from the mid-line.

Intracerebral inoculation of suckling mice less than

2 days old is achieved by holding the mouse between the finger and thumb on the bench and inserting the needle of a tuberculin syringe into the pad of fat between the shoulder blade, first injecting 0·01 ml there, then making the point of the needle track up towards the foramen magnum into the cerebrum and injecting a further 0·01 ml there. This procedure is used in the isolation of some viruses such as the enteroviruses, including Coxsackie viruses.

Common diseases

These include salmonellosis and virus diseases, including ectromelia (mousepox), *Streptobacillus moniliformis* infection and worms.

Other animals, such as rabbits and rats, are less commonly used in routine microbiology and are therefore not described.

BIBLIOGRAPHY

1. Worden, A.N. and Lane-Petter, W. (Eds.) (1972) *The U.F.A.W. Handbook on the Care and Management of Laboratory Animals* (4th Edition). London: The Universities Federation of Animal Welfare.
2. Short, D.J. and Woodnott, D.P. (Eds.) (1969) (Reprint 1978) *The I.A.T. Manual of Laboratory Animal Practice and Techniques* (2nd Edition). London: Crosby Lockwood.
3. Lane-Petter, W. and Pearson, A.E.G. (1971) *The Laboratory Animal—Principles and Practice.* London: Academic Press.

PART THREE

Histology and Cytology

19. General outline of procedures in a routine histopathology department

Histology is the study of tissue structure at microscopic level. Histopathology is the examination of the tissues for the presence or absence of changes in their structure due to abnormal conditions. This study is made possible by the preparation of thin slices or sections of the tissues which are coloured differentially by the use of various dyes and chemicals. It is not possible to demonstrate all the normal and abnormal components of the tissues in a single preparation. Because of this numerous techniques are used, even in the routine department. These methods range from those devised for the demonstration of the general structure of the tissues to those which are designed to visualise one specific component.

When examining a finished section with the microscope some of what is seen will have occurred during the preparation of the material. These appearances are known as artifacts and have been well described by Wallington.[1] Distortion of tissue structures, displacement of tissue constituents and the addition of various foreign materials are examples. Some artifacts result from necessary treatment in the fixation and processing of tissues for cutting and are unavoidable, but many, such as damage caused by a poor knife-edge, stain deposits and various foreign bodies, can and should be avoided. The collection of a set of slides illustrating various artifacts is a useful exercise.

This is an outline guide to the treatment of routine histopathology specimens. Details of these procedures may vary from laboratory to laboratory, but the basic principles will be the same. Where necessary, detailed explanations of the different stages are given in later chapters.

Reception

When specimens arrive at the department the following points must be checked at the earliest opportunity:

1. That the specimen is for histological examination.
2. That the specimen container is labelled and is accompanied by a correctly completed request form.
3. That sufficient fixative is in the container. If the specimen is not in fixative or is in a fluid other than that supplied by the laboratory this should be noted on the request form and appropriate action taken.

The request form is now date-stamped, and it and the specimen container are identified with a serial number. A stiff card label is made on which this serial number is written with lead pencil. This label remains with the specimen during the whole of the following treatment.

Trimming and block selection

It is desirable to have a set time each day when the pathologist will examine the specimens, where necessary describe their macroscopic appearance, and then select the pieces from which he wishes sections to be prepared. This is best done in an area away from the main laboratory. A sink and running water are essential. The specimens, together with their request forms and card labels, are arranged in this area. For the trimming session the pathologist should have available rubber gloves, sponge, small scalpel, large ham knife, plain and rat-tooth forceps, probes, scissors, bowel scissors, small bone saw, steel rule and some means of weighing the specimens. Other instruments may be accumulated according to the individual preferences of each pathologist. It is usually convenient for the technician to write the description of the specimen together with a note of the number of pieces taken for processing on the back of the request form.

The pieces selected for processing are placed into small jars of fresh fixative together with their card label. Should it be necessary to distinguish blocks from different areas of the specimen, these are placed in separate containers and suffixes 'a', 'b', 'c', etc., added to the serial number as necessary. In the case of a small biopsy that is to be processed in its entirety a note to this effect is made on the back of the form.

Processing

As most diagnostic departments now use automatic processing machines, this procedure will be described.

Hand processing involves the use of the same fluids and materials but takes considerably longer. The selected pieces of tissue are loaded into the processing machine containers. The number of pieces loaded is checked against the number recorded on the request form and any discrepancy dealt with before proceeding further. The machine schedule is set as required, checked by a second technician, and the machine switched on. The details of each specimen are now entered in numerical order in a daybook. This book serves primarily as a technician's check system, and the following illustrates a useful layout.

20th January 19—

174	BLOGGS Joseph	4√ Stomach	PAS
175	SMITH Frederick	2√ L. Node	ZN: Retic.
1976	JONES Hilda	7√ Rectum etc.	

21st January 19—

| 177 | BROWN William | AE√Biopsy oesophagus | Levels |
| 178 | GREEN Charles | 2√ Appendix | |

The columns record from left to right: serial number, name, number of blocks (AE means all embedded), number correct when embedded, nature of specimen and any special stains or other treatment used.

Embedding

At the end of the processing cycle the machine is unloaded and the tissues embedded in paraffin wax. This may be done either in conventional embedding moulds or in one of the various plastic moulds now available. At this time the technician checks that the number of pieces embedded tallies with the number recorded in column three of the day book, and if correct ticks column four. This continual checking of the blocks may seem tedious but experience has shown that it minimises errors.

Cutting and staining

Sections are now cut from the wax blocks. Sometimes it may be apparent from the information on the request form or from the macroscopic appearance of the specimen that certain extra stains will be necessary. Sections for these can be cut at this time. The cut sections are mounted on glass slides on which the serial number is scratched with a diamond pencil. They are then dried. When dry they are stained, mounted under a cover glass, labelled and checked against the information on the request form. Then, together with the request form, they are handed in to the pathologist.

Reporting and filing

After examining the sections the pathologist will usually give in his report for typing and despatch. He may, however, require further sections, special stains, or more blocks to be taken from the gross specimen before he gives his report. When he has finished with the slides they should be dried for at least 2 weeks at 37°C. They can then be filed away. It is advisable to keep the gross specimens for at least one month after the report has been completed. By then it should be apparent whether any further material needs to be sectioned or if the specimen is suitable for museum or teaching purposes. If not, it should be disposed of.

In this summary of the routine processing of histological material, emphasis has been placed on the need for constant cross-checking of the selected tissues in order to avoid loss or confusion. It is essential that the histopathological technician fully realises the implications of his work. Whereas it is possible, though doubtless undesirable, to repeat a throat swab, urine sample or blood sample, this is not the case with regard to tissues taken from a patient at operation.

REFERENCE

1. Wallington, E.A. (1979). *Med. Lab. Sci.*, **36**, 3–61.

20. Fixation

Fixation is the term used in histology to describe the process of rendering the tissues resistant to changes in structure. Such changes may result from the action of substances such as enzymes normally present in the tissues themselves, and this process is known as autolysis or self-destruction. Other changes can result from external influences such as bacteria causing decomposition, putrefaction, drying and shrinkage. Even after a fixing fluid has halted these changes distortion can occur during the subsequent treatment of the tissues which is necessary for the preparation of sections. Many chemicals and chemical mixtures are capable of preventing some of these changes but they have other qualities which make them unsuitable for use in the laboratory. Modern fixatives are expected to fulfil other requirements in addition to stabilisation. The ideal fixative would have all of the following properties:

1. Prevention of autolysis and decomposition.
2. Neither adding to nor removing from the tissue constituents.
3. Causing no shrinkage or swelling.
4. Preventing distortion by any reagents used subsequently.
5. Penetrating tissues rapidly, evenly and deeply.
6. Imparting a suitable hardness and texture to allow the easy cutting of sections.
7. Rendering the tissues receptive to stains.
8. Non-toxic, non-corrosive, non-inflammable.
9. Cheap and easy to prepare.
10. Stable.
11. Suitable for long-term storage of specimens.
12. Allowing restoration of some natural colour for museum work and photography.

At present there is no fixative which fulfils all of the above requirements and it is for this reason that such an abundance of formulae is to be found in the literature. Several mixtures have become established as routine general fixatives, but the majority have been devised for a specific purpose and are unsuitable for routine use. Examples of established fixatives are 10% formalin which has many of the requirements of the ideal

mixture and Carnoy's fluid which has few and is retained for special purposes only.

Considerable improvement over the results obtained by the use of 10% formalin alone can be achieved by the technique of secondary fixation. This method has been comprehensively studied and described by Wallington.[1] All specimens are collected in 10% formalin and the blocks selected by the pathologist for processing are then treated with a second, more specialised, fixative for the appropriate time. This time will be less than if the fixative were primary. In this way the suitability of formalin for bulk use, distribution outside the laboratory, frozen-section work, storage of gross specimens etc., is supplemented by the improved fixation, cutting texture and staining given by some of the other fixatives. Wallington recommends the use of 10% formal-sublimate as the second fixative and suggests 4 hours' immersion at the first station on the processing machine as a suitable time. This method does, however, introduce some complications into the processing schedule such as the preparation of saturated mercuric chloride solution, the extreme care with which such solutions must be handled and the need to remove mercury pigment from the sections. These considerations have probably prevented the more widespread use of this method.

Whichever method of fixation is used it is important that the tissues should be immersed in the fixative as soon as possible following removal from the body. The volume of fluid needed is often quoted as being 20 times that of the tissue. In the case of large specimens such as whole spleens this is impractical, and these large specimens should be sliced at intervals of 2 cm or less to allow proper penetration of the fixative. Hollow structures such as bowel and stomachs should be cut open for the same reason.

Smaller blocks from these specimens should be selected as soon as possible and placed in fresh fixative in separate containers. The surface area of the selected blocks will to some extent be governed by the type of microtome to be used, but the thickness of the blocks should be kept to between 2 and 4 mm. If delay in fixation is unavoidable the tissues should be kept moist and chilled. Some fixing mixtures will introduce artifacts in the form of deposits in the tissue and these must be removed before the sections are stained. Methods for the removal of these deposits are given at the beginning of the chapter on staining. The fixatives described below will cover practically all the requirements of the routine department. The name 'formalin' refers to the commercially available solution of approximately 40% formaldehyde gas in water. In the formulae some of the components are in brackets. Comparative studies with many different tissues over a number of years have shown that these components may be omitted without discernible effect on the resulting preparations.

GENERAL ROUTINE FIXING MIXTURES

10% formalin

Formalin	100 ml
Water	900 ml
(Sodium chloride	8·5 g)

Pieces of tissue not thicker than 4 mm and of a size suitable for machine processing will be adequately fixed in 18 hours. Improvement in fixation will continue for up to 72 hours. Larger specimens will require longer, but delay in obtaining a result can be avoided by the selection of smaller pieces for separate fixation as soon as the specimen is received. This fixative is probably the most widely used, certainly in Great Britain, for routine work. It fulfils many of the criteria of the ideal fixative. It is suitable for frozen-section work, photography and museum work. It can be followed by secondary fixation in a more specialised fluid if required. Contact with the fluid may cause dermatitis and rubber gloves should be worn when handling material in formalin. Splashes on the skin should be washed off with cold water. The concentrated vapour causes irritation to the eyes and respiratory tract, so efficient ventilation is essential in the specimen trimming and disposal areas. Commercial formalin becomes acid owing to the formation of formic acid, and stock solutions of prepared fixative should be stored over a layer of calcium carbonate in the form known as marble chips. This acidity is responsible for the formation of a brown deposit in the tissues, particularly in areas containing much blood. This deposit may be referred to as formalin pigment or acid formaldehyde haematin. It is easily removed prior to staining but can be avoided by the use of a buffered fixing mixture.

Buffered 10% formalin (pH 7·0)

Formalin	100 ml
Water	900 ml
Sodium dihydrogen phosphate, either	
anhydrous	3·5 g
or hydrated	4·0 g
Disodium hydrogen phosphate, either	
anhydrous	6·5 g
or hydrated	16·4 g

This is an extravagant fluid for routine use and is not generally necessary. It is used in exactly the same way as ordinary 10% formalin. It is recommended for specimens where there is much blood and where cellular details are of prime importance as with bone-marrow biopsies. It also allows a more complete demonstration of ferric iron deposits, again of importance with bone-marrow specimens.

10% formol-sublimate

Saturated aqueous mercuric chloride	
(approx. 7%)	900 ml
Formalin	100 ml

This mixture fixes in approximately half the time taken by 10% formalin alone, gives better protection during processing, better cutting consistency and brighter staining. The trouble and expense of preparing large quantities of saturated mercuric chloride solutions, together with the corrosive and toxic properties of this substance, make it unsuitable for issue to other departments outside the laboratory. For these reasons it cannot be recommended as a routine primary fixative. Excellent results can be obtained by using this fluid on the processing machine following the collection of specimens in 10% formalin. Here it is acting as a secondary fixative and a 4-hour immersion is sufficient. The tissues can go direct into 90% alcohol as the next stage of the processing schedule. The mercuric chloride produces a deposit in the tissues and this must be removed before staining the sections.

The technician should also be aware of the following four fixatives which, for practical purposes, duplicate results obtainable with those already described, but are nevertheless to be found in the literature. Tissues may be received from other departments in these fluids and methods may be published which recommend their use, and for these reasons they are included here.

Bouin's fluid[2]

Saturated aqueous picric acid	75 ml
Formalin	25 ml
Glacial acetic acid	5 ml

This solution keeps well. Fixation of selected blocks is complete in 8–24 hours, depending on size. The tissues must be transferred direct to 90% alcohol as the next stage of the processing schedule in order to avoid the loss of some water-soluble protein picrates. Nuclear fixation is good and the use of this fluid has been recommended for the study of mitotic figures in, for example, testicular biopsies. It should not be used for mammalian kidneys which are poorly preserved.

Zenker's fluid[3]

Stock solution:

Saturated aqueous mercuric chloride	100 ml
Potassium dichromate	2·5 g
(Sodium sulphate	1·0 g)
Immediately before use add	
Glacial acetic acid	5 ml

Fixation times vary from 8 hours for small biopsies to 24 hours for ordinary-sized blocks. After fixation the tissues must be washed for at least 6 hours in running water to remove the chrome salts. Failure to do this will result in the formation in the tissues of an insoluble brown pigment. The mercuric chloride deposit must also be removed before staining the sections. Nuclear details are well preserved, but some of the cytoplasmic contents may be removed. Red blood cells are lysed. Staining by most routine methods is quite good, but metallic impregnation techniques may prove difficult.

Helly's fluid[4]

Zenker stock solution	100 ml
Immediately before use add	
Formalin	10 ml

Fixation times are the same as for Zenker's fluid and the treatment necessary after fixation is identical. Nuclear detail is possibly slightly inferior to that given by Zenker's fluid, but cytoplasmic granules are not destroyed and the red blood cells are not lysed. Staining, particularly with acid dyes, is good and this fixative is often recommended for specimens of bone marrow. Metallic impregnation methods may give poor results.

Heidenhain's fluid[5] (usually referred to as Susa)

Mercuric chloride	4·5 g
Sodium chloride	0·5 g
Trichloracetic acid	2·0 g
Glacial acetic acid	4·0 ml
Formalin	20·0 ml
Distilled water	80·0 ml

Fix tissues for 8–24 hours according to the size of block and transfer direct to 90% alcohol. This is quite a good general fixative for both nuclei and cytoplasm, and preserves the micro-anatomical picture well. Staining with most routine methods is clear and bright. Although containing mercuric chloride, it is an odd fact that sometimes no deposit is formed in the tissues. However, this phenomenon is not consistent, and sections must either be examined microscopically before staining or treated for the removal of mercury pigment as a routine. A further disadvantage of this fluid is the slightly complicated formula.

SPECIAL FIXING MIXTURES

There are very many fixing fluids which have been devised for special techniques. Three examples are given. They are usually prepared as required, though all three will keep well.

Carnoy's fluid[6]

Absolute alcohol	60 ml
Chloroform	30 ml
Glacial acetic acid	10 ml

The fluid is very useful when the rapid preparation of a paraffin block is necessary. Small biopsies are fixed in 30 minutes and ordinary blocks 2–4 mm thick in 1–3 hours. Nuclear details are well preserved, but red blood cells are lysed and there is considerable shrinkage resulting in distortion of micro-anatomical structure. Fixation is accompanied by partial dehydration and tissues are transferred direct to absolute alcohol which further speeds processing.

Orth's fluid[7]

Potassium dichromate	2·5 g
Water	100 ml
(Sodium sulphate	1·0 g)
Immediately before use add	
Formalin	10 ml

Small blocks are fixed in 12–24 hours. Tissues must be washed in running water for at least 6 hours after fixation. The chromaffin cells of the adrenal medulla react with the dichromate to form a brown pigment. As these cells are present in certain tumours known as phaechromocytomas or chromaffinomas this fluid should be used if such a tumour is suspected.

Schaudinn's fluid[8]

Saturated aqueous mercuric chloride	60 ml
Absolute alcohol	30 ml
Glacial acetic acid	5 ml

This is a rapid fixative which can be recommended if smears of sputum, pleural effusion, etc, are to be examined. The smears are made and, without being allowed to dry, are immersed in fixative for 10–20 minutes. Mercury deposits must be removed before staining. Cells rarely appear to become detached from the slide when this fluid is used.

REFERENCE

1. Wallington, E.A. (1955). *J. Med. Lab. Technol.*, **13**, 53.
2. Bouin, P. (1897). *Arch. Anat. Microsc.*, **1**, 225.
3. Zenker, K. (1894). *Münch. med. Wschr.*, **41**, 532.
4. Helly, K. (1903). *Z. Wiss. Mikr.*, **20**, 413.
5. Heidenhain, M. (1916). *Z. Wiss. Mikr.*, **33**, 232.
6. Carnoy, J.B. (1887). *Cellule*, **3**, 276.
7. Orth, J. (1896). *Berl. klin. Wschr.*, **33**, 273.
8. Schaudinn, F. (1900). *Zool. Jahrb. Abth. Anat.*, **13**, 211.

21. Decalcification

Methods exist which make possible the preparation of sections of bone and other tissues containing calcium salts without special treatment, but it is the usual practice in the routine laboratory to remove these hard deposits before attempting to cut sections. This process is known as decalcification. It is usually done between fixation and processing, although it is possible to remove small deposits from the surfaces of prepared paraffin blocks. The tissues must be completely fixed before decalcification is begun. Immersion of unfixed tissues in decalcifying fluids will result in gross tissue damage and impairment of staining. After complete fixation small bone biopsies can be immersed entirely in decalcifying fluid. Selection of blocks from larger bone specimens is done by using a fine-toothed saw. After decalcification is complete, the rough surfaces of these sawn blocks are trimmed smooth with a fine scalpel. This is done to remove any bone dust left in the surface of the block by the saw.

Several methods have been suggested for the removal of calcium salts from tissues. As a general rule the more rapid the method the greater the damage to the tissues and a balance has to be struck between speed and quality of preparation.

ACIDS

Many different acids have been used, either as simple solutions or as quite complicated mixtures. The addition of a fixative, usually formalin, to the decalcifying fluid makes no discernible difference to the results.

20% aqueous formic acid

This fluid causes little tissue disruption and staining results are generally good. It is rapid enough for most routine work, the average size of surgical block being decalcified in 2–4 days. It is not as rapid as nitric acid but causes less damage to tissues should they be left in it longer than is absolutely necessary for complete decalcification. Removal of calcium can be confirmed by X-ray or by the chemical test.

5% aqueous nitric acid

This fluid removes calcium salts more rapidly than the formic acid solution described above, but material must not be left in it for any longer than is absolutely necessary or considerable maceration of the tissues, together with very poor staining, will result. Decalcification can be confirmed by X-ray or the chemical test.

CHELATING AGENTS

Ethylenediamine tetra-acetic acid (EDTA)

When in solution this substance will combine with calcium ions to form soluble compounds. As this reaction can occur in a neutral solution, tissues can be left in the fluid for several days without maceration or loss of staining qualities occurring. The method is usually far too slow for diagnostic surgical histology but is suitable for post-mortem or research materials. The results are superior to those obtained by any other method and this technique is recommended where time permits its use.

Dissolve 250 g ethylenediamine tetra-acetic acid in 1750 ml distilled water.

Adjust to pH 7·0 using sodium hydroxide.

Change the fluid every 5 days. Decalcification should preferably be confirmed by X-ray as the chemical test is unreliable when used with this method.

PROPRIETARY FLUIDS

R.D.C.

A fluid known as R.D.C. is now obtainable in Great Britain. Its formula is not disclosed by the makers and there must be considerable reluctance to use any such unidentified chemicals in the laboratory. However, after many comparative studies and thorough testing this fluid has proved very valuable for all routine work. It is more rapid than any of the conventional fluids and,

179

if used correctly, preservation of structure and staining results are excellent. Cortical bone is decalcified in 6–10 hours in blocks not thicker than 5 mm and small deposits of calcium are removed in 1–4 hours. If, as is usually the case, only one batch of fluid is necessary to decalcify the specimen the chemical test is of no value, and completeness of decalcification should be checked by X-ray. R.D.C. *must not* be mixed with formaldehyde in an attempt to simultaneously decalcify and fix. It is obtainable from Bethlehem Instruments Ltd.*

ION-EXCHANGE RESINS

Techniques involving the addition of ion-exchange resins to the decalcifying fluid are based on the theory that the absorption of the calcium ions from the fluid by these resins will speed decalcification. In practical terms the improvements, if any, are so marginal as to be of little value and the method has nothing to recommend it.

ELECTROLYTIC DECALCIFICATION

This method is based on the idea that the calcium ions in the acid electrolyte are attracted to the negative electrode thus speeding decalcification—a similar theory to that involving ion-exchange resins. Any increase in the speed of decalcification is due to the increase in temperature of the fluid and is accompanied by a related increase in tissue damage and loss of staining quality.

TESTING FOR DECALCIFICATION

Whichever method is chosen to decalcify the tissues, complete removal of the calcium salts must be established before the tissues are processed.

X-ray

Where facilities are available, X-raying of the specimen at 24-hour intervals is the method of choice except

* Bethlehem Instruments Ltd., 45 Bedmond Rd., Hemel Hempstead, Herts.

when using R.D.C. fluid, when the interval would have to be perhaps as short as 1 hour.

Chemical testing

Unfortunately, X-ray facilities are not always available and the chemical test is the best alternative. It may be used after formic acid, nitric acid, or R.D.C. It can be tried after EDTA, but may prove unreliable.

Method. 5 ml of decalcifying fluid from the specimen pot are made neutral to litmus paper using strong (0·880) ammonia solution. Turbidity at this stage indicates the presence of considerable calcium. If the fluid remains clear add 5 ml of saturated aqueous ammonium oxalate. Turbidity within 5 minutes indicates the presence of calcium. If the result is positive the specimen and container are rinsed with distilled water and the specimen immersed in fresh decalcifying fluid. The test is repeated daily or more frequently if using R.D.C. The first sample of decalcifying fluid is not tested as it must obviously be positive.

Other methods

Testing for decalcification by bending the tissues or by sticking needles into them are unreliable methods which can only damage the tissues, and must be condemned.

SURFACE DECALCIFICATION

Occasionally when trimming the surface of a paraffin block before cutting the sections small deposits of calcium salts, hitherto unsuspected, may become apparent. To avoid damage to the knife edge and unsightly scores in the finished sections, these small deposits can be removed by treating the block surface with decalcifying fluid. The block is inverted in a shallow dish and kept slightly off the bottom by resting it on a matchstick. Sufficient fluid is poured into the dish to just wet the under-surface of the block. Formic acid, nitric acid, and R.D.C. are all suitable, and in 20–60 minutes sufficient surface calcium will be removed to allow several sections to be cut. Before cutting the sections the block surface should be rinsed in weak ammonia solution to remove any acid. This will minimise staining of, and damage to, the knife edge.

22. Processing

In order that thin sections of the body tissues may be cut, these tissues must have a suitable hardness and consistency when presented to the knife edge. These properties can be imparted by infiltrating and surrounding the tissues with paraffin wax; celloidin or low-viscosity nitrocellulose (LVN); various types of resins; or by freezing. Each of these methods has special uses. Celloidin or LVN are used mainly for work with central nervous system tissues and with organs with greatly differing textures such as eyes, embryos and sometimes bone. Plastic embedding media such as acrylic, polyester and epoxy resins are used for sectioning of undecalcified bone; preparation of ultra thin sections (50–80 nm) for electron microscopy and increasingly for semi-thin sections (1–2 μm) for light microscopy, especially of lymph nodes, renal biopsies and bone marrow biopsies. Frozen tissue techniques are used for urgent diagnostic work, the demonstration of fats and certain enzymes, and for some staining techniques requiring free-floating sections. Practically all routine diagnostic work is done with material embedded in paraffin wax. The stages between fixation and section-cutting are usually referred to as 'processing' and can be subdivided into dehydration, clearing, infiltration and embedding. In the case of frozen-section work no processing in this sense takes place, and the preparation of sections by this method is dealt with in Chapter 26.

PARAFFIN WAX METHOD

In the majority of histopathology departments the technique of embedding the tissues in paraffin wax is the method of choice for routine work. It is relatively uncomplicated and inexpensive. The finished blocks are permanent and convenient for storage, and almost every type of tissue structure can be demonstrated in sections prepared in this way. Examples of important exceptions are fats and some enzymes. The principle of the method is the infiltration of the tissues by a firm paraffin wax. In order to make this possible all water must first be removed from the tissues. This is done by replacing it with alcohol and is referred to as dehydra-

tion. The alcohol is then replaced by a wax-miscible reagent which in turn is replaced by molten paraffin wax which is finally allowed to set. Many of these alcohol-wax miscible reagents render the tissues transparent and so this stage is often referred to as 'clearing'. Because of the wide margin of timing permissible in each stage of the paraffin wax method it is ideally suited to automatic machine processing where different schedules will be necessary to cope with daily and week-end specimens, and for some special treatments.

Dehydration

This is done by taking the tissues through increasing strengths of alcohol. Routinely, 70% alcohol is sufficiently dilute for the first bath but lower concentrations may be used for very delicate tissues in order to avoid excessive shrinkage and distortion. After fixation in Bouin's fluid or Heidenhain's Susa the tissues should be placed directly into 90% alcohol, and after Carnoy's fluid they should go directly into absolute alcohol.

Clearing

Many different reagents have been used for clearing the tissues. Many of them give comparable results and attempts to give a list of advantages and disadvantages for each and every one are pointless. However, some of them are sufficiently different to warrant description and to make them of value in the different processing schedules that may be required.

*1. Inhibisol** (1,1,1-trichlorethane with patented inhibitor system)

The use of this reagent was suggested by Maxwell.[1] It is suitable for all routine materials and for hand or machine processing schedules. Tissues tend to float and are not rendered transparent. It is not inflammable and the vapour is less toxic than that of xylene, toluene or chloroform. It evaporates more rapidly than toluene and so there is less carry-over and contamination of the

* Bestobell Chemical Products Ltd., 131 Western Road, Mitcham, Surrey CR4 3YQ.

paraffin wax baths when it is used on a processing machine. It is recommended for use in all processing schedules.

2. *Toluene*

Suitable for all routine material. The tissues are rendered transparent. It is ideally suited for machine processing schedules as the tissues are cleared in 4–6 hours. This relatively short time may prove inconvenient for hand processing schedules. Tissues left in toluene for longer periods than necessary may become brittle. Toluene is inflammable, and the vapour is harmful in high concentration.

3. *Xylene*

Very similar to toluene but may cause more brittleness.

4. *Benzene*

Again very similar to toluene in practical terms though said to cause less brittleness. It is inflammable. Of greater importance, the inhalation of benzene vapour is associated with severe liver damage and aplastic anaemias, and its use for routine work cannot be recommended.

5. *Chloroform*

Suitable for processing schedules where the timing is such that the tissues must be left in clearing reagent overnight. Normal-sized blocks require 10–14 hours' treatment, but tissues may be left in chloroform for several days without becoming excessively brittle. The tissues do not become transparent. Chloroform is difficult to replace with molten paraffin wax and a useful procedure is to follow it with a 30–60 minute bath in toluene. Chloroform is not inflammable, but the vapour is harmful and it is an expensive reagent.

6. *Cedar-wood oil*

Of little use in routine histopathology, although for certain special purposes it may be of value. It is very slow-acting and is difficult to replace with paraffin wax, but tissues may be left in it for months without suffering damage or becoming brittle.

Paraffin wax infiltration

After the tissues are cleared they are transferred to molten paraffin wax. The melting point of wax usually falls within the range of 54–60°C and it is kept molten at a temperature of approximately 4°C higher than its melting point. A wax with a melting point of 56°C will cope with nearly all conditions in Great Britain, but in the event of very hot summer weather a harder wax may prove useful. In recent years paraffin waxes with a proportion of microcrystalline wax or plastic polymers incorporated have become available and these, while being slightly more expensive, have less tendency to crumble, and make cutting, in particular the preparation of ribbons of sections, much easier. Waxes may be purchased in slab or pastillated form and a melted stock is kept in jugs in the wax oven. After melting, the wax should be passed through a coarse filter paper into clean jugs. When filtered it can be used directly from the jug in the oven or, more conveniently, transferred to a wax dispenser. This is a heated container with a fine outlet tap from which easily controlled amounts of wax can be run. Infiltration of the tissues by wax will usually be complete after four changes of 1 hour each, but this time can be shortened and infiltration improved by using the wax baths under a reduced pressure of from 600–700 mm of mercury (75–95 kPa). This is done by placing the tissues in a container of molten wax in a vacuum oven. The tissues are given 30 minutes in wax at normal pressure, two changes of wax of 30 minutes each at reduced pressure followed by a further 30 minutes at normal pressure. This procedure reduces the total time in wax to 2 hours. By reducing the pressure, the evaporation of the clearing agent is hastened owing to a lowering of its boiling point and also any trapped air bubbles are removed from the tissues. This latter point is of importance with tissues, such as lung, which contain many air spaces. Reduction of pressure and subsequent return to normal should be done slowly in order to avoid damage to any delicate tissue structures. Automatic processing machines have provision for at least two molten-wax baths and some models allow these to be used under a partial vacuum. Tissues that have been processed on machines without this vacuum facility should be given 30 minutes under vacuum before embedding.

Embedding

This is the process of casting the tissues in paraffin wax which is then allowed to set and form a firm supporting block. The traditional Leuckhart moulds are simple to use and consist of two L-shaped pieces of metal, usually brass, and a metal or plate-glass base plate. The L-pieces are laid on the plate and can be adjusted to give various sizes of mould. A 7-in square plate and L-pieces made of ½-in square brass rod, some sets with 6 in arms and some with 3 in arms have been found most useful. The mould is filled with molten paraffin wax, the tissue placed in it with the surface to be cut facing downwards, the corner of the identifying label immersed in the wax and the wax allowed to set. Several blocks may be embedded together, but at least a half inch must be left between them and great care must be taken when attaching their labels. The setting of the wax can be hastened if, as soon as a skin has formed over the surface of the wax, the complete unit is immersed in cold water. This rapid cooling also minimises crystallisation of the wax. When the wax is completely set the tissues are separated into individual blocks, each with a 5 mm wax border around the edges of the tissue. When large numbers of tissue blocks have been embedded this trimming into separate blocks is time-consuming and tedious, and this consideration has led to the introduction of various types of individual moulds. A very convenient type consists of a disposable plastic tray divided into separate compartments. Various sizes are available. Each compartment is filled with wax and the pieces of tissue embedded in the same way as with the Leuckhart moulds. When set, the blocks are shelled out and require no further preparation other than levelling of the base.

The time necessary in each processing reagent will be reduced if the tissues are suspended and continuously agitated. The transfer of the tissues from reagent to reagent then becomes possible at shorter intervals. The use of automatic machines allows these transfers to take place during hours when the department is normally closed. Various models of automatic machines are available, but the features of suspension with agitation and automatic transfer of the tissues from fluid to fluid at pre-selected times are common to all. Most machines have twelve stations, one of which can accommodate a siphoning container for washing the tissues in running water, and at least two others which will hold heated wax baths. Some models allow partial vacuum to be used during processing. A mechanism allowing the start of the actual processing cycle to be delayed for up to 24 hours after switching on the machine is usually incorporated and it is also sometimes useful to be able to by-pass the stop mechanism to allow the cycle to be longer than 24 hours. The selected blocks of tissue are placed, together with their labels, into individual containers which in turn are loaded into a large carrier basket. Very small pieces of tissue may first be wrapped in gauze or cotton bandage to prevent loss from the perforated container. The large basket is suspended from an arm which provides the means of agitation and of transfer from fluid to fluid. This transfer is controlled by some type of programming mechanism such as the use of a notched card on a timer. Details of construction and method of operation of individual machines can be obtained from the various makers (*see* Fig. 22.1).

The following manual and machine-processing schedules have given satisfactory results over many years, but the times given in them may be varied within quite wide limits to suit the requirements of individual departments.

Manual processing schedules

1. Standard day schedules taking approximately 3½ days including fixation

10% formalin	at least 24 hr
70% alcohol	9.00 am to 5.00 pm
90% alcohol	5.00 pm to 9.00 am
Absolute alcohol 1	9.00 am to 11 am
Absolute alcohol 2	11.00 am to 1.00 pm
Absolute alcohol 3	1.00 pm to 3.00 pm
Absolute alcohol 4	3.00 pm to 5.00 pm
Inhibisol or chloroform	5.00 pm to 9.00 am
Inhibisol or toluene	9.00 am to 9.30 am
Then either:	
Paraffin wax 1	1 hr
Paraffin wax 2	1 hr
Paraffin wax 3	1 hr
Paraffin wax 4	1 hr
or better:	
Paraffin wax 1	30 min
Paraffin wax 2 under vacuum	30 min
Paraffin wax 3 under vacuum	30 min
Paraffin wax 4	30 min

Embed tissues in fresh wax and allow to set.

2. Rapid schedule taking 3 hours including fixation

This schedule is suitable for pieces of tissue not exceeding $6 \times 6 \times 3$ mm in size. All the reagents are kept in screw-capped bottles in an oven at 60°C. They are used once only and then discarded.

Carnoy's fixative	1 hr
Equal parts absolute alcohol and acetone	30 min
Equal parts acetone and Inhibisol or xylene	30 min
Inhibisol or xylene	15 min
Paraffin wax 1	15 min
Paraffin wax 2 under vacuum	15 min
Paraffin wax 3	15 min

Embed tissues in fresh wax and allow to set.

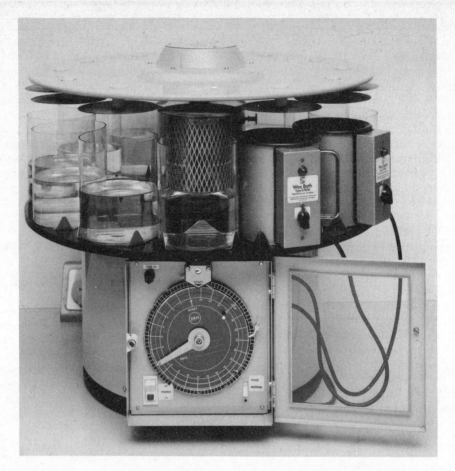

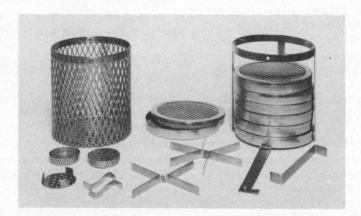

Fig. 22.1. Tissue processing machine with carrier basket and tissue containers (British American Optical Co.)

3. Week-end schedule covering non-working days

The 'standard' day schedule (1. above) is used but the timing is arranged so that the long stay in reagent necessary during the non-working days does not occur in absolute alcohol, toluene or paraffin wax.

Automatic processing machine schedules

The two daily schedules are for specimens taken from patients during the previous day. This means that they will have been in fixative at least overnight. Fresh specimens can be processed on the week-end schedules as they will receive adequate fixation on the machine.

1. Day schedule taking 22 hours

Stations 1, 2	10% formalin	2 hr each
Station 3	70% alcohol	2 hr
Station 4	90% alcohol	2 hr
Stations 5, 6, 7, 8	Absolute alcohol	1½ hr each
Stations 9, 10	Inhibisol or toluene	2 hr each
Stations 11, 12	Paraffin wax	2 hr each

Remove from machine.

Paraffin wax under vacuum	30 min

Embed in fresh paraffin wax and allow to set.

2. Day schedule with secondary fixation taking 21 hours

Station 1	10% formalin	2 hr
Station 2	10% formal-sublimate	4 hr
Station 3	90% alcohol	2 hr
Stations 4, 5, 6, 7	Absolute alcohol	1½ hr each
Stations 8, 9, 10	Inhibisol or toluene	1 hr each
Stations 11, 12	Paraffin wax	2 hr each

Remove from machine.

Paraffin wax under vacuum	30 min

Embed in fresh paraffin wax and allow to set.

3. Schedules incorporating one non-working day

Either of the above schedules may be used provided that the 'delay' mechanism is put into operation. According to the time at which the machine is switched on, the delay is set so that the actual processing cycle will start on the non-working day and finish at the required time on the following day.

4. Schedules incorporating two non-working days

In this case the use of the 'delay' mechanism is supplemented by processing schedules taking 48 hours and by cutting out the stop mechanism which normally operates after one revolution of the timing disc. The following examples can be varied to suit particular requirements. However, it is essential that whatever variations are introduced the cycle must not finish before a member of the staff has arrived in the department. With the automatic switch-off mechanism inoperative the machine must be switched off manually at the end of the cycle. Failure to do this will result in the specimens being transferred from the last wax bath into the first beaker of the schedule.

(a) Schedule taking 48 hr plus the selected delay time

Stations 1, 2	10% formalin	4 hr each
Station 3	70% alcohol	4 hr
Station 4	90% alcohol	4 hr
Stations 5, 6, 7, 8	Absolute alcohol	4 hr each
Stations 9, 10	Inhibisol or toluene	4 hr each
Stations 11, 12	Paraffin wax	4 hr each

Remove from machine.

Paraffin wax under vacuum	30 min

Embed in fresh paraffin wax and allow to set.

(b) Schedule with secondary fixation taking 48 hr plus selected delay time

Exactly as given under (a) above but substituting 10% formal-sublimate for the second 10% formalin bath.

After embedding is completed the used tissue capsules and lids should be cleaned of wax by overnight immersion in Inhibisol or toluene. The used reagent from the processing machine is suitable for this purpose.

CELLOIDIN OR LOW-VISCOSITY NITROCELLULOSE METHOD

Low-viscosity nitrocellulose (LVN) has practically replaced celloidin in those areas of histology where their use is recommended. LVN dissolves more readily than celloidin and solutions of higher concentration can more easily be prepared. These stronger solutions infiltrate the tissues as rapidly as the weaker celloidin solutions. Their use, however, results in the formation of firmer blocks which will allow thinner sections to be cut if required. Probably the largest users of this material are the departments specialising in neuropathology and orthopaedic and dental work. Only rarely will routine departments find it either necessary or of value. Some of the reasons for its use in the specialist departments mentioned are as follows:

(a) No clearing agents or heat are used during processing. Shrinkage and distortion to which brain and spinal cord are particularly susceptible are thus kept to a minimum.

(b) Relative ease of preparation of very large sections.

(c) Ease of preparation of comparatively thick (30 μm) sections. These thick sections are of value when following the processes of nerve and glial cells.

(d) Greater ease of sectioning blocks of tissues of widely differing hardness such as compact bone enclosing marrow, than with the paraffin wax methods.

In the routine diagnostic department time is usually at a premium and the LVN method is far too slow for general use. The distortion caused to tissues by the paraffin wax method, whilst wholly undesirable, seldom prevents a diagnosis being made. It is almost always advantageous to have thinner sections than are easily obtainable from LVN-embedded material. Staining of large numbers of free-floating sections taken from a number of different blocks such as are encountered in the routine department is difficult and time-consuming. A further problem associated with the LVN method is the storage of the blocks of tissue after sectioning is completed. To prevent drying and cracking they must be stored wet, usually in 70% alcohol, and this makes a heavy demand on space. Both celloidin and LVN are highly inflammable. They are supplied, and should be kept dampened with *n*-butyl alcohol. Because of the high concentration of the LVN solution used for embedding there is a tendency for the sections to crack. This can be avoided by the incorporation of a plasticiser in the solution. Castor oil, celloidin, and tricresyl phosphate have all been used successfully.

The following processing schedule is suitable for most tissues, but the times may be altered to deal with special cases involving, perhaps, very large blocks or particularly difficult specimens such as eyes.

Standard LVN processing schedule

Stock LVN solution:

    Add 200 g LVN to 500 ml absolute alcohol.
    Shake until thoroughly wetted and then add 500 ml diethyl ether. When completely dissolved add 50 ml tricresyl phosphate.

Wash fixed tissue blocks for 24 hr in running water.
Place in 70% alcohol for 24 hr.
Transfer to 90% alcohol for 24 hr.
Three changes of absolute alcohol of 24 hr each.
Equal parts of absolute alcohol and diethyl ether for 48 hr.

A mixture of:

absolute alcohol	3 parts	
diethyl ether	3 parts	for 7 days.
stock LVN	2 parts	

A mixture of:

absolute alcohol	2 parts	
diethyl ether	2 parts	for 7 days.
stock LVN	4 parts	

Stock LVN solution for 7 days.

Embed the tissues either in small paper boxes or in glass dishes. Place the dishes or boxes in an airtight container until all bubbles have risen to the surface. Ensure that no air bubbles are trapped under the blocks. Slowly harden the LVN by exposure to the air for short intervals daily. This hardening can be hastened by exposing the LVN to chloroform vapour, but this is not recommended as it may cause a very tough skin to form on the surface of the LVN. When fully set remove from the container, trim off the excess LVN to a border all round the tissues of at least 0·5 cm and store the blocks in 70% alcohol.

REFERENCE

1. Maxwell, M.H. (1978). *Med. Lab. Sci.*; **35**, 401–3.

23. Microtomes and microtome knives

Having fixed, processed and embedded the tissues it is now necessary to cut sections from the blocks. This is done on a machine called a microtome into which is fitted a special microtome knife.

MICROTOMES

Many types of microtome are available, but all should fulfil the following requirements:

(a) Rigid support of the knife and the tissue block.

(b) Means of moving either the tissue block across the fixed knife-edge or the knife-edge across the block.

(c) Means of accurately advancing the tissues to cut each section at the selected thickness.

The following descriptions of the various microtomes are limited to the general features and manufacturers should be consulted for fuller details of their particular models. To repeatedly cut slices of a variety of materials at a thickness of perhaps as little as 2 micrometres (μm) requires a precision instrument, and the degree of precision built into the machine is largely reflected in the price.

Cambridge rocking microtome

A simple machine in which the tissue block is swung across the fixed knife-edge in an arc. The force of the movement is governed by a spring and is actuated by a handle attached to a piece of cord. The movement of this handle also automatically advances the tissue block after each cutting stroke. The size of the blocks to be cut is best limited to approximately 2 cm square. The whole structure is not very rigid and this makes the cutting of tough tissues very difficult, if not impossible. The application of this machine is usually confined to paraffin wax embedded material, although it may sometimes be used in the cold chamber or cryostat for cutting frozen sections.

Rotary microtome (Fig. 23.1)

A mechanically complicated machine in which the

tissue block is moved up and down in a flat plane across the knife-edge. The movement is controlled by the turning of a handle at the side of the machine which at the same time advances the block after each section is

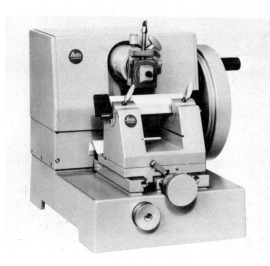

Fig. 23.1. Rotary microtome (E. Leitz).

cut. The rotary microtome is ideally suited to the preparation of serial sections from paraffin blocks of relatively soft tissues. Although it is far more rigid and sophisticated than the rocking microtome, difficulty is still found with tough materials and the block size is best limited to approximately 3 × 4 cm.

Base sledge microtome (Fig. 23.2)

A heavy-duty rigid machine in which the tissue block holder is attached to a sledge resting on precision machined runners. This sledge is pushed beneath a fixed knife. The advance of the block after each section is cut may be manual or automatic. The knife can be slanted in relation to the tissue block and this makes possible the cutting of very hard tissues, and is also useful when dealing with material embedded in celloidin or LVN. Special large tissue stages can be

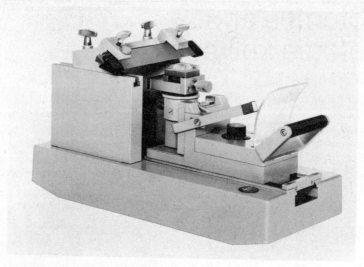

Fig. 23.2.   Base sledge microtome (E. Leitz).

attached which allow blocks up to approximately 8×12 cm to be cut, and it is also possible to attach freezing stages to these microtomes. The base sledge is the most versatile of microtomes and is the machine of choice in any department dealing with a wide variety of tissues and block sizes.

Freezing microtome

With these machines the tissue stage is fixed and the knife swung across the surface of the block which is held in place by freezing it to the stage. Having the stage fixed allows the attachment of a supply of carbon dioxide gas under pressure to the expansion chamber incorporated in the stage. This allows rapid freezing of the tissues to the stage and the consistency obtained makes the use of embedding materials such as paraffin wax unnecessary. The knife can also be cooled by carbon dioxide gas. The movement of the knife back across the block after the section has been cut automatically advances the tissue. The block size is usually limited to approximately 2×2 cm. The freezing microtome is not usually used for routine work but is essential, in one form or another, for the demonstration of such materials as fats and enzymes.

MICROTOME KNIVES

These knives are available in various lengths and blade profiles. The length is chosen to suit the particular

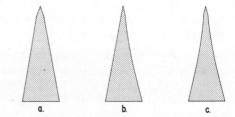

Fig. 23.3.   Knife profiles
(a) Wedge; (b) plano-concave; (c) biconcave.

microtome in use and the profile of the blade to suit the materials being cut (Fig. 23.3).

Wedge profile

This profile of blade is used for almost all paraffin section work with the sledge and rotary microtomes and for frozen section cutting with the bench freezing microtome. It is also used in cryostats fitted with microtomes other than the Cambridge rocking machine. Because of its shape, the edge is relatively vibration-free and this enables the toughest materials to be cut. It maintains its edge longer than the other types of knife but may take slightly longer to sharpen. The combination of a wedge knife and a base sledge microtome will enable almost any paraffin-embedded material to be cut.

Plano-concave profile

A useful type of knife which, when used with a base sledge microtome, will cut all but the toughest material embedded in paraffin wax and is also ideally suited to celloidin and LVN material. It is used with the concave surface of the blade facing upward. Although not as vibration-free as the wedge blade it is easier and quicker to sharpen to a very good edge.

Bi-concave profile

A shape which is almost entirely confined to the rocking microtome, generally in the form known as the Heiffor knife which has an integral handle. The bi-concave knife can also be used for celloidin and LVN work on the base sledge microtome, but has no advantage over the more rigid plano-concave pattern.

KNIFE SHARPENING

The technique of preparing a sharp microtome knife to enable high-quality sections to be cut represents the first major demand on the manipulative skills of the histopathology technician. Success in section cutting hinges on the quality of the microtome knife-edge, and it is essential that each technician should have his own knife or, preferably, knives which he learns to sharpen and look after. The preparation of the microtome knife can be considered in two stages; honing or the removal of metal in order to obtain a straight cutting edge free from nicks; and stropping which is the process of polishing this edge. Before describing these processes the terminology used to identify the parts of a knife should be understood (Fig. 23.4).

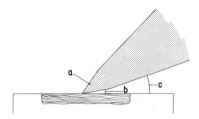

Fig. 23.4.   *(a)* Knife edge; *(b)* bevel; *(c)* angle of tilt.

The heel is the end of the blade nearest the handle and the other end is called the toe. The back and the edge are self-explanatory terms. The tilt of the knife refers to the angle made between the blade and the cut surface of the block. The bevel of the blade is that part of the edge which is in direct contact with the hone when sharpening. When honing and stropping wedge profile knives by hand it is necessary to attach a knife back in order to obtain this bevel. The knife back is usually a tubular steel device which slides over the back of the knife and thus raises the back up from the surface of the hone or strop (Fig. 23.5).

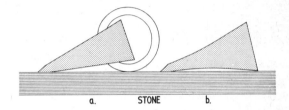

Fig. 23.5.   *(a)* Wedge knife with tubular honing back; *(b)* biconcave knife, honing back unnecessary.

A knife back is not required with a bi-concave blade, but is usually used with a plano-concave knife. Since during honing the knife back will also be ground away it is necessary for each knife to have a back of its own. With automatic machine sharpening the desired bevel is obtained by adjusting the knife support and a back is not necessary except for stropping. As the back will not be worn away by stropping one tubular back will serve several knives. Some automatic sharpening machines have a stropping facility and this enables knife backs to be dispensed with.

Honing (Fig. 23.6)

1. Manual honing

Although many laboratories will use automatic machines for knife honing the technician should be familar with the process of sharpening a knife by hand. The grinding away of the metal can be achieved by using a rough surface in the form of a hone or by applying a grinding paste to a flat surface such as a glass plate which has a very finely ground surface. Excellent commercially available hones are the Belgian yellow stone and the Arkansas stone. For sharpening, a mixture of fine oil and xylene is ideal, and xylene is used to clean the stone afterwards. With glass plates a paste of fine machine oil mixed with various grades of grinding powder is used to produce the cutting edge. To remove a bad edge aluminium oxide Optical 50 powder should be used. This is followed, after cleaning the plate, with Bauxilite 1200 powder and oil, and finally with oil alone. If the microtome knife is looked after the last two stages will normally be sufficient. To sharpen the knife, it is placed on the surface of the hone with the cutting edge leading and pushed with firm but gentle

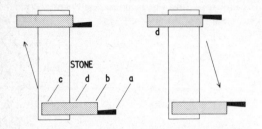

Fig. 23.6.   Honing
        (a) Knife handle; (b) heel of knife; (c) toe of knife; (d) cutting edge.

pressure across the surface moving from toe to heel. It is then rolled over on its back and brought back moving from heel to toe. In the case of plano-concave blades the knife is honed with the concave side kept downwards until the edge is satisfactory, and then a few strokes on each side are used to remove the metal burr.

The amount of honing necessary is usually determined by experience, and although examination of the knife-edge with a low-power microscope objective will reveal the presence of any nicks in the blade and can act as a guide to the need for further honing, the final test is always whether or not the blade will cut good sections.

2. Automatic machine honing

Various automatic knife-sharpening machines are available. Some use ground-glass plates with the oil and powder mixtures described above, and others use various roughened surfaces similar to hones. An improvement in automatic knife sharpening has been the introduction of copper plates to replace the glass used previously. The surface of these copper plates is relatively soft and is impregnated with diamond lapping compound applied sparingly to the surface. One application is sufficient to sharpen from four to six knives. Two grades of compound are available, one having $8\,\mu$m and the other $3\,\mu$m particles, and each is used with its own plate. Sharpening times are much shorter than with the glass and powder method, 5–10 minutes being

sufficient for all but badly damaged knives. Usually the knife is fixed in position while the sharpening surface moves across its edge. On the better machines the bevel, the pressure on the knife edge, and the duration of sharpening time can be set, the machine switched on and left. The knife automatically turns over from edge to edge, but this control can be overridden thus allowing one edge only to be ground. This facility is essential when sharpening plano-concave knives.

Stropping (Fig. 23.7)

When a sharp edge free from nicks has been obtained by honing, the edge of the blade is polished on a leather strop. The strop may be either hanging or fixed to a supporting base, usually of wood. The hanging strop is attached by one end to bench or wall at a suitable height for the individual user and held taught in one hand by the other end. The knife is held in the other hand and pushed along the strop from toe to heel with the cutting edge trailing, that is the reverse of the honing position. It is then rolled over on its back by a combination of wrist and finger movement and pulled back from heel to toe.

Any tendency for the strop to sag must be avoided. The mechanics of using the block strop are the same except that it is rested on the bench surface and has the

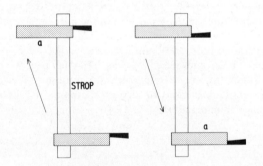

Fig. 23.7.   Stropping
        (a) Cutting edge.

advantage of having no sagging problem. As with microtome knives it is to be strongly recommended that each technician should have his own strop. Stropping is done with knife backs in position where appropriate and, unlike the honing procedure, the plano-concave knife is stropped on both sides.

24. Microtomy

PARAFFIN WAX EMBEDDED MATERIAL

Before cutting sections from paraffin wax blocks it is usual to attach the blocks to suitable supporting holders. These may be special attachments as is the case with the Cambridge rocking microtome, or pieces of hard material, commonly wood, made to be clamped in the microtome chuck. The surface of the block holder should be at least as large as the surface of the paraffin block and should have several shallow scores in the face to ensure a firm adhesion between it and the paraffin block. With blocks of above-average size, it may be necessary to use a stepped block holder so that the surface can be large but the base can still be clamped in the jaws of the microtome chuck. For very large blocks special platform stages are available for use with sledge microtomes. These have surface areas of up to 14×10 cm and are bolted on to the microtome in place of the standard chuck. The rocking microtome block holder is in the form of a metal tube which is slid over a rod on the microtome and clamped in place. Some patterns have a movable head which allows accurate positioning of the block in relation to the knife. To attach the wax block to a holder a palette knife is heated and then rested on the surface of the holder. The paraffin block is placed on top of the palette knife, and as soon as the base of the wax block melts the palette knife is slid away and the wax block and holder pressed firmly together. The paraffin wax sets almost at once, but should be allowed to harden for at least 10 minutes before cutting is attempted. When ready, the block holder is fixed in place on the microtome and the surface pared away in 15–$25\,\mu$m slices to expose the tissue face prior to taking the sections. This rough trimming is done either using one end of the cutting knife or, preferably, on a microtome knife that has seen better days and is kept specifically as a trimming knife. On most microtomes some orientation of the chuck is possible. This can prove useful when dealing with small fragments of tissue, sent, perhaps, from another department in the form of a wax block which has already been cut on a different machine. By using the chuck movement it is possible to avoid having to lose tissue in levelling the block surface. However, if the tissue has been correctly embedded, the paraffin block trimmed square and attached in a flat position to the block holder, this orientation device, once set level, need seldom be used. Apart from being convenient, this technique allows blocks to be removed and replaced repeatedly on the microtome and sections cut with the minimum of tissue loss.

Sections for staining can be cut from wax blocks at thicknesses of from $3\,\mu$m to $10\,\mu$m without difficulty, but for most routine purposes a thickness of $5\,\mu$m is suitable. The actual cutting of the sections is essentially a practical exercise and can only be mastered by constant practice and close observation of the results, but the following points are important.

1. Knife sharpness

The need for a sharp knife is obvious. To struggle to cut sections with a knife which is below standard is a pointless exercise. Two faults may be present in the knife edge, either singly or together. If the edge has nicks in it, scores or even tears will be seen in the sections. Minor faults of this nature can sometimes be cured by stropping, but generally honing will be necessary. If the knife tilt is correct but the sections are smaller than the block surface, then the edge of the knife is probably rounded. This can result from over-stropping and the knife must be honed.

2. Fixing of the knife and block

All clamping screws must be firmly tightened on the knife holder as also must the screws of the block holder. Failure in this respect will result in vibration, and chattering will occur as the block passes across the knife-edge. This appears in thick and thin zones in the stained section running parallel to the knife edge.

3. Tilt of the knife (Fig. 24.1)

This refers to the angle between the flat of the blade and the block surface. Some machines have a scale on the side of the knife clamps to enable the setting to be noted and obtained repeatedly. When the knife tilt is

191

correct the sections will be of constant thickness and of the same surface size as the paraffin block. If the tilt is too shallow the block will be compressed as it passes under the knife and the sections will be alternately thick and thin. If the tilt is too steep a scraping rather than a cutting action will result in the sections being smaller than the surface of the block, and in the case of tough tissues a chattering action will occur giving alternate thick and thin bands and a striped appearance in the stained sections.

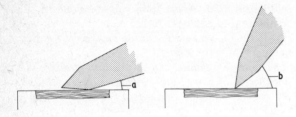

Fig. 24.1.   Tilt of knife
(a) Angle too shallow; *(b)* angle too steep.

4. *Speed of cutting action*

The correct speed for the block to pass across the knife edge will vary from tissue to tissue, and is an important factor in the cutting of good sections. A point in favour of the base sledge microtome is the direct control which the operator has over this speed of cutting.

5. *Slant of the knife* (Fig. 24.2)

With most routine material the cutting edge of the knife can be kept at right angles to the direction of travel of the block, but with very tough material it is often helpful to present the block to a slanted knife blade. Only the base sledge microtome allows this adjustment to be made.

Once suitable sections are being cut they are then attached to glass slides prior to being stained. There are several methods of getting the section from the microtome knife on the slide and each technician will develop his own modification of whichever technique he adopts. The following method is simple and reliable. Place a drop or two of 10% alcohol on the surface of a clean slide. Manipulate the section from the knife blade using forceps and a small paint brush, and lay it on to the alcohol. Do not allow the section to turn over. Carefully float the section on to a water-bath by lowering the slide away from underneath the section. The temperature of the water in the bath should be 2–3°C

below the melting point of the wax. The section will flatten out and it is then picked up on a clean slide by immersing the slide at the side of the section, bringing it to touch the section and then withdrawing it from the water with the section attached. The section and slide are then drained and put to dry in an incubator at a temperature of 40–45°C. Ideally they should be left overnight, but if essential after 1 hour at this temperature they may be transferred to a wax oven at 60°C for a further hour when the section can be stained. If this latter procedure is to be followed it is advsiable to use a section adhesive with certain tissues such as bone and brain to avoid sections floating off the slides during staining. On no account should the wax supporting the cut section be melted until all traces of water have been removed, and techniques involving such melting should be avoided whenever possible.

In some circumstances it may be necessary to examine several consecutive sections through a piece of tissue. The preparation of these sections is known as serial sectioning. The sections are cut in the normal manner but instead of floating out each section as it is cut, they are manipulated up the blade of the knife in a continuous ribbon. The number of sections that will fit on to a slide is ascertained and when this number is cut

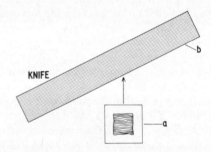

Fig. 24.2.   Slant of knife
(a) Tissue block; *(b)* knife edge slanted to direction of block travel.

they are transferred to a slide ready for floating out, and another set is cut. Alternatively a longer ribbon of sections is cut, laid on to a clean surface, separated into strips of a suitable length and then floated out. The slides on which the sections are finally mounted must be numbered in sequence.

A less time-consuming practice which is sometimes as useful to the pathologist is that of preparing step sections or levels. The first section is cut and kept, and the next ten or so sections are discarded. This process is repeated as many times as required. Several of these 'step' sections may be mounted on to one slide but they must be kept in order and their sequence indicated on the slide.

Section adhesives

With clean slides and thin, flat sections which are allowed sufficient drying time the use of section adhesives is seldom necessary. Nevertheless, occasions will arise, either when a quick result is required, or perhaps with certain tissues such as brain or bone, or with certain staining methods, when the use of such an adhesive will save much time and trouble. Many different substances have been used, usually in the form of a protein which is coagulated between section and slide either chemically or by heat. The most commonly used adhesive is a mixture of equal parts egg white, glycerine and water which is filtered and a crystal of thymol added as a preservative. This mixture is commercially available in small dispensing tubes which are very convenient and easy to use. Prior to picking up the section from the warm water a drop of adhesive the size of a pinhead is smeared over the surface of the slide. The section is then picked up and dried in the usual manner. An excess of adhesive must be avoided or it will pick up stains and spoil the final preparation. Adhesives should generally be avoided in any histochemical investigations.

CELLOIDIN OR LVN-EMBEDDED MATERIAL

The details are the same for both celloidin and LVN material and, as with wax blocks, the first stage of section cutting is the attachment of the block to a support. Wooden blocks as used for paraffin work are suitable, but they must not be contaminated with paraffin wax. The base of the LVN block must rest level on the surface of the support, and it can be made flat by first trimming with a scalpel blade and then smoothing with a medium-grade sandpaper. The LVN block is then rested, base downwards on two matchsticks in a Petri dish and sufficient of a mixture of equal parts ether and absolute alcohol poured in to come 1 or 2 mm up the sides of the block. This is left for 20 minutes. The suface of the block support is thoroughly wetted with the ether/alcohol mixture and liberally coated with the strong LVN solution used for processing. When the base of the block is sufficiently tacky it is placed on top of the coated block holder and firm pressure applied for at least 5 minutes. The pressure is then removed and after a further 5 minutes the block and support are placed in chloroform to harden the LVN. After 30 minutes they are transferred to 70% alcohol where they can remain until required for cutting. A sledge microtome with either a moving knife or a moving block should be used for section cutting and the knife should be fixed in the machine with the blade edge at an angle to the line of travel. A plano-concave knife is ideal and is used with the concave side upwards. Although some LVN can be cut dry it is easier to keep the block surface and the knife blade moistened with 70% alcohol. The sections are cut with a slow continuous movement. Any jerking or hesitation can result in transverse ridges in the sections. The sections may be cut from $10-30\,\mu m$ thickness, although those over $20\,\mu m$ thick may be difficult to flatten and mount after staining. As the sections are cut they are guided up the blade of the knife with a fine paint brush and then transferred to a dish of 70% alcohol where they can be stored until staining is commenced. The preparation of serial sections of LVN-embedded material is time-consuming, although small series can be collected in separate numbered containers. Large series can be collected in a single container by alternating the sections with leaves of thin paper. Fluffless toilet paper is ideal for this purpose. After cutting is completed the LVN blocks are stored in 70% alcohol, preferably remaining on their support blocks.

25. Section staining and mounting

In order to distinguish between the different structures present in the cut sections it is necessary to colour them. Although the term 'staining' is generally used to describe this process the actual colouring may be achieved by techniques other than that of using a dye or dyes. Examples of such methods are the coating of reticulin and nerve fibres with metallic silver and the use of various chemical reactions having a coloured end-product as in Perls' method for ferric iron. No single method will demonstrate all the tissue structures present and it may often be necessary to perform several different techniques on consecutive sections from a block of material in order that a diagnosis can be reached.

PARAFFIN WAX SECTIONS

In order to avoid repetition in the staining schedules certain procedures have been condensed into short phrases, the meanings of which are given below. Because of its lower toxicity Inhibisol (*see* page 181) is preferred to xylene for the de-waxing baths and for the first de-alcoholising bath in schedules *(a)* and *(b)* below. However, the higher evaporation rate may cause problems if used in the pre-mounting bath. Large sections or long ribbons of small sections may dry before the mountant has covered them and for this reason xylene is retained in this final dish.

(a) To remove paraffin wax and hydrate section:

'Section to water'
= Inhibisol (1)   2 min.
  Inhibisol (2)   2 min.
  Absolute alcohol (1)   2 min.
  Absolute alcohol (2)   2 min.
  70% alcohol   2 min.
  Water.

(b) To dehydrate, clear and protect sections:

'Dehydrate, clear and mount'
= Agitate continuously and gently through:
  Absolute alcohol (1)   30 sec.
  Absolute alcohol (2)   30 sec.

Inhibisol   30 sec.
Xylene at least   1 min.
Mount in 'Terpene resin' or 'Ralmount'.

(c) If formalin pigment is formed in the tissues owing to acidity of the fixative it should be removed before staining. This can be done by treating the sections as follows:

'Remove formalin pigment'
= Sections to 70% alcohol
  0·2% potassium hydroxide in 80% alcohol   30 min.
  Wash in running tap water   10 min.

(d) With tissues which have been fixed in a mercury-containing fixative such as Helly, Zenker, or formal-sublimate it will be necessary to remove the mercury pigment in the following way:

'Remove mercury pigment'
= Sections to 70% alcohol
  0·5% iodine in 70% alcohol   5 min.
  Rinse in water
  3% sodium thiosulphate   5 min.
  Running tap water   5 min.

(e) 'Differentiate.' This term refers to the removal of excess stain from the sections leaving only the required structures coloured with the particular dye. It may be done simply by washing the section in water or by the use of special reagents such as acid-alcohol.

In the staining schedules which follow, the times are for tissues fixed in 10% formalin. All the methods will work very well on tissues fixed in other fluids but it may be necessary to alter some of the staining times slightly in order to obtain optimum results. The method of applying stains and reagents to sections depends to a large extent on the number of slides to be stained. Single slides may be supported on a rack resting across a sink and the reagents applied from dropping-bottles. Where evaporation of a particular reagent is likely to occur it should be kept in a Coplin jar with a lid. When large numbers of slides are to be stained they may be put in special racks which hold up to 24 slides, and these racks are taken through the various fluids which are kept in large glass troughs. Washing in running tap water is done by placing the slide rack or the individual slides in a tray connected to the water supply by rubber tubing. The use of a photographic siphon device makes a convenient arrangement for this purpose and ensures an even and regular changing of the water.

A few of the methods given are suitable for use on automatic staining machines, but the timing of the schedules is very critical and requires careful calculation to suit conditions prevailing in individual departments.

After staining is completed it is usual to cover the section with a coverslip or coverglass in order to make the preparation as permanent as possible. Coverslips are obtainable in a large variety of sizes and several thicknesses. For routine use the thickness known as No. 1 (0·15 mm) is recommended. The coverslip is attached to the slide with an adhesive made from natural or synthetic resins dissolved in an organic solvent, usually xylene. These mountants are mixed to achieve a refractive index near to that of glass. It is convenient to obtain these mountants from commercial sources and excellent examples are 'Terpene resin'* and 'Ralmount'†. Each technician should keep a small quantity of mountant in a glass container with a lid which is designed to allow a glass dropping-rod to remain in the container when the lid is on. This will minimise thickening of the mountant due to evaporation of the solvent.

When the section is ready for mounting a coverslip is selected and polished with a dust-free cloth. The coverslip should be of a size sufficient to leave a 3 mm border around the edges of the section. The slide is removed from the xylene, the excess xylene is wiped from around the section and a small quantity of mountant applied directly to the section. The slide is immediately inverted over the coverslip and lowered until the blob of mountant touches the coverslip. On no account should the section be allowed to dry. The slide is then turned back over so that the section is uppermost. With practice in this manoeuvre the mountant will now run outwards to cover the whole of the area under the coverslip without either the formation of air bubbles under the coverslip or the presence of excess mountant around the edges. Should air bubbles be formed over the section it is advisable to remove the coverslip, wash off the mountant with xylene and remount the section. The alternative technique of squeezing out the air bubbles by applying pressure to the coverslip may result in displacement of parts of the

* Difco Laboratories, PO Box 14B, West Molesey, Surrey.
† R.A. Lamb, 6 Sunbeam Road, London NW10 6JL.

section and will almost certainly result in a mess of mountant around the edges of the coverslip and on its surface.

Haematoxylin and eosin

1. Purpose

To demonstrate the general structure of tissues. Recommended as a standard reference method to be done on all tissues.

2. Demonstration tissues (to show the results obtained by the method)

Stomach; prostate; skin; kidney.

3. Solutions

(a) Cole's haematoxylin[1]:
Dissolve 1·0 g haematoxylin powder in 250 ml of distilled water by warming gently. Add 50 ml of 1·0% iodine in 70% alcohol and 750 ml of saturated aqueous aluminium ammonium sulphate. Bring rapidly to the boil, cool and store in a dark bottle in a cool place. This stock solution will keep for several months. For use, filter into a staining dish. This smaller amount should be discarded after 2 weeks.

(b) Acid-alcohol:
1·0% hydrochloric acid in 70% alcohol

(c) Eosin:
1·0% eosin Y in distilled water.

4. Method

Bring sections to water and stain in solution (a) for 20 min.
Wash in running tap water for 2 min.
Differentiate in solution (b) with continuous agitation for 15 sec.
Wash in running tap water for at least 5 min.
Stain in solution (c) for 5 min.
Wash in running tap water for 30 sec, dehydrate, clear, and mount.

5. Results

Nuclei: bright blue.
Collagen and cytoplasm: pale pink.
Muscle, keratin, and colloid: bright, strong pink.
Erythrocytes: orange-red.

Haematoxylin and Van Gieson

1. Purpose

To facilitate the differentiation between collagen and other tissues.
Areas of scar tissue and fibrosis are well shown.

2. Demonstration tissues

Skin; prostate; breast.

3. Solutions

   (a) Celestine blue:
Grind 1·0 g celestine blue to a smooth paste in 1·0 ml sulphuric acid. Add 100 ml of 2·5% aqueous ammonium ferric sulphate and 10·0 ml glycerol and mix thoroughly. Add 0·5 ml sulphuric acid. This solution keeps indefinitely but must be filtered just before use.

   (b) Cole's haematoxylin (p. 195)

   (c) Van Gieson solution, Unna's modification:[2]
Dissolve 0·25 g acid fuchsin in 90·0 ml distilled water. Add 10·0 ml glycerol, mix well and add 0·5 ml nitric acid.
Mix thoroughly and add picric acid to saturation. Filter before use.

4. Method

Bring sections to water.
Stain in freshly filtered solution *(a)* for 3 min.
Rinse in distilled water and stain in solution *(b)* for 3 min.
Wash in running tap water for at least 5 min.
Stain in solution *(c)* for 5 min.
Rinse rapidly in distilled water and blot with filter paper.
Dehydrate, clear, and mount.

5. Results

Nuclei: blue-black.
Muscle: brownish yellow.
Erythrocytes: yellow.
Young collagen: pale pink.
Old collagen and bone: red.

Connective tissue trichrome[3]

1. Purpose

For differentiation between collagen and muscle. Fibrin is also well shown. With the Van Gieson method the collagen is picked out strongly against the background while with this method the muscle is shown most clearly. It is a more precise method than the Van Gieson and less subject to fading.

2. Demonstration tissues

Prostate; uterine myometrium; tongue; stomach.

3. Solutions

   (a) 5% chromium trioxide in distilled water

   (b) Celestine blue (*see* above)

   (c) Cole's haematoxylin (p. 195)

   (d) 1% chromazone red in 1% acetic acid

   (e) 1% phosphomolybdic acid in distilled water

   (f) 6 parts 1% light green in 1% acetic acid
      4 parts solution *(e)*
      2 parts solution *(d)*

   (g) 1% acetic acid in distilled water.

4. Method

Bring sections to water.
Treat with solution *(a)* for 10 min.
Wash in running tap water for 10 min.
Stain in solution *(b)* for 3 min.
Rinse with distilled water and stain in solution *(c)* for 3 min.
Wash in running tap water for at least 10 min.
Stain in solution *(d)* for 5 min.
Rinse with distilled water and place in solution *(e)* for 10 min.
Drain and stain in solution *(f)* for 10 min.
Wash off stain with solution *(e)*.
Treat with solution *(g)* for 2 min.
Dehydrate, clear, and mount.

5. Results

Muscle, fibrin, keratin, erythrocytes: red.
Collagen, cell cytoplasm: green.
Nuclei: blue-black.

Phosphotungstic acid haematoxylin

1. Purpose

Usually to demonstrate muscle striations, neuroglial fibres or fibrin. Many other tissue components such as nuclei, erythrocytes and mitochondria are also stained.

2. Demonstration tissues

Voluntary and cardiac muscle. Rhabdomyosarcoma. Late lobar pneumonia. Brain, preferably with areas of gliosis.

3. Solutions

(a) Mix fresh for use equal parts of 0·3% potassium permanganate and 0·3% sulphuric acid.

(b) 5% oxalic acid in distilled water.

(c) Phosphotungstic acid haematoxylin.[4]
In a glass mortar grind together 0·08 g of haematein and 1·0 ml of distilled water. Slowly add 100 ml of 0·9% aqueous phosphotungstic acid continuing grinding until a uniform purplish solution is obtained. Transfer to a beaker, bring quickly to the boil and allow to cool.

4. Method

Bring sections to water and treat with solution (a) for 5 min.
Rinse with distilled water and treat with solution (b) for 5 min.
Wash in several changes of distilled water.
Stain in solution (c) for from 3 hr to overnight.
Rinse quickly in distilled water, dehydrate, clear and mount.

5. Results

Muscle, fibrin, neuroglial fibres, nuclei, erythrocytes: deep blue.
Collagen, mucin: red to reddish brown.

Orcein and methylene blue

1. Purpose

To demonstrate fine and delicate elastic fibres.

2. Demonstration tissue

Skin.

3. Solutions

(a) Dissolve 1·0 g synthetic orcein in 100 ml of 70% alcohol. Add 1·0 ml hydrochloric acid. This solution keeps well and may even improve with age.

(b) 0·5% methylene blue in 1·0% acetic acid.

4. Method

Bring sections to 70% alcohol.
Stain in solution (a) in a covered jar for 30 min.
Rinse off excess stain with 70% alcohol.
Stain in solution (b) for 2 min.
Rinse off excess stain with distilled water and blot with filter paper.
Dehydrate, clear, and mount.

5. Results

Elastic fibres: light to deep brown.
Nuclei: blue.

Resorcin-fuchsin elastic stain

1. Purpose

Suitable for the demonstration of all elastic fibres, but of particular value when connective tissue stains such as the Van Gieson or the trichrome are required on the same section as the elastic. Better than the orcein method when coarse elastic fibres are to be shown and also when photography is required.

2. Demonstration tissues

Aorta; lung; skin.

3. Solutions

(a) Mix fresh for use equal parts 0·3% potassium permanganate and 0·3% sulphuric acid.

(b) 5% oxalic acid in distilled water

(c) Stock elastic stain.
Bring to the boil 200 ml distilled water.
Add very slowly:
1·0 g crystal violet
1·0 g basic fuchsin
4·0 g resorcin
0·5 g dextrin.

Continue boiling gently until dissolved and then slowly add 25 ml of 10% ferric chloride solution. Boil for a further 5 minutes, allow to cool, and filter. Add the precipitate and the filter paper to 100 ml of 95% alcohol and leave overnight. Simmer gently for one hour, cool and add 100 ml 95% alcohol and 6 ml hydrochloric acid. This stock solution will keep indefinitely.

(d) Working elastic stain:

Mix 3 parts solution *(c)* and 7 parts 1% hydrochloric acid in 70% alcohol.

This staining mixture also keeps well, but will slowly evaporate when kept in an ordinary staining jar with a loose-fitting lid.

4. Method

Bring sections to water.
Treat with solution *(a)* for 5 min.
Rinse with distilled water and treat with solution *(b)* for 5 min.
Wash thoroughly with distilled water and place in 70% alcohol for 1 min.
Place in solution *(d)* for from 6 hr to overnight.
Wash off all loose stain with 70% alcohol.
Wash in running tap water for 2 min.
Counterstain with the Van Gieson method, the trichrome method, or with a simple red nuclear stain as given in the Perls' method for haemosiderin. Dehydrate, clear, and mount.

5. Results

Coarse and fine elastic fibres: jet black.
Background according to counterstain.

Silver impregnation for reticulin fibres

1. Purpose

The differentiation of reticulin and collagen fibres.

2. Demonstration tissues

Liver; spleen; lymph nodes.

3. Solutions

(a) Mix fresh for use equal parts 0·3% potassium permanganate and 0·3% sulphuric acid

(b) 5% oxalic acid in distilled water

(c) 5% silver nitrate in distilled water

(d) To 20 ml of 10% aqueous silver nitrate add strong ammonia until the precipitate dissolves. Add one drop of 10% silver nitrate and 20 ml distilled water. Filter and store in a dark bottle

(e) 5% formalin in distilled water

(f) 5% sodium thiosulphate in distilled water

(g) Cole's haematoxylin (p. 195).

4. Method

Bring sections to water and treat with solution *(a)* for 5 min.
Rinse in distilled water and treat with solution *(b)* for 5 min.
Rinse 3 times with distilled water.
Flood slide with solution *(c)* for 5 min.
Rinse 3 times with distilled water.
Flood slide with solution *(d)* for 5 min.
Rinse 3 times with distilled water.
Flood slide with solution *(e)* for 5 min.
Rinse slide with distilled water and flood with solution *(f)* for 5 min.
Wash well in running tap water.
Stain in solution *(g)* for 5 min.
Wash in running tap water for at least 5 min.
Dehydrate, clear, and mount.

5. Results

Reticulin fibres: black.
Collagen fibres: brownish yellow.
Nuclei: blue.

Note: Care must be taken to prevent a mixture of the vapours of formalin (used in this method) and hydrochloric acid (used in Perls' method, page 201). This mixture results in the formation of bis-chloromethyl-ether (bis-CME) which is carcinogenic.

Periodic acid–Schiff

1. Purpose

Mainly used to demonstrate 'epithelial' mucins, glycogen and some fungi. It is classed as a histochemical method and may be used in conjunction with various other techniques for the detailed investigation of carbohydrates in tissues. When the presence of glycogen is being considered a duplicate section treated with diastase must be stained. If the demonstration of mucin or fungi is required these steps may be omitted.

2. Demonstration tissues

Infant liver for glycogen (with diastase control).
Stomach; salivary gland.

3. Solutions

(a) 1% periodic acid in distilled water

(b) Schiff's reagent:

To 200 ml boiling distilled water <u>slowly</u> add 1·0 g basic fuchsin. When dissolved, cool and add 2·0 g sodium metabisulphite and 2·0 ml hydrochloric acid.
Stopper flask with cotton wool and stand in a dark cupboard overnight. Add 0·5 g decolorising charcoal. Shake well, filter and store at 0–5°C. As long as the solution remains water white it is usable. Any suggestion of a pink colour means it must be discarded.

(c) Freshly prepared 0·1% malt diastase in distilled water

(d) Cole's haematoxylin (p. 195)

(e) 1% hydrochloric acid in 70% alcohol.

4. Method

Bring two sections to water.
Place one section (control) in solution *(c)* at 37°C for 30 min.
Wash control and test section in distilled water for 5 min.
Treat both sections with solution *(a)* for 10 min.
Wash in running tap water for 5 min.
Wash in at least 3 changes of distilled water.
Treat both slides with solution *(b)* for 10 min.
Wash thoroughly in several changes of distilled water.
Stain in solution *(d)* for 3 min.
Rinse in tap water and then in solution *(e)* for 5 sec.
Wash in running tap water for 10 min.
Dehydrate, clear, and mount.

5. Results

Nuclei: blue.
PAS-positive materials: deep purple red.
Glycogen: test section: positive.
               control section: negative.

Alcian blue

1. Purpose

Demonstration of acid mucopolysaccharides which occur in 'connective tissue' mucins and mucoid degeneration and also mixed with 'epithelial' mucins.

2. Demonstration tissues

Umbilical cord; stomach; large bowel.

3. Solutions

   (a) 1% alcian blue 8GX in 3% acetic acid

   (b) 0·2% safranin O in 1% acetic acid.

4. Method

Bring sections to water.
Stain in solution *(a)* for 10 min.
Rinse in distilled water.
Stain in solution *(b)* for 2 min.
Rinse with distilled water and blot with filter paper.
Dehydrate, clear, and mount.

5. Results

Acid mucopolysaccharides: green-blue.
Nuclei: red.

Alcian blue/periodic acid-Schiff

1. Purpose
A screening method which demonstrates most mucins in a single preparation. It may be preceded by glycogen removal with diastase (*see* periodic acid-Schiff method, above), but this is seldom necessary.

2. Demonstration tissues

Stomach. Large bowel.

3. Solutions

   (a) 1% alcian blue 8GX in 3% acetic acid.

   (b) 1% periodic acid in distilled water.

   (c) Schiff's reagent (above).

   (d) Cole's haematoxylin (p. 195).

4. Method

Bring sections to water.
Stain in solution *(a)* for 10 min.
Rinse with distilled water.
Treat with solution *(b)* for 10 min.
Wash well with several changes of distilled water.
Treat with solution *(c)* for 10 min.
Rinse with distilled water and wash in running tap water for 10 min.
Stain nuclei in solution *(d)* for 30 sec.
Blue in running tap water for 10 min.
Dehydrate, clear and mount.

5. Results

Acid mucins: blue green.
Neutral mucins: red.
Mixtures of above mucins: reddish purple green.
Nuclei: blue.

Martius scarlet blue (MSB) modified for formalin fixation

1. Purpose

To demonstrate fibrin in contrasting colour to erythrocytes.

2. Demonstration tissues

Late lobar pneumonia. Placenta. Organising thrombi.

3. Solutions

(a) 10% aqueous chromium trioxide.

(b) Celestine blue (p. 196).

(c) Cole's haematoxylin (p. 195).

(d) Yellow stain:

Martius yellow	0·5 g
Phosphotungstic acid	2·0 g
95% ethanol	100 ml

(e) Red stain:

Brilliant cresyl scarlet 6R	1·0 g
2·5% aqueous acetic acid	100 ml

(f) 1% aqueous phosphotungstic acid

(g) Blue stain:

Methyl blue	0·5 g
1% aqueous acetic acid	100 ml

4. Method

Bring sections to water.
Treat with solution (a) for 10 min.
Wash in running tap water for 10 min.
Stain in solution (b) for 3 min.
Rinse with distilled water.
Stain in solution (c) for 3 min.
Wash in running tap water for 10 min.
Rinse in absolute ethanol.
Stain in solution (d) for 2 min.
Rinse in tap water.
Stain in solution (e) for 10 min.
Rinse in tap water and treat with solution (f) for 5 min.
Rinse in tap water.
Stain in solution (g) for 10 min.
Rinse in tap water, dehydrate, clear and mount.

5. Results

Fibrin: bright red.
Muscle: dull red.
Collagen: blue.
Erythrocytes: yellow.
Nuclei: blue grey.

Azure A[5]

1. Purpose

The selective demonstration of mast cells.

2. Demonstration tissues

General connective tissue. Skin with urticaria pigmentosa.

3. Solutions

(a) 1% aqueous potassium permanganate.

(b) 5% aqueous oxalic acid.

(c) 0·2% aqueous azure A (MacNeal) or toluidin blue.

(d) 0·2% aqueous uranyl nitrate.

4. Method

Bring sections to water.
Treat with solution (a) for 5 min.
Rinse with distilled water.
Bleach with solution (b) for 5 min.
Wash in several changes of distilled water for 2 min.
Stain in solution (c) for 2 min.
Rinse with distilled water.
Differentiate with solution (d), agitating constantly until section appears a pale blue.
Rinse with distilled water and blot.
Dehydrate, clear and mount.

5. Results

Nuclei: blue.
Mast cell granules: red-purple.
Most acidic mucins: purple.

Methyl green–pyronin

1. Purpose

Usually to selectively demonstrate plasma cells. With appropriate enzyme digestion or chemical extraction methods claims of specificity for deoxyribonucleic acid (DNA) and ribonucleic acid (RNA) may be valid.

2. Demonstration tissues

Nasal and aural polyps. Sites of chronic inflammation.

3. Solutions

(a) Acetate buffer pH 4·8:

0·2 M acetic acid	8 parts
0·2 M sodium acetate	12 parts

(b) 0·8% methyl green in above buffer and kept over chloroform.

Before bottling, contaminating methyl violet must be removed by extracting with several changes of chloroform. This is to ensure green nuclear staining.

(c) 0·25% pyronin Y in above buffer and kept over chloroform.

Before bottling, contaminating dyes must be removed by extracting with chloroform. This is to avoid pink background staining.

Chloroform extraction. Thoroughly shake together equal parts of dye solution and chloroform in a separating funnel. Allow mixture to separate out when the chloroform will be the lower fraction. Run this off. Repeat with fresh chloroform until it remains almost colourless.

4. Method

Bring sections to distilled water.
Stain for 30 min. in freshly mixed:

solution (a)	30 ml
solution (b)	10 ml
solution (c)	10 ml.

Rinse rapidly in distilled water.
Blot, dehydrate, clear and mount.

5. Results

Cell nuclei (DNA): green.
Plasma cell cytoplasm (RNA): red.

Azoeosin–haematoxylin

1. Purpose

The selective demonstration of eosinophils.

2. Demonstration tissues

Chronic inflammation of gall bladder. Hodgkin's granuloma of lymph node. Bronchial asthma lung.

3. Solutions

(a) Cole's haematoxylin (p. 195).

(b) 1% hydrochloric acid in 70% ethanol.

(c) 1% aqueous azoeosin.

4. Method

Bring sections to water.
Stain in solution (a) for 5 min.
Rinse in tap water.
Differentiate in solution (b) with continuous agitation for 10 sec.
'Blue' in running tap water for 10 min.
Stain in solution (c) for 10 min.
Rinse in water, dehydrate, clear and mount.

5. Results

Nuclei: pale clear blue.
Eosinophil granules: bright red.

Perls' method[6]

1. Purpose

For the demonstration of ferric iron or haemosiderin deposits.

2. Demonstration tissues

Liver of haemachromatosis; sites of infarcts or haemorrhages.

3. Solutions

(a) Just before use mix together equal parts of 2% aqueous hydrochloric acid (Analar) and 2% aqueous potassium ferrocyanide (Analar).

(b) 0·2% safranin O in 1% acetic acid.

4. Method

Bring test section and a positive control section to distilled water.
Treat with solution (a) for 20 min.
Wash thoroughly with distilled water.
Stain with solution (b) for 2 min.
Rinse with distilled water and blot with filter paper.
Dehydrate, clear, and mount.

5. Results

Ferric iron deposits: blue-black.
Nuclei: red.

Note: See note following 'Silver impregnation for reticulin fibres' on p. 198.

Von Kossa's method[7]

1. Purpose

Demonstration of deposits of calcium salts. Urates may also react.

2. Demonstration tissues

Atheromatous blood vessels; senile prostate.

3. Solutions

(a) 10% aqueous hydrochloric acid

(b) 5% silver nitrate in distilled water

(c) 3% sodium thiosulphate in distilled water

(d) 0·2% safranin O in 1% acetic acid.

4. Method

Bring two sections to water.
Place one section (control) in solution (a) for 20 min.
Wash both sections in 3 changes of distilled water.
Place in a staining jar of solution (b) in bright daylight or artificial light for 2–4 hr.
Rinse in 3 changes of distilled water.
Treat with solution (c) for 2 min.
Wash in running tap water for 5 min.
Stain with solution (d) for 2 min.
Rinse with distilled water and blot with filter paper.
Dehydrate, clear, and mount.

5. Results

Calcium deposits: black in test section and absent in control.
Nuclei: red.

Gram's method[8]

1. Purpose

Demonstration of bacteria and some fungi.

2. Demonstration tissues

Acutely inflammed appendix; pneumococcal lung.

3. Solutions

(a) Dissolve 2·0 g crystal violet in 30 ml absolute alcohol. Dissolve 1·0 g ammonium oxalate in 70 ml distilled water. Mix the two solutions. This mixture keeps indefinitely but must be filtered before use.

(b) Dissolve 2·0 g potassium iodide in 300 ml distilled water and add 1·0 g iodine crystals. Shake well to dissolve.

(c) 0·2% safranin O in 1% acetic acid.

4. Method

Bring sections to water.
Stain in freshly filtered solution (a) for 3 min.
Rinse off excess stain with distilled water.
Treat with solution (b) for 3 min.
Rinse with distilled water.
Agitate vigorously in a staining jar of acetone for 5 sec.
Plunge immediately into running tap water and leave for 5 min.
Stain in solution (c) for 2 min.
Rinse with distilled water and blot with filter paper.
Dehydrate, clear, and mount.

5. Results

Gram-positive organisms (sometimes keratin and fibrin): blue-black.
Gram-negative organisms and nuclei: red.

Ziehl-Neelsen method[9]

1. Purpose

Demonstration of acid- and alcohol-fast organisms.

2. Demonstration tissues

Any tissues, but usually lung or lymph nodes, from a positive case of active tuberculosis or from an animal inoculated with positive material.

3. Solutions

(a) Carbol-fuchsin:
 (i) 9·0% basic fuchsin in absolute alcohol
(ii) 5·0% phenol in distilled water
For use mix 10 ml of (i) with 90 ml of (ii). This mixture keeps well but must be filtered on to the slides.

(b) 1% hydrochloric acid in 70% alcohol

(c) 0·2% methylene blue in 1% acetic acid.

4. Method

Bring test section and known positive control to water.

Place slides on a staining rack and flood with solution *(a)*.

Heat to steaming twice. This is done by holding with forceps a small plug of cotton wool dipped in alcohol and ignited below the slides.

Allow to cool, rinse in tap water and remove excess stain in solution *(b)* by gentle agitation. When the section appears colourless, wash in tap water and examine under the microscope when the erythrocytes should appear pale pink.

Wash for a further 10 min. in running tap water.

Stain in solution *(c)* for 2 min.

Rinse with distilled water and blot with filter paper.

Dehydrate, clear, and mount.

5. Results

Acid–alcohol-fast organisms: strong red.
Erythrocytes: pale pink.
Nuclei: blue.

Hexamine silver[10]

1. Purpose

A screening method for fungi.

2. Demonstration tissue

Any showing fungal infection.

3. Solutions

(a) 5% aqueous chromium trioxide.

(b) 1% aqueous sodium bisulphite.

(c) Mix fresh for use in the order given:

5% aqueous silver nitrate	2·5 ml
3% aqueous hexamine	50 ml
distilled water	50 ml
5% aqueous sodium tetraborate	4 ml

(d) 0·1% aqueous yellow gold chloride.

(e) 2% aqueous sodium thiosulphate.

(f) 0·1% light green SF in 0·1% aqueous acetic acid.

4. Method

Bring test section and known positive control to water.
Oxidise in solution *(a)* for 1 hr.
Rinse with distilled water.
Bleach in solution *(b)* for 1 min.
Wash in several changes of distilled water.

Place in solution *(c)* pre-heated to 60°C and keep at this temperature (in wax oven). Inspect after 20 min. and thereafter at 10 min. intervals until sections are yellow–brown. Fungi in the control section should now be dark brown.

Rinse in three changes of distilled water.
Tone in solution *(d)* for 5 min.
Rinse in three changes of distilled water.
Treat with solution *(e)* for 5 min.
Wash in running tap water for 10 min.
Stain in solution *(f)* for 1 min.
Rinse in water, dehydrate, clear and mount.

5. Results

Fungi, mucins, glycogen: black.
Background: green.

CELLOIDIN AND LVN SECTIONS

It will be remembered from the chapter on section cutting that as celloidin and LVN sections are cut they are collected in 70% alcohol where they remain until required for staining. During staining the sections are transferred from reagent to reagent by gripping the LVN border with a broad-ended pair of forceps. This must be done with care to avoid tearing the LVN. The staining solutions are kept in shallow containers such as Petri dishes with lids to prevent evaporation. In the case of strongly coloured solutions such as haematoxylin or crystal violet, finding the sections is made easier if the dish is held above a bright light. When staining is completed the sections are dehydrated through two changes of propan-2-ol of 1 minute each and then placed into a mixture of equal parts propan-2-ol and xylene.

From here they are picked up on to clean microscope slides, arranged neatly in the centre of the slide and any wrinkles or folds removed by gentle manipulation with a dissecting needle and forceps. The sections must be kept moistened with the propan-2-ol and xylene mixture. When suitably arranged the excess LVN border is trimmed away from the section, using a sharp scalpel or razor blade, and the section is covered with smooth paper and blotted flat, keeping the paper wet with xylene from a dropping bottle. Fluffless toilet paper cut into strips is ideal for this purpose. This flooding and blotting is repeated with fresh pieces of paper until the section is completely cleared.

A generous quantity of mountant is applied to the section, the slide is immediately inverted over a clean coverslip and lowered to pick up the coverslip. The slide is turned the right way up and the mountant allowed to cover the section.

Because of the thickness of LVN and celloidin sections and the fact that they are not fixed to the slide, there is a tendency for them not to remain flat as the mountant dries. This tendency can be lessened if a small weight is applied to the centre of the coverslip until the mountant has set. The weight used must not be excessive or too much mountant will be squeezed from under the coverslip resulting in the formation of large air spaces as the mountant finishes hardening.

The tendency to limit the use of celloidin and LVN embedding to special tissues means that the staining methods used also tend to be somewhat specialised. However, most of the methods described in the paraffin section pages can be applied to cellulose nitrate sections if slightly modified.

It should be noted that in methods where the celestine blue–haematoxylin sequence is described this technique should not be used. This is because celestine blue colours celloidin and LVN quite strongly and cannot subsequently be removed. The problem is overcome by substituting an iron haematoxylin such as Weigert's mixture.[8] This is prepared and used as follows:

Solution (a): 1% haematoxylin in absolute alcohol

Solution (b):

30% aqueous ferric chloride	4 ml
Distilled water	95 ml
Hydrochloric acid	1 ml

Mix equal parts of (a) and (b) just before use and stain sections for 10 minutes. Wash in running tap water for 10 minutes.

This is used in the staining sequence in place of the celestine blue–haematoxylin stages and the method is then proceeded with according to the schedule given.

REFERENCES

1. Cole, E.C. (1943). *Stain Technol.*, **18**, 125.
2. Lillie, R.D. (1976). *Histopathological Technic and Practical Histochemistry*. New York: McGraw Hill, p. 694.
3. Badloo, I. and James, K.R. (1975). *Basic Medical Laboratory Technology*. Tunbridge Wells: Pitman Medical, p. 186.
4. Shum, M. and Hon, J. (1969). *J. Med. Lab. Technol.*, **26**, 38–42.
5. Hughesdon, P.E. (1949). *J. Roy. Mic. Soc.*, **69**, 1.
6. Perls, M. (1867). *Virchows Arch. Path. Anat. Physiol.*, **39**, 42.
7. Kossa J. von (1901). *Beitr. Path. Anat.*, **29**, 163.
8. Gram, C. (1884). *Fortschr. Med.*, **2**, 185.
9. Ziehl, F. (1882). *Dt. Med. Wschr.*, **8**, 451.
10. Groscott, R.G. (1955). *Am. J. Clin. Path.*, **25**, 975–9.
11. Weigert, C. (1904). *Z. Wiss. Mikr.*, **21**, 1.

26. Frozen sections

There are three main occasions when the use of frozen-section techniques is necessary. First, constituents such as certain enzymes and fats may be removed from the tissues either by fixation or by the subsequent processing required in the preparation of paraffin or LVN sections. Secondly, some of the methods used to demonstrate certain tissue elements, particularly in the central nervous system, require free-floating sections. Thirdly, and of major importance in the modern diagnostic department, a frozen section can be prepared and a report given while the patient remains in the operating theatre. The report on this rapid-frozen section can help the surgeon decide on the course of action to be taken.

SECTION CUTTING

Frozen sections can be prepared on fixed or unfixed tissues, and if unfixed the cut sections may be fixed before staining or left unfixed, according to the requirements of the method. Frozen sections are prepared either on a freezing microtome or with an instrument called a cryostat.

Freezing microtome

A description of this instrument has been given on page 188. The selected block of tissue is placed on the microtome stage in a pool of a 50% solution of crystalline gum arabic in water or a commercial product such as Tissue-Tek OCT Compound* or Bright Cryo-M-Bed.* It is held in position with the tip of a pair of forceps and rapidly frozen with short bursts of carbon dioxide gas supplied to the stage from a cylinder. It is best to slightly overfreeze the tissue and then cut the sections as the block warms to optimum temperature. Several sections can be cut while the block is maintained at this temperature by the use of short bursts of gas. As each section is cut it is removed from the knife edge with a downward movement of either the fingertip

* Obtainable from R. A. Lamb, 6 Sunbeam Rd., Acton, NW10 6JL.

or a fine paint brush and transferred to fixative, distilled water, or other reagent as necessary.

Gelatin embedding

Porous tissues such as lung, and tissues which are liable to fragment such as muscle, may require support before cutting if they are to be handled as free-floating sections. This support can be provided by embedding the tissues in gelatin. The selected blocks must first be thoroughly washed to remove all traces of fixative. They are then immersed for 24 hours each in 5%, 15%, and 25% aqueous solutions of gelatin maintained at 37°C. After the final 24 hours they are placed in an embedding mould filled with 25% gelatin which is then allowed to cool and set. When set, the excess gelatin is cut away with a scalpel and the embedded block of tissue is immersed in 10% formalin to harden for 2 days. This gelatin block can then be sectioned in the manner described above.

Cryostat (Fig. 26.1)

Although described many years ago this instrument has only recently become established as an essential part of the equipment of the routine laboratory. Basically it consists of a microtome inside a refrigerator. The chamber may be kept at temperatures ranging from 0°C to −30°C, but a temperature of −20°C will enable most tissues to be sectioned. The microtome may be operated with the lid of the chamber open or, more commonly, by means of external controls connected through the top and sides of the cold chamber to the microtome. In the past the microtome was usually an adapted standard machine, but with the increased use of cryostats specially designed microtomes are now fitted to most models. A popular example works on the same principle as the Cambridge rocking microtome but is more robust, the controls are purpose designed and it uses a sturdier wedge-profile knife. The tissue is frozen to the microtome chuck outside the cold chamber either by plunging it into a beaker of 2-methylbutane kept in a vacuum flask of liquid nitrogen, or by using compressed

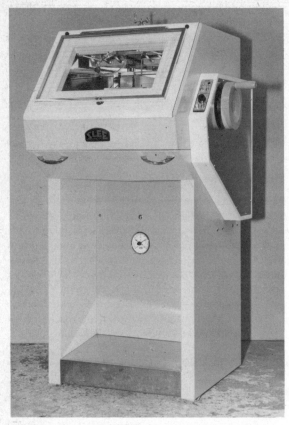

Fig. 26.1.   Cryostat (SLEE).

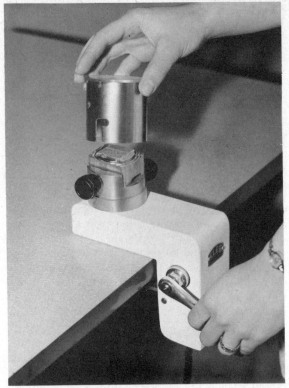

Fig. 26.2.   Rapid freezer (SLEE).

carbon dioxide gas from a cylinder attached to a special chuck holder with an expansion chamber similar to that of the freezing microtome (Fig. 26.2).

When dealing with unfixed tissues it is essential that the freezing process should be rapid in order to prevent the formation of ice crystals which cause considerable distortion to the cells. For this reason the tissue blocks must be kept as small as possible. After attaching the tissue to the microtome chuck the front window of the cryostat is opened and the chuck fixed in position on the microtome. Resting on the front of the knife is an attachment known as the guide plate. This consists of a piece of glass, the vertical edges of which are bound with an adhesive cellulose tape. This tape keeps the top horizontal edge of the glass approximately $50\,\mu$m away from the cutting edge of the knife and so leaves a slot through which the section passes as it is cut. This ensures that the section remains flat on the knife blade. The adjustment of this guide plate is the most critical factor in the production of good cryostat sections. The manufacturer's handbook devotes considerable space

to the details of its setting and to descriptions of the various faults which occur if it is not positioned correctly. Once the guide plate is correctly set sectioning is straightforward (Fig. 26.3).

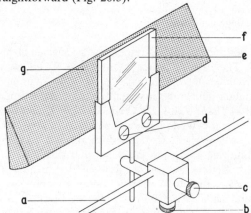

Fig. 26.3.   Guide plate assembly
(a) Connecting rod to external control; *(b)* adjustment for guide plate tilt; *(c)* coarse height adjustment; *(d)* fine adjustment screws; *(e)* glass guide plate; *(f)* cellulose tape spacer; *(g)* knife.

Depending upon the requirements of the method to be used the cut sections can either be delivered down a stainless-steel chute direct into the reagent or they can be picked up from the knife blade on to a coverslip or microscope slide. In the latter case the guide plate is swung aside and the slide or coverslip is pressed gently on to the section which is lying flat on the knife blade. Because the slide or coverslip is at room temperature the section will attach itself to the glass. This is then withdrawn from the cabinet and immersed in the required reagent.

SECTION STAINING

Free-floating sections

These are stained by transferring them from reagent to reagent using a glass 'hockey' stick. This is made by drawing one end of a 15 cm length of 5 mm diameter glass rod to a diameter of 1–2 mm and then bending the last 15 mm to an angle of 45°. The sections may be very fragile and must be handled carefully. When stained they are manipulated on to a slide and, depending upon the staining method being used, either mounted in a water-miscible mountant or blotted with filter paper, dehydrated, cleared and mounted in 'Terpine resin' or 'Ralmount'.

Cryostat sections

When these have been attached to slides or coverslips they are stained by passing through the reagents in the usual way. If the tissues are cut unfixed, immersion in a protein precipitant fixative will cause them to adhere to the glass. Alternatively they may be dried at 37°C. If the tissues are fixed prior to sectioning it is advisable to smear a small amount of albumin adhesive on to the slide or coverslip as described on page 193. These sections can then be immersed in a protein precipitant fixative or dried at 37°C. Sections of tissue which must not be fixed or dried prior to staining should be handled as free-floating.

STAINING METHODS

Oil red O for neutral fats

This method is best done on free-floating sections of formalin-fixed tissues cut at 8μm on either the freezing microtome or the cryostat.

1. Purpose

Demonstration of triglycerides or neutral fats.

2. Demonstration tissues

Fatty liver, normal adrenal.

3. Solutions

(a) Cole's haematoxylin (p. 195)

(b) Oil red O:

Saturated (0·6%) oil red O in propan-2-ol	6 parts
Distilled water	4 parts

Mix when required, allow to stand for 10 min and filter into a small staining dish. Keep covered to prevent evaporation and precipitation.

(c) Water mountant:

Clean gum Arabic crystals (not powder)	50 g
Sucrose	50 g
Potassium acetate	50 g
Distilled water	50 ml
Thymol	0·05 g

Dissolve with gentle heat and allow to cool.

4. Method

Cut the sections into distilled water.
Rinse in 60% alcohol for 5 sec.
Stain in oil red O solution for 10 min.
Rinse off excess stain in 60% alcohol for 5 sec.
Transfer to a deep dish of tap water and hold the section below the surface for a few seconds to prevent spinning and disintegration.
Stain in Cole's haematoxylin for 1 min.
Using occasional gentle agitation, blue the haematoxylin in tap water for 5 min.
With the 'hockey' stick manipulate the section on to a clean glass slide. Stand the slide on end and allow most of the water to drain off, then mop up any remaining drops around the edges of the section with a filter paper. Leave the section until almost dry and then place a generous amount of water mountant in the centre of the section. Tilt the slide to allow the mountant to run over the whole of the section and then invert over a clean coverslip and lower until the coverslip is picked up. Turn the slide the right way up, place on a flat surface and allow to set. Do not press out the mountant as this will at worst cause the section to disintegrate and at best will displace some of the fat

globules. With care and practice, bubbles can be avoided and the excess mountant can be cleaned away later with a damp rag.

5. Results

Triglycerides or neutral fats: orange-red.
Nuclei: blue.

RAPID HAEMATOXYLIN AND EOSIN

Freezing microtome method

1. Solutions

(a) Harris's haematoxylin:[1]
Dissolve 1 g haematoxylin in 10 ml absolute alcohol.
Dissolve 20 g aluminium ammonium sulphate in 200 ml distilled water.
Mix these two solutions and warm to 100°C.
Add 0·5 g mercuric oxide and maintain at 100°C for 10 min.
Cool and add 8 ml glacial acetic acid.
This solution is ready for immediate use.

(b) 0·5% hydrochloric acid in 70% alcohol

(c) Distilled water containing 3 drops of strong ammonia per 50 ml

(d) 0·5% eosin Y in absolute alcohol.

2. Method

Select a block of tissues not larger than $1 \times 1 \times 0.5$ cm and fix it by plunging it into boiling distilled water for 1 min.
Transfer to the microtome chuck, freeze, and cut sections at 6–8 μm into distilled water.
Stain in Harris's haematoxylin for 1 min.
Rinse well in tap water and dip in acid-alcohol for 3 sec.
Rinse in ammoniated water for 30 sec.
Dip in 20% alcohol and transfer to a deep dish of water. The section will spin out flat. Pick up on to an albuminised slide. Blot firmly with filter paper, smooth side towards section. Keeping the paper in place, flood with alcoholic eosin from a drop bottle and blot by smoothing a finger firmly across the paper. Repeat twice.
Peel away the paper and replace with a fresh piece.
Repeat the blotting process first with absolute alcohol and then with xylene or preferably Inhibisol.
Remove the paper and mount the section in Terpene resin or 'Ralmount'.

Cryostat method

1. Solutions

(a) Fixative: 5% glacial acetic acid in absolute alcohol

(b) Harris's haematoxylin (see preceding method)

(c) 0·5% hydrochloric acid in 70% alcohol

(d) Distilled water containing 3 drops of strong ammonia per 50 ml

(e) 1% aqueous eosin Y.

2. Method

Attach the block of unfixed tissue to the microtome chuck and cut sections at 5–6 μm, picking them up on a coverslip and transferring them immediately to fixative for 1 min.
Rinse in tap water for 10 sec.
Stain in Harris's haematoxylin for 1 min.
Rinse off excess stain in tap water.
Agitate gently in acid–alcohol for 3–5 sec, rinse in tap water and blue in ammoniated water for 5 sec.
Rinse in tap water for 5 sec.
Stain in eosin for 30 sec.
Wash in 70% alcohol for 5 sec.
Dehydrate in three changes of absolute alcohol for 5 sec each.
Clear in three changes of xylene or preferably Inhibisol for 5 sec each.
Mount in 'Terpene resin' or 'Ralmount'.
This method produces sections of better quality than the freezing microtome technique and is slightly quicker.

REFERENCE

1. Harris, H.F. (1900). *J. Appl. Micr.*, **3**, 777.

27. Cytology

Cytology is the study of more or less discrete cells from various organs of the body. These cells may be shed by the body itself; aspirated by tube or needle; or scraped, brushed or washed from the surfaces. They may be suspended in fluid in variable concentrations as with urine, ascites, pleural effusions and washings, or they may be relatively fluid-free as with cervical and buccal smears.

The greatest demand in cytology is for an early indication of malignant change but other information may be obtained about, for example, infestations and infections, chromosomal abnormalities and hormonal states. Collection of specimens is less traumatic than even minor surgical procedures but a diagnosis of malignancy usually requires confirmation by histological procedures.

It is emphasised that all fresh specimens are possibly infectious and must be treated with the same care as is observed in a microbiology department. All work stations must be provided with containers of disinfectant solutions and clearly identified incinerator bags, all of which should be renewed daily. There should be one container of disinfectant such as Hycolin for the disposal of specimens and another for any glassware or apparatus which is to be washed and re-used. The incinerator bags are used for such things as disposable specimen containers, Petri dishes, spatulas, contaminated gowns and protective gloves. A 10% solution of hypochlorite disinfectant such as Domestos should be kept for use when any virus-infected material has been handled but this should not be used on any metal surfaces or equipment. Details of other suitable disinfectants and their use should be studied in the 'Code of Practice for the Prevention of Infection in Clinical Laboratories and Post-Mortem Rooms'.

SPECIMEN COLLECTION AND PREPARATION

In almost all cases it is essential that smears be placed into fixative before the cells dry. An exception to this rule is when preparations are to be stained by the May-Grunwald–Giemsa method and the smears are then air-dried before fixation.

Fluids

Effusions

Specimens such as pleural fluid and ascitic fluid have a tendency to form clots. This can be prevented by collecting them in a sterile container with approximately 5 ml of 3·8% sodium citrate solution to each 20 ml of specimen. If clotting has occurred the clot should be processed and sectioned for histology.

Decant the well-mixed fluid into one or more disposable sealed centrifuge tubes and spin at 2000 rpm for 5 min.

Note the appearance of both the supernatant and the deposit. Invert the tube and discard the supernatant. Keep the tube inverted to prevent any fluid from running back into the deposit. Prepare six smears from the deposit. Fix two in 95% ethanol before they dry. Allow the other four to air-dry and then fix them in methanol. The two ethanol-fixed smears are for Papanicolaou staining. Two of the air-dried smears are for May-Grunwald-Giemsa staining. The two remaining smears are kept for any special stains that may be required. Should the deposit appear to be mainly blood and a 'buffy' coat be visible this can be carefully pipetted off and smears of it made as described above. If no 'buffy' coat can be seen the deposit should be prepared as for blood smears (page 228).

Urines

If specimens of urine are being collected in the laboratory or are being delivered there without delay they may be centrifuged and the deposit smeared and fixed. If there is any likelihood of a delay the specimen should be mixed with an equal volume of a fixative such as 95% ethanol. Smears of specimens already fixed in this way should be made on albuminised slides (page 193) to provide adhesion of the cells.

As an alternative to ordinary centrifugation, cells in non-viscous fluids may be concentrated by filtration through special membranes. These are made from cellulose acetate or a similar material and are available with various pore sizes, 5 μm being the most useful for cytology. Purpose-designed holders are used with these membranes. The holder may fit onto the end of a syringe and the specimen be forced from the syringe through the membrane by gentle positive pressure. Alternatively the filter may be positioned in a vacuum system and the specimen drawn through the membrane by gentle negative pressure. A third method utilises two containers joined at the necks where the membrane is gripped. The specimen is transferred from one container to the other by centrifuging at 700 rpm for 5 min. In all cases the cells are firmly attached to the membrane which is then clipped to a microscope slide, fixed, stained and then mounted between a slide and coverslip.

Sputa

These specimens are usually spread directly onto slides but if, for example, they are to be examined for suspected oat cell carcinoma or asbestos bodies it is advantageous to digest the mucous content and concentrate the rest of the material. All sputum specimens must be prepared in an approved exhaust protective cabinet and the operator must wear protective clothing.

1. Direct method. Transfer the specimen to a disposable Petri dish, examine and describe the macroscopic appearance, for example, mucoid, purulent, blood-stained, etc.

Tease out the sputum with a wooded applicator to obtain suitable pieces for spreading—white flakes or threads, black specks, blood flecks—and make four smears. Fix immediately for staining with the Papanicolaou method or with haematoxylin and eosin.

2. Concentration method. Examine and describe the specimen as for the direct method.

Add an equal volume of Cytoclair* (methyl cysteine) in physiological saline to the specimen and place the container in a water bath at 37°C for 2–12 hr.

Transfer to a disposable centrifuge tube and spin at 3000 rpm for 5 min. Pour off the supernatant fluid into disinfectant. With a disposable Pasteur pipette resuspend the deposit in the small amount of fluid remaining in the centrifuge tube.

Place two drops of suspension on each of four slides, spread evenly and place in fixative immediately.

* Sinclair Pharmaceuticals Ltd., 8 Oakford Road, Godalming, Surrey.

Stain with Papanicolaou or haematoxylin and eosin, and if suspecting asbestos bodies, Perls' method (page 201).

FIXATION

Most cytological fixatives contain alcohol and are inflammable. They must not be sent through the mail. Smears for mailing can be fixed in the usual way and then allowed to dry or they can be coated with a 'dry' fixative. Several of these fixatives are available commercially as fluids or as aerosol sprays. Alternatively a mixture can be prepared in the laboratory.

When using aerosol sprays care must be taken not to blast the smear from the slide by holding the spray too close. Another danger arises from using the aerosol when it is empty of fixative but is still under gas pressure. This results in an air-dried smear.

Fixatives

1. 95% ethanol

Fix for 20 min. Widely used good general purpose fixative.

2. Absolute methanol

Fix for 10 min. Used prior to staining with May-Grunwald–Giemsa.

3. 'Dry' fixative

Carbowax 1500	3·0 g
glacial acetic acid	0·2 ml
absolute ethanol	100·0 ml.

Cover smear from a drop-bottle and allow fluid to evaporate (approx. 10 min). Before staining remove Carbowax film by immersion in ethanol for at least 10 min.

*4. Cytofix**

A commercial version of (3), supplied as a 25 ml drop-bottle containing the acetic acid and Carbowax. Industrial spirit is added before use. These containers can be sent by mail to outside clinics and the alcohol added by the clinic staff. The fluid is used in the same way as (3) above.

* McCarthy's Laboratories, Romford, Essex.

5. 5% acetic acid in 95% ethanol

Fix for 20 min. A good general fixative giving better nuclear preservation than (1) above and sometimes brighter Papanicolaou staining.

6. Schaudinn's fluid (page 178)

Fix for 15 min. Useful for sputa and pleural effusions if haematoxylin and eosin staining is required. Mercury pigment must be removed before staining (page 194).

7. Carnoy's fluid (page 177)

Fix for 20 min. Sometimes very helpful with specimens containing a large amount of blood. The erythrocytes are lysed resulting in a much clearer picture of the remaining material.

MOUNTING

Because of the variable thickness of some smear preparations, in particular from lumpy specimens such as sputa, the mounting media recommended in the histology section of this book may be too thin and so give rise to problems such as air bubbles and mountant drying back under the coverslip leaving the smear unprotected. Examples of mountants which avoid these problems are 'Styrolite'* and 'Eukitt'*. They are much thicker than either Ralmount or terpene resin and dry sufficiently for microscopy within 20–30 min. Eukitt is the thickest and is particularly suitable for mounting membrane filters. After clearing in xylene the filter is placed in a Petri dish of mountant and left to soak for 10 min before mounting.

STAINING METHODS

Where large numbers of specimens are being dealt with it is convenient to purchase some of the staining solutions ready made. In the methods given below staining solution formulae are given to aid understanding of the results. Staining times may require small changes to suit local conditions such as laboratory temperature and quality of water and also the personal preferences of those responsible for screening the preparations.

---

* R. A. Lamb, 6 Sunbeam Road, London NW10 6JL.

Papanicolaou

1. Purpose

To provide clear nuclear detail together with differential staining of the cytoplasm of squamous cells, in particular those from the female genital tract. It can also indicate response to hormones. Cytoplasm has a transparent appearance which facilitates screening very cellular specimens such as some sputa.

2. Demonstration material

A good scrape from mid-cycle cervical epithelium, preferably from a non-hormone receiver. A cellular sputum preparation.

3. Solutions

(a) Harris's haematoxylin with acetic acid (page 208). For use dilute two parts to one part distilled water.

(b) 0·5% hydrochloric acid in 70% ethanol.

(c) Orange G (OG 6)

0·5% orange G in 95% ethanol	500 ml
phosphotungstic acid	0·075 g

(d) Eosin-azure (EA 36 or EA 50)

0·1% light green SF in 95% ethanol	225 ml
0·5% Bismark brown in 95% ethanol	50 ml
0·5% eosin Y in 95% ethanol	225 ml
phosphotungstic acid	1·0 g
saturated aqueous lithium carbonate	5 drops

N.B. Solutions (a), (c) and (d) may be purchased ready-made. A reliable source is Ortho Pharmaceuticals.* The solutions should all be kept in dark bottles and must be well shaken and then filtered before use.

4. Method

I. Manual schedule

Bring fixed smears to water	
Solution (a)	3 min
Wash briefly in tap water	
Solution (b)	few seconds
Wash in running tap water	5 min
70% ethanol	30 sec
95% ethanol	30 sec
Solution (c)	2 min
Rinse in two changes of 95% ethanol	
Solution (d)	3 min

---

* Ortho Pharmaceuticals Ltd., Saunderton, High Wycombe, Buckinghamshire.

Rinse in two changes of 95% ethanol
Dehydrate, clear and mount.

II. Machine schedule

Because of the large number of slides being stained by Papanicolaou's method in most cytology departments it is usual to take advantage of the convenience and the uniformity of results obtained by staining on an automatic machine. As previously mentioned the schedule given here may require slight changes to suit local conditions. It is arranged for a 23-station cycle.

Fix smears	
70% ethanol	1 min
50% ethanol	1 min
Distilled water	1½ min
Solution (a)	4 min
Distilled water	1 min
Distilled water	30 sec
70% ethanol	30 sec
Solution (b)	20 sec
70% ethanol	2 min
70% ethanol with a few drops of ammonia added	1 min
70% ethanol	1 min
70% ethanol	1 min
95% ethanol	30 sec
95% ethanol	30 sec
Solution (c)	2 min
95% ethanol	30 sec
95% ethanol	30 sec
Solution (d)	3 min
95% ethanol	1 min
95% ethanol	1 min
Absolute ethanol	2 min
Absolute ethanol	2 min
Inhibisol	2 min

Remove from machine into xylene and mount.

5. Results

Nuclei: blue.
Cytoplasm—superficial cells: pink
                intermediate cells: blue green
                parabasal cells: deep green.
Erythrocytes: pink to green.
Candida albicans: red to pale pink.
Trichomonads: grey green.

Notes

When staining membrane filters all absolute ethanol baths should be replaced by absolute propan-1-ol as the filters may wrinkle and distort in ethanol.

May-Grunwald–Giemsa

1. Purpose

For use with air-dried smears. Nuclear state, for example, mitotic figures, and cytoplasmic morphology such as vacuolation are clearly shown. Cell types such as eosinophils and mast cells are well demonstrated.

2. Demonstration material

Air-dried smears from serous effusions. Smears from 'buffy' coats of bloody specimens. Blood films.

3. Solutions

(a) pH 6·8 buffer
    M/15 disodium hydrogen phosphate (Na_2HPO_4)
                                          496 ml
    M/15 potassium dihydrogen phosphate (KH_2PO_4)
                                          504 ml

    OR use commercial buffer tablets

(b) May-Grunwald
    Commercial stock solution   25 ml
    Solution (a)   25 ml
    Prepare fresh each day and filter into a Coplin jar.

(c) Giemsa
    Commercial stock solution   5 ml
    Solution (a)   45 ml
    Prepare fresh each day and filter into a Coplin jar.

4. Method

Fix air-dried smears in methanol   10 min
Rinse in solution (a)
Stain in solution (b)   8 min
Drain off excess fluid and stain in solution (c)   10 min
Wash for a few seconds in solution (a)
Blot carefully and allow to completely air-dry.
Mount in Styrolite.

5. Results

Nuclei: purple.
Cytoplasm: blue to mauve.
Erythrocytes: pink.
Eosinophil granules: red.
Mast cell granules: blue.

Cresyl fast violet

1. Purpose

The demonstration of the sex chromatin or Barr body present on the nuclear membrane of cells. This body is characteristic of the female cell and represents the inactive X chromosome. It is not present in the normal male possessing an XY complement but may be seen in Klinefelter's syndrome where XXY chromosomes are found. It is missing in the female with Turner's syndrome.

2. Demonstration material

A good scrape from the buccal mucosa of a normal female.

3. Solutions

   (*a*) 1% aqueous cresyl fast violet.

4. Method

Firmly scrape the inside of the mouth with the blunt rounded end of a spatula and smear the material onto two clean slides. Fix immediately in acetic-alcohol (page 211) for 20 min

70% ethanol	2 min
50% ethanol	2 min
Distilled water	2 min
Solution (*a*)	5 min

Differentiate in 95% ethanol until cytoplasm of the majority of the cells is colourless.   2–5 min
Dehydrate, clear and mount.

5. Results

Sex chromatin: deeply stained purple against a slightly paler nuclear membrane.
Cytoplasm: very pale purple to colourless.

PART FOUR

Haematology

28. Introduction to haematology

THE NATURE OF BLOOD

Blood is a transportation system which visits all the organs and tissues of the body and in obedience to the body's requirements its constitution is altered. The elements of blood, erythrocytes, leucocytes and platelets, are suspended in plasma and can, in their size, number and chemical content reflect many of the physical changes occurring in the body. These reflections are not always specific to a particular disease but taken in conjunction with other physical signs they can be a reliable aid to diagnosis.

On its travels through the cardiovascular system blood transports oxygen from the lungs, absorbs nutriments from the small intestine and passes through the kidneys where its salt concentration is regulated and harmful substances are removed. Oxygen provided by the blood is used by the liver in the oxidative metabolism of the amino acids. The liver also synthesises the blood plasma proteins as well as converting ammonia from the de-amination of amino acids into urea prior to its being transported by the blood to the kidneys. Blood also acts as a temperature regulator and a defence mechanism against invasion by foreign bodies and infection. The endocrine glands use blood for the rapid transport of their hormones. Enzymes present in blood promote the clotting process which prevents excessive loss whenever a blood vessel is injured.

HAEMOPOIESIS

The sites of blood formation in the adult are the bone marrow and the lymphatic system. In the fetus it occurs in the liver with the marrow playing an increasing role as the time of birth approaches. In the neonate active, red marrow occupies all the marrow spaces. This marrow is gradually replaced by yellow inactive marrow until in the normal adult red marrow is mainly found in the sternum, ribs, vertebrae, pelvic bones and the proximal ends of the long bones.

The bone marrow is the source of erythrocytes, granulocytes, monocytes and platelets. Lymphocytes also originate in the bone marrow but, as will be described later, the thymus has a prime function in the production of mature lymphocytes along with the spleen, lymph nodes and lymphoid tissues of the gut.

The precursors of these cells can be differentiated morphologically into blast cells, i.e. erythroblast, lymphoblast, etc.; but the more primitive the cells the more difficult is the task of differentiation. At their most primitive they exist as undifferentiated 'stem' cells. These stem cells are called pluripotential cells because of their capacity to produce different cell lines in response to regulator mechanisms in the haemopoietic system.

The basis of haematological diagnosis is the blood count. This may range from haemoglobin estimation and examination of a stained film to a fully automated procedure producing a further six measurements. After the blood count, of course, a wider range of haematology investigations may be considered; but the blood count is a stage which should never be omitted.

ANTICOAGULANTS

When blood is shed it clots, and the cells become enmeshed in a web of fibrin strands. To prevent this occurring, and to enable a satisfactory count to be performed, the blood must be added to a substance which will prevent the clotting process from taking place. This substance is called an anticoagulant. The most suitable anticoagulants for haematological purposes are sequestrene, sodium citrate and heparin.

Sequestrene

The potassium salt of ethylenediaminetetraacetic acid (EDTA) is more conveniently known as sequestrene. Blood cannot coagulate without the presence of calcium ions. Sequestrene acts as a chelating agent (Gk. 'chele'–a claw) and binds calcium so that it is not available for the coagulation process. Sequestrene is the anticoagulant of choice for blood counts and films. It is ideal for platelet counts as it prevents them from clumping. However, it is not suitable for coagulation studies because it destroys factors v and vIII.

Method

Add 0·1 ml of a solution of the salt (100 g/litre) to the sample tube and allow to evaporate at room temperature. This is sufficient for 5 ml of blood.

Trisodium citrate

Trisodium citrate is used in coagulation studies because it is the anticoagulant which most satisfactorily preserves the coagulation factors in blood. It is also used in the estimation of the erythrocyte sedimentation rate (ESR). It acts by binding calcium in an un-ionised form so that it is not available for the coagulation process.

Method

For coagulation studies add 9 volumes of blood to 1 volume of 0·109 mol/litre (32 g/litre) trisodium citrate dihydrate in a plastic container.

For ESR estimation add 4 volumes of blood to 1 volume of 0·105 mol/litre (30·88 g/litre) trisodium citrate dihydrate.

Heparin

Heparin is a natural substance which is synthesised by the liver. It is derived commercially from mammalian viscera, e.g. intestinal mucosa of pigs. With the aid of a co-factor in plasma, heparin neutralises thrombin which is an essential factor involved in the coagulation process. Heparin may be used for osmotic fragility tests, LE cell preparations and G-6-P-D estimations. It is not satisfactory for leucocyte counts because it clumps the cells, and blood films from heparinised blood have a blue background when stained by Romanowsky dyes. It is used at a concentration of 0·1–0·2 g/litre of blood.

Method

Add 0·25 ml of a solution of sodium heparin (4·0 g/litre) to a sample tube and allow to dry at 37°C. This will be sufficient to prevent 10 ml of blood from clotting.

Defibrination

Another method of maintaining blood in liquid form is defibrination. As the term implies fibrin is removed during the coagulation process so that the cells do not become enmeshed.

Method

Paper clips, glass beads, pieces of capillary tubes or anti-bumping granules are placed in a tube. The blood is added and gently agitated for about 5 min. when fibrin will collect around the paper clips, etc. The blood may then be decanted and the serum separated from the cells if necessary. The method's main use in haematology is for the preparation of LE cells.

Degenerative changes occur in cells as soon as they leave the circulation. Blood films made from the same anticoagulated sample over a period of 24 hours will show progressive changes in the appearance of the white cells. At the end of the 24 hour period the changes can be so bizarre as to bear no resemblance to their original morphology. Anticoagulants vary in their effect on cell morphology and as sequestrene has least effect on the cells it is the anticoagulant of choice. However, it is still recommended that blood films be made within an hour of collection.

COLLECTION OF BLOOD

An essential prerequisite to the satisfactory completion of a blood count is a sample which has not been adversely affected by the technique used in its collection. For haematological purposes capillary or anticoagulated venous blood may be used. Venous blood is more convenient for handling at the bench because of its larger volume, and the results from it are considered to be more representative of the blood as a whole. However, satisfactory results may be obtained from capillary blood provided meticulous care is taken in sampling.

Capillary blood from finger-prick

Select the site—the ball of the middle finger is usually satisfactory—and rub with dry cotton wool. This helps to promote the circulation. Cleanse the site with 70% alcohol and allow to dry. Prick the finger to a depth of 2–3 mm with a sterile disposable lance. Wipe away the first few drops of blood, which will contain an excess of tissue fluid, then take off the blood as required. Squeezing the finger will result in dilution with tissue fluid.

It is worthwhile perfecting the technique of obtaining blood from the earlobe. Some patients prefer it because they do not see the complete procedure and they maintain it is less painful than the finger-prick! The technique is similar to the above. The site should be warm and well filled with blood. Rubbing with dry cotton wool will promote circulation before cleansing with alcohol.

Capillary blood by heel-prick

This technique is used solely for the collection of blood from infants and is not easily mastered. The heel should be warm and to achieve this it may be immersed in warm water. The heel is pricked on the plantar surface with the intention of producing a small cut rather than the hole which would be obtained with a straight jab. This may be effected by a sideways motion of the needle after it has entered the skin. A counsel of perfection would be to refrain from squeezing the heel to promote the flow of blood; but one must be realistic. Remember that every squeeze increases the unreliability of any tests.

Blood by venepuncture

The equipment needed is a syringe, needle (21 gauge), tourniquet, cotton wool, antiseptic and containers for the sample. There is rarely any necessity for a needle of finer gauge than 21. It is sometimes recommended for children but this tends to prolong the procedure and speed promotes happiness on both sides of the needle! The preferred site of venepuncture is inside the bend of the elbow (the antecubital fossa). Apply the tourniquet to the upper arm sufficiently tightly to obstruct the venous flow. Ask the patient to clench his fist and straighten his arm. If a vein cannot be seen or felt light slapping on the skin may help. It is always advisable to feel the vein. Pressure with a finger will often disclose a substantial vein which does not wish to advertise itself. Time taken in finding the most suitable vein reduces the need for repeating the procedure (Fig. 28.1). Cleanse the skin with a suitable antiseptic—70% alcohol or 0·5% hibitane. Press just below the vein with the thumb to draw the skin tight. Insert the needle smoothly into the skin to a depth of a few millimetres with the

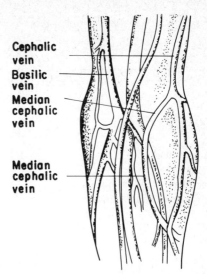

Fig. 28.1. Veins suitable for venepuncture in the left antecubital fossa.

bevel uppermost. The needle should be at an angle of about 20° to the surface of the arm. However, this angle will depend on the depth of the vein selected. When the needle has entered the vein and blood can be withdrawn the tourniquet should be released and the syringe filled. On completion place a wad of cotton wool over the wound and withdraw the needle. Detach the needle and discard it into a box provided for the purpose. Fill sample tubes as required. At this point a strip dressing may be applied.

QUALITY CONTROL

The usefulness of any laboratory and, indeed, its credibility, depends upon an ability to eliminate gross error from its reports and maintain a consistent standard of service. Techniques for controlling the quality of results are described in Chapter 39, and these techniques can and should be applied to haematology.

The following national quality control schemes are recommended in the United Kingdom:

(a) National Reference Laboratory for Anticoagulant Reagents and Control, Withington Hospital, Manchester, M20 8LR.

(b) UK National External Quality Assessment Scheme for Haematology, Royal Postgraduate Medical School, London, W12 OHS.

Many reporting errors, however, are clerical rather than technical and will not be revealed by the quality control systems referred to above. It is therefore important that every care is taken to avoid transcription errors. Keeping a cumulative record for each patient is an additional aid to accurate reporting, as unexpected changes in values may point to an error.

DOCUMENTATION

Laboratory report

Once a satisfactory format has been established a laboratory report should remain unchanged for as long as possible. The identification, date, results and comment should be always in the same position so that the recipient, by relying on pattern recognition built up over a long period, may quickly evaluate the whole report. When designing a report form consideration should be given to its appearance in the patient's notes. The 'tiling method' of presentation is useful in that any change in results may be rapidly assessed (Fig. 28.2). The latest report is fully displayed because it is placed on top. All previous reports have their bottom edges protruding with only date, identification and results visible. However, all the information is readily accessible (Fig. 28.3).

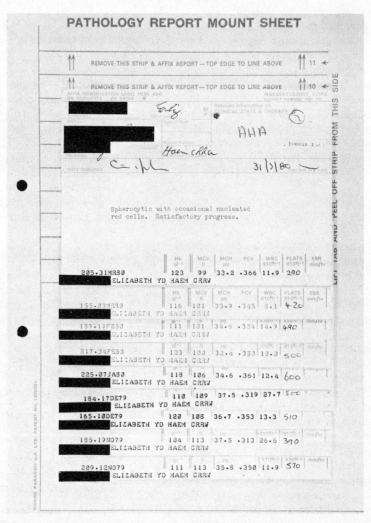

Fig. 28.2.   Haematology reports as arranged in patients' notes.

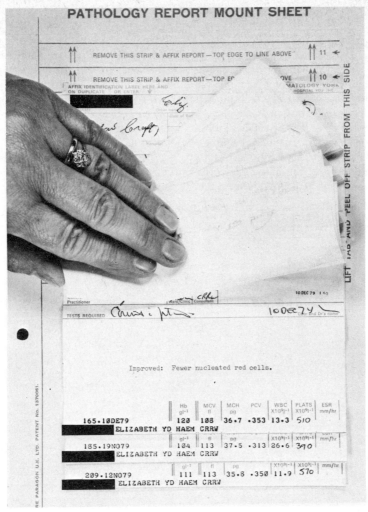

PATHOLOGY REPORT MOUNT SHEET

↑↑ REMOVE THIS STRIP & AFFIX REPORT—TOP EDGE TO LINE ABOVE ↑↑ 11 ←

↑↑ REMOVE THIS STRIP & AFFIX REPORT—TOP E_____ ___VE ↑↑ 10 ←

Improved: Fewer nucleated red cells.

	Hb gl⁻¹	MCV fl	MCH pg	PCV	WBC X10⁹l⁻¹	PLATS X10⁹l⁻¹	ESR mm/hr
165·10DE79	120	108	36·7	·353	13·3	510	
ELIZABETH YD HAEM CRRW							
185·19NO79	104	113	37·5	·313	26·6	390	
ELIZABETH YD HAEM CRRW							
209·12NO79	111	113	35·8	·350	11·9	570	
ELIZABETH YD HAEM CRRW							

Fig. 28.3. Patients' notes showing easy access to previous film reports.

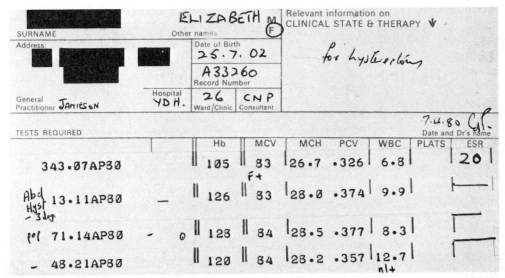

SURNAME	Other names ELIZABETH M Ⓕ	Relevant information on CLINICAL STATE & THERAPY ▼
Address:	Date of Birth 25.7.02	for hysterectomy
	A33260 Record Number	
General Practitioner JAMIESON	Hospital YDH.	26 Ward/Clinic	CNP Consultant	

7.4.80 Date and Dr's name

TESTS REQUIRED		Hb	MCV	MCH	PCV	WBC	PLATS	ESR
343·07AP80		105	83 F+	26·7	·326	6·8		20
Abd Hyst 13·11AP80 – 3 day		126	83	28·0	·374	9·9		
Pol 71·14AP80	– 0	128	84	28·5	·377	8·3		
– 48·21AP80		120	84	28·2	·357	12·7 nl+		

Fig. 28.4. A cumulative laboratory record.

Laboratory record

A cumulative record should be kept for each patient. This provides information on progress and plays a useful role in the quality control programme by indicating sudden changes in levels which may be due to errors. Periodically record cards may be culled of those which have not been used within a defined period.

The format may be a 6 × 4 in. card with each day's results entered in columns and the blood film comments noted in shorthand form (Fig. 28.4). Once again discipline is needed in positioning dates and figures so that the evaluation of past results may be rapidly achieved. In Fig. 28.4 'nl+' entered in the WBC column indicates neutrophil leucocytosis. An abbreviated clinical comment appears on the extreme left of one entry indicating an abdominal hysterectomy 3 days ago. Abbreviations such as these may be invented, and will provide much information in a small space. If, with each entry, their relative positions are maintained, a cumulative record will result which may be assessed in a very short time.

29. The blood count

HAEMOGLOBIN

Haemoglobin is the red-coloured substance contained in the red cell. Its main purpose is to provide oxygen to those tissues which require it and to remove waste carbon dioxide. To achieve this it must necessarily be able to combine loosely with oxygen in order to take up or release it according to the concentration of oxygen surrounding the red cell. In its transport of oxygen and carbon dioxide it also plays an important role in maintaining the pH of the blood.

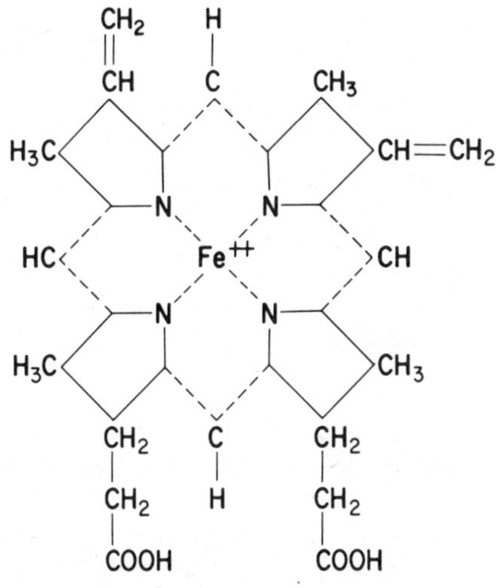

Fig. 29.1. Diagram of haem group.

The haemoglobin molecule consists of a protein portion—globin, and an iron-containing pigment—haem (Fig. 29.1). Globin is composed of two identical pairs of closely linked polypeptide chains termed α and β. There are 141 amino acids in the α chain and 146 amino acids in the β chain. The haem portion contains iron and protoporphyrin, the protoporphyrin which provides the red colouring of haemoglobin, being linked in the form of four pyrrole rings to one atom of divalent iron. One haem group is attached to each polypeptide chain.

The haemoglobin molecule therefore has four atoms of ferrous iron, each of which will combine with one molecule of oxygen.

The ease with which the haem group can surrender or combine with oxygen is related to the shape of the molecule. The four polypeptide chains are interlocked to form an egg-shaped molecule and the haem groups lie in pockets on the surface. When the first atom of ferrous iron becomes saturated with oxygen there is a spatial rearrangement of the molecule so that other haem pockets become more accessible. When oxygen is taken up in the molecule ionisation occurs which in turn affects the pH, making it more acidic, a situation which is reversible and accounts for the buffering power of haemoglobin. The association of pH and oxygen affinity is known as the Bohr effect.

1·0 g of haemoglobin will bind 1·34 ml of oxygen. A litre of normal blood is therefore capable of carrying 200 ml of oxygen.

ESTIMATION OF HAEMOGLOBIN

The several methods of estimating haemoglobin vary in their reliability and will be discussed briefly below. The method to be described in detail is the cyanmethaemoglobin method recommended in 1966 by the International Committee for Standardisation in Haematology (ICSH). Methods in general use involve the measurement of the colour of haemoglobin, those employing photoelectric colorimeters being superior to visual procedures which are subject to individual variance.

The ICSH established a specification for a cyanmethaemoglobin standard based on a molecular weight of 64 458 and an optical density, measured at 540 nm, of a solution of haemoglobin containing 223 ng/litre. The solution is stable for a year. These standards are available commercially at a concentration of approximately 0·6 g/litre, the exact concentration of each batch being stated on the label.

Principle

The iron in haemoglobin is converted to the ferric state by potassium ferricyanide forming methaemoglobin.

This in turn combines with potassium cyanide to form cyanmethaemoglobin. All forms of haemoglobin except sulphaemoglobin are converted to cyanmethaemoglobin. The optical density of this solution is measured in a photoelectric colorimeter at 540 nm (Ilford green filter 625).

Reagent

Drabkin's solution (Van Kampen and Zijlstra modification)

Potassium ferricyanide	0·2 g.
Potassium cyanide	0·5 g.
Potassium dihydrogen orthophosphate	0·14 g.
Distilled water to	1 litre.

The pH should be 7·0–7·4.
Store in a black-painted bottle and discard if turbidity develops. The solution keeps for several months.

Method

Add 20 μl of blood to 4·0 ml of reagent, mix and allow to stand for 3 min to allow complete conversion of pigment. Using diluent as a blank read the test against a known standard at 540 nm. Haemoglobin concentration may be calculated as follows:

Haemoglobin (g/dl) =

$$\underbrace{\frac{\text{abs. of test}}{\text{abs. of standard}}}_{} \times \underbrace{\text{conc. of standard}}_{\text{(g/dl)}} \times \underbrace{201}_{\text{(dilution factor)}}$$

Reference range

Men	13·0–18·0 g/dl
Women	11·5–16·5 g/dl
Infants	13·5–19·5 g/dl
Children	10·0–14·8 g/dl

Calibration of photoelectric colorimeter

It is convenient to calibrate a colorimeter so that readings may be converted, by means of graph or chart, directly into haemoglobin concentration in g/dl. This is easily done by preparing dilutions of a cyanmethaemoglobin standard. Three dilutions should be sufficient (1 in 2, 1 in 3, 1 in 4) since the solution obeys Beer's Law and a straight line should be obtained. Knowing the concentration of the reference standard and the dilution factor chosen for the method, concentrations corresponding to the colorimeter readings may

be calculated and a graph drawn on mathematical paper. The line drawn should cover the range 0–18·0 g/dl.

Example of calculation for colorimeter calibration

Stated concentration of standard	= 0·062 g/dl
Concentration of a 1 in 2 solution	= 0·031 g/dl
Dilution factor of method	= 1 in 201.
	(20 μl in 4·0 ml)
Final concentration of 1 in 2 dilution	= 0·031 × 201 = 6·23 g/dl
Similarly a 1 in 3 dilution	= 4·154 g/dl
Similarly a 1 in 4 dilution	= 3·112 g/dl

These concentrations are plotted against their readings (absorbances) in the colorimeter (*see* Fig. 29.2).

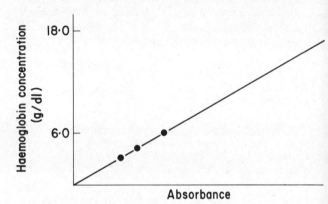

Fig. 29.2.   Calibration of photoelectric colorimeter.

The cyanmethaemoglobin method is rapid and simple to use. It has an easily prepared, relatively stable reagent and a standard which is stable for 12 months. All forms of haemoglobin are converted to cyanmethaemoglobin except sulphaemoglobin which is present in inconsiderable amounts in normal human blood. It is also recommended by the ICSH and has become the method of choice for most laboratories resulting in a standardised approach to haemoglobinometry with a consequent improvement in comparability between centres.

Concentrated lysing/cyanide reagents are available commercially which, when added in small amounts to saline dilutions of blood, lyse the red cells and rapidly convert haemoglobin to cyanmethaemoglobin leaving white cells in suspension for later counting (p. 226), one such reagent is Zapoglobin.*

---

* Coulter Electronics Ltd., Coldharbour Lane, Harpenden, Herts.

Alternative methods of haemoglobinometry

Haemoglobin may be converted to carboxyhaemo-globin, acid haematin, or alkaline haematin and the pigment measured, or it may be simply diluted in water and measured as oxyhaemoglobin. The methods have their attendant disadvantages.

Oxyhaemoglobin is not a stable solution and the standard is therefore unsatisfactory. A diluent consisting of 0·4 ml/litre ammonia (sp.gr. 0·88) helps to stabilise the pigments for approximately 24 hours. The usual standard is an artificial one consisting of a solution of inorganic salts which at a suitable dilution produce an absorbance equivalent to a haemoglobin concentration of 14·6g/dl. This method is the quickest of the alternatives.

Carboxyhaemoglobin is produced by bubbling coal gas through an aqueous solution of blood. It is a slightly smelly business and the gas is toxic. The standard is a sealed ampoule of a similarly produced solution. Interest in the method is purely historical.

Acid haematin is a brown pigment produced when blood is diluted in 0·1 M hydrochloric acid. The haemoglobin is calculated after water has been added to the acid haematin, drop by drop, until the resultant brown colour matches a coloured glass standard; this was the method of Sahli. It is time-consuming and does does not measure all haemoglobin pigments.

The alkaline haematin method, although converting all pigments by the addition of alkali, is again time-consuming.

VISUAL METHODS OF COUNTING CELLS

The visual method of cell counting can produce an inherent error of approximately 10% even when performed with scrupulous care by an experienced operator. Using the method involves acceptance of this error and the need to make allowances in the interpretation of the results. The method, now superseded by electronic methods which are more convenient and have a smaller inherent error, will be described because the need to perform a visual count will arise occasionally in every laboratory.

The most frequently used counting chamber is the Improved Neubauer chamber (Fig. 29.3). It has a total ruled area of 3 × 3 mm producing a central area which is divided into 25 groups of 16 small squares. This central area is used for red-cell counts and the four corner squares, which are divided into 16 squares only, are used for white-cell counts. The depth of the central

platform is 0·1 mm. Other counting chambers exist with different rulings and depths designed to accommodate fluids with only few cells. They will not be described. The British Standard Specification for the Improved Neubauer chamber is BS 748.

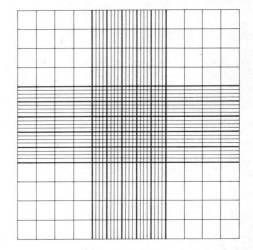

Fig. 29.3.   Improved Neubauer counting chamber.

Red-cell count

Dacie's formol-citrate fluid is recommended as a diluting fluid. It consists of 31·1 g/litre trisodium citrate to which has been added 10 ml/litre 40% formaldehyde. The citrate prevents coagulation of the red cells and the formalin prevents the growth of moulds and fixes the red cells.

20 μl of well-mixed blood are added to 4·0 ml of diluting fluid and the tube gently mixed for 2 min. This results in a dilution of 1 in 201 (for ease of calculation the dilution is taken to be 1 in 200). The counting chamber is prepared, the cover slip having been centrally positioned over the ruled area. The chamber is now filled with the diluted blood using a capillary or Pasteur pipette. A smooth action is used and the blood should not be allowed to overflow into the trough. 2–3 min should now be allowed for the cells to settle. If the chamber is left too long the edges of the fluid will evaporate causing currents which will alter the positions of the red cells.

The central square of the ruled area is surveyed with a ×40 objective and the cells in 5 of the 16 smaller squares are counted, i.e. a total of 80 small squares (Fig. 29.4).

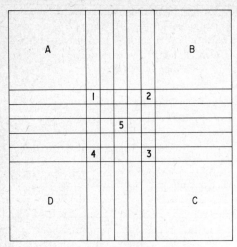

Fig. 29.4. Representation of counting chamber
For white blood cells (WBC) count squares A, B, C and D.
For red blood cells (RBC) count squares 1, 2, 3, 4 and 5.

Calculation

As there are 400 small squares in the centre occupying $1\,mm^2$, 80 squares are equivalent to $0\cdot02\,mm^2$. The depth is $0\cdot1\,mm$ therefore the volume is $0\cdot02\,\mu l$.

The number of cells counted (N) per μl would be $N \times 50$. The dilution was 1 in 200 therefore the number of cells in $1\,\mu l$ of blood would be $N \times 50 \times 200$. The red-cell count would therefore be $N \times 10,000$.

Reference ranges

Men $4\cdot5–6\cdot5 \times 10^{12}$/litre
Women $4\cdot0–5\cdot5 \times 10^{12}$/litre
Infants (newborn) $4\cdot0–6\cdot0 \times 10^{12}$/litre
Children (3 months) $3\cdot2–4\cdot8 \times 10^{12}$/litre
Children (1–12 years) $3\cdot6–5\cdot4 \times 10^{12}$/litre.

Technical errors

These may be caused by:
(*a*) Bad sampling due to stasis caused by prolonged use of the tourniquet or a poor flow of blood from a peripheral sample.
(*b*) Insufficient mixing of sample and dilution.
(*c*) Failure to wipe off excess blood from side of pipette.
(*d*) Incorrect pipetting of blood or diluent.
(*e*) Poor technique in filling counting chamber.
(*f*) Counting before cells have settled.

(*g*) Counting after dilution has been allowed to dry in the counting chamber.
(*h*) Inaccurate counting which may be caused by fatigue or inexperience.
(*i*) Incorrect calculation.

These are operator errors which can be eliminated. A further technical error is that which is caused by inaccurately calibrated pipettes. The accuracy of pipettes must be established before attempting to use them for blood counts. In the case of $20\,\mu l$ and $50\,\mu l$ pipettes mercury is drawn up to the mark, expelled on to a watch glass and weighed. $20\,\mu l$ of mercury weigh $272\,mg$ and $50\,\mu l$ weigh $680\,mg$.

Inherent error

Even in a perfectly mixed sample the cells in a counting chamber settle in an irregular pattern. This random distribution occurs according to a mathematical distribution—Poisson series—and if the mean of the cells counted in similar areas is M then the standard error will be $\sqrt{M}$. This is an indication of the variation in counts that can be expected between areas of the same size. If we take twice the standard error we can expect that in 95 out of 100 areas the count would fall within the range $\pm\sqrt{2M}$. If we assume that in the 80 small squares quoted above the mean of the cells counted (M) is 500:

Standard error $= \sqrt{M} = \sqrt{500} = 22$.
In 95% of the areas the counts would fall within the range $\pm2\sqrt{M} = 500 \pm 44$ which is the same as saying that there would be a 95% chance that the number of cells actually counted would be between 456 and 544. The red-cell count would be $5\cdot0 \pm 0\cdot44 \times 10^{12}$/litre.

Clearly inherent error has a considerable influence on visual cell counting. The only way to reduce the error is to count more cells. If 160 small squares were counted one would arrive at a mean of 1000.

$2\sqrt{1000} = 64$, i.e. a range of 936–1064.
The red-cell count would be $5\cdot0 \times 10^{12}$/litre $\pm 6\cdot4\%$.

White-cell count

The diluting fluid used for white-cell counts is 20 ml/litre acetic acid coloured pale violet with gentian violet. The acetic acid lyses the red cells and leaves the white cells intact and faintly stained. A dilution of 1 in 20 is made by washing $50\,\mu l$ of blood into 0·95 ml of diluting fluid. The subsequent steps are the same as for the red-cell count until the counting stage is arrived at. The cells in the four outer corner squares are counted. This is equivalent to an area of $4\,mm^2$ (Fig. 29.4) and as the depth is 0.1 mm, the volume is $0.4\,\mu l$.

If the number of cells counted in $0.4\,\mu l = N$ then the number of cells in $1\,\mu l = N/0.4 \times 1 = N \times 2.5$
but the dilution of blood was 1 in 20
therefore the number of cells in $1\,\mu l$ of blood $= N \times 2.5 \times 20 = N \times 50$
and the number of cells in 1 litre of blood $= N \times 50 \times 10$.

Reference range

$4.0–11.0 = 10^9$/litre.

Causes of error

The causes of error in the white-cell count are the same as in the red-cell count. The inherent error is, however, greater because of the smaller number of cells normally expected in the areas counted. Assuming the count is performed in the manner described above, one can expect in a normal count in the upper range (say 10×10^9/litre) to count a mean of 200 cells. The standard error would be $M = \sqrt{200} = 14$ approximately. The range that one would expect 95 times out of 100 would be $2\sqrt{200} = 2 \times 14 = 28$, i.e. 172–228.

The result of the white-cell count could be reported as low as 8.6×10^9/litre and as high as 11.4×10^9/litre.

This is alarming and the only way to improve on this inherent error is to count more cells. It is fortunate that the error in white-cell counts is not as important as the error in a red-cell count, although in the sample quoted the result may fall inside or outside the reference range!

Platelet count

The diluting fluid for platelet counts should be free of all particulate matter which might be mistaken for platelets. It should maintain the platelets without clumping and render the erythrocytes less conspicuous. In the ammonium oxalate reagent below, the red cells appear as ghosts.

Ammonium oxalate   10 g
Distilled water up to 1 litre
Filter before use

To prevent the platelets clumping the blood should be collected with EDTA anticoagulant. Plastic tubes and siliconed pipettes should be used throughout the proce-

dure because platelets rupture on contact with a water-wettable surface.

The preliminary stages of the platelet count are the same as the white-cell count. Once the chamber has been filled it is placed in a Petri dish containing damp cotton wool and left for 20 min. Platelets take this time to settle because they are small and of low density. The damp cotton wool keeps the chamber moist and prevents evaporation of the diluting fluid. The platelets are counted with a ×40 objective. They are best observed with only a small amount of light passing through the microscope's substage condenser when they will appear as small, round, refractile bodies. The central square of the chamber is counted in the same manner as the red-cell count. The calculation, however, is different because the dilution is 1 in 20. The calculation now becomes:

$N \times 5 \times 10 \times 20 = N \times 1000$

Reference range

150–400 $\times$ 10^9/litre.

Technical errors

The platelet count suffers from the same technical errors as the red-cell count but in addition the following must be considered.

(a) Some platelets are destroyed on contact with glass.

(b) Anticoagulants other than EDTA cause clumping.

(c) Particulate matter in diluting fluids can resemble platelets.

(d) If counts are performed on capillary blood platelets are lost due to adherence to the wound. Clumping also occurs.

Inherent error

In a normal platelet count one can expect to count, for example, a mean number of 225 cells. This would mean a platelet count which would range between 195 and 255 $\times$ 10^9/litre; an inherent error of $\pm 13\%$.

It is clear that visual counting methods are inaccurate. However, if great care is taken to avoid technical errors, and large numbers of cells are counted to reduce inherent error, a result can be achieved which may be a reasonable reflection of the true count. The result must always be considered in the light of the method's weaknesses.

30. The blood film

Having counted the white cells, red cells or platelets the next step is the examination of a stained blood film to establish their morphology and distribution; an essential part of any haematological investigation.

PREPARATION OF BLOOD FILMS

Blood films should be made as soon as possible after the sample has been taken. The preferred anticoagulant is sequestrene which has the least effect on cellular morphology. Use chemically cleaned, grease-free slides. Place a drop of blood on the centre of the slide about 15 mm from one end (Fig. 30.1). Another glass slide is used as a 'spreader'. Place the end of the spreader (which must be smooth and free from chips) in the middle of the glass slide and draw it back until it touches the drop of blood which will run along the edge. Push the spreader forward smoothly and the blood will be drawn along, forming a film on the slide. The angle at which the spreader should be held is about 40–45°. The thickness and length of the film will depend on the angle of the spreader, the size of the drop of blood and the speed at which the spreader is pushed forward. The spreader may have a bevelled end so that the film will be narrower than the slide. Dry the film immediately by waving the slide in the air. The stream of air from an electric fan may also be used. The film will be thick at the head and thin at the tail. The aim is to spread a film, about 35 mm long, which has all the white cells evenly dispersed throughout. Unfortunately the tendency in blood films made on slides is for the larger cells, monocytes and granulocytes, to move towards the edges and the tail. This concentration is greater in a badly prepared film and is particularly evident in the long thin ragged tails produced by a spreader with a worn or dirty edge. If the film is allowed to dry slowly the red cells will be distorted and stick together giving the appearance of piles of coins (rouleaux). Once made the film may be identified by writing in soft pencil on the film itself the name of the patient and any other information such as date or number.

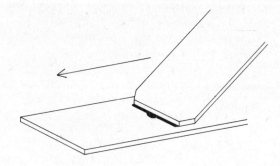

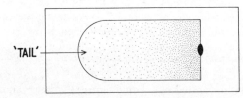

Fig. 30.1.   Preparation of a blood film.

STAINING

The affinity of a cell for particular stains depends upon the nature of its constituents. The acidic structures take up basic dyes, and the basic structures take up acidic dyes. The acidophilic or basophilic property of the cell is subject to the reaction of the medium in which it is suspended and staining will therefore vary with the pH of buffers used for the staining procedure.

The Romanowsky group of stains in general use for the staining of blood films produce their delicate nuances of colour as the result of a combination of methylene blue and eosin dyes. Romanowsky used an old solution of methylene blue which had oxidised producing methylene blue azure compounds. He combined this 'polychromed' methylene blue with eosin and produced a precipitate of neutral dye. Leishman, Wright and Giemsa are stains in the Romanowsky group which vary in their method of polychroming the methylene blue. Jenner and May–Grunwald stains do not belong to this category as they do not contain polychromed methylene blue. The particular compounds responsible for the staining effect are azure B and eosin Y.

The type of stain used, and the details of the method employed, are subject to preference and prejudice; but popular choice seems to lie between Leishman's stain used on its own, and Giemsa's stain used in combination with Jenner's or May–Grunwald's stains.

Fixation

As soon as possible after its preparation the blood film should be 'fixed'. This is a process which fixes the cells so that they do not deteriorate by chemical or putrefactive change. The agent (fixative) used precipitates protein and inactivates the enzymes which promote the degeneration of the cells. It also prevents the cells being lysed when treated with aqueous stains.

Buffers

The acidophilic or basophilic properties of cells depend on the reaction of their surroundings. With the Romanowsky stains a slightly acid solution will accentuate the eosin character of the dye and a slightly alkaline reaction will favour azure B. The pH of distilled water used must be stabilised, and for this purpose buffers are used. A suitable buffer is Sörenson's phosphate buffer. Two solutions are prepared:

Solution A: potassium dihydrogen phosphate
20·4 g/litre
Solution B: disodium hydrogen phosphate
21·3 g /litre

From these solutions a working solution is made containing 50·8 ml of solution A and 49·2 ml of solution B. 50 ml of this solution added to 1 litre of distilled water will maintain a pH of 6·8.

May–Grunwald Giemsa method

The combination of the two stains compensates for the poor nuclear staining which is characteristic of May–Grunwald stain when used on its own.

May–Grunwald stain

Add 3·0 g of the powdered stain to 1 litre of acetone-free methanol. Bring the solution up to a temperature of 50°C, remove the source of heat and allow to cool slowly. Incubate at 37°C for 24 hours. Shake at intervals. Filter before use.

Giemsa stain

Add 1 g of powdered stain to 66 ml of glycerol. Heat the mixture at 50°C for 2 hours then add 66 ml of acetone-free methanol. Mix well and allow to stand at room temperature for a week. Filter before use.

Procedure

Fix the blood film by placing it in a staining jar of methanol (5 min), transfer to a jar of May–Grunwald stain which has been diluted 1 in 2 with buffered water. Stain for 5 min. Allow to drain and transfer to a jar of Giemsa stain diluted 1 in 10 with buffered water. Stain for 15 min. Transfer to a jar of buffered water for 5 min. This last stage washes out excess stain and is known as differentiation. Remove the slide from the buffered water and allow to drain and dry in air.

Leishman's method

This method does not require prior fixation of the blood film as the stain is dissolved in methanol and used undiluted in the first stage.

Leishman's stain

Weigh out 1·5 g of powder and place in a flask. Add 1 litre of methanol and heat the mixture to a temperature of 50°C for 15 min. Allow to stand at room temperature for 1–2 weeks. Filter before use.

Procedure

Place the blood film on a staining rack and cover the slide with the stain. After 2 min add twice the volume of buffered water. Mix carefully with a Pasteur pipette. After 7–10 min wash off the stain with buffered water. Leave the buffered water on the slide for 1–2 min. Wipe excess stain off the back of the slide and allow the film to drain and dry in air.

In each of the above procedures the correct staining times are arrived at by experimentation. A cover slip may be placed on the film to complete the preparation. This is a rectangle of glass large enough to cover the whole film. It is stuck to the glass slide with a drop of neutral mountant which will preserve the staining for many years. Alternatively the film may be left un-mounted and immediately prior to examination a thin film of immersion oil should be spread over its surface. This has the advantages of speed—neutral mountant takes time to dry—whilst still allowing the use of a low-power dry lens and an oil-immersion lens.

The importance of the blood film in haematological diagnosis cannot be over-stressed. A satisfactory pre-paration requires attention to the technique of spread-ing, the quality of stain, the choice of stain, staining times, pH and an awareness of the possibility of batch variation. A standardised staining procedure increases the confidence of the observer at the microscope. Automatic staining machines, as well as being conve-nient to use, have an advantage over manual proce-dures in the production of uniformly stained films.

The examination of a blood film requires the observation of three elements—erythrocytes, leuco-cytes and platelets. These will be briefly considered.

ERYTHROCYTES (RED CELLS)

Erythrocytes are the end-product of a system which starts with an undifferentiated pluripotential stem cell, progresses to the next stage—a committed erythroid cell—through to a recognisable proerythroblast and onward to the mature cell. Throughout these stages the nucleus gradually decreases in size to the reticulocyte which has no nucleus at all. The final stage is the red cell. A substance called erythropoietin, formed in the kidney, is one of the humoral factors which have an influence on the formation of the erythrocyte. As the cell matures its content of haemoglobin increases.

Under the microscope the mature red cell appears as a biconcave disc without a nucleus. Its function is to protect and transport haemoglobin (p. 223) and it is therefore an agent for supplying oxygen to, and remov-ing carbon dioxide from, the tissues.

A reduction in haemoglobin or red cell numbers would result in a shortage of oxygen available for the tissues. In this situation a patient could be considered to be 'short of breath'—a symptom of anaemia.

Many complex chemical changes occur in the red cell to enable it to survive, change shape, maintain haemo-globin and allow the passage of gases across its mem-brane. The average life-span of the mature red cell in the circulation is 120 days, after which it disintegrates and is ingested by the large phagocytic cells (macro-phages) of the reticuloendothelial system. The iron

from the haemoglobin is stored in the marrow and the pigment is excreted in the faeces as stercobilinogen.

The number of red cells which we would expect to find in normal blood is

Men	$4 \cdot 5 – 6 \cdot 5 \times 10^{12}$/litre.
Women	$4 \cdot 0 – 5 \cdot 5 \times 10^{12}$/litre.
Infants (newborn)	$4 \cdot 0 – 6 \cdot 0 \times 10^{12}$/litre.
Children (3 months)	$3 \cdot 2 – 4 \cdot 8 \times 10^{12}$/litre.
Children (1–12 years)	$3 \cdot 6 – 5 \cdot 4 \times 10^{12}$/litre.

Reticulocytes

As red cell maturation proceeds it arrives at a stage where all the nuclear material has disappeared leaving ribosomes—material derived from the cytoplasm of the precursor cell. This material is dispersed by the metha-nol used in Romanowsky stain and takes up the basic portion of the stain resulting in a blue-grey appearance known as polychromasia.

Ribosomes may be stained by a special technique known as 'supravital' staining (*see* p. 235); a reaction which takes place only in unfixed preparations. The cell is called a reticulocyte. A count of circulating reticulo-cytes is an important indication of the rate of red-cell production in the bone marrow. A count above the normal (1–2%) will indicate that the marrow is re-sponding to a call for the replacement of lost red cells.

LEUCOCYTES (WHITE CELLS)

These cells derive their name from their greyish-white appearance when they are concentrated together to form a layer on the top of a column of blood. Leuco-cytes exist to defend the body against the invasion of foreign particles or bacteria. This defence is provided by the process of phagocytosis (engulfing or 'eating' the invading foreign substance) or by the production of an immune response. An immune response is the produc-tion of substances (antibodies) which will react against and destroy the foreign invader. The term antigen is applied to a substance which will stimulate the produc-tion of antibodies.

The number of white cells in the peripheral blood of normal adults falls within the range $4–11 \times 10^9$/litre, and in children within the range $8–16 \times 10^9$/litre. An increase in the total count is termed a leucocytosis and a decrease a leucopenia. There is a rhythmical variation in the count during the day (diurnal variation) depend-ing on various factors such as physical exercise, emo-tional stress and eating; but when these factors are taken into consideration the levels are remarkably constant in each individual. The cells in the circulation are replaced several times each day; some, the lymphocytes, recirculating via the lymph nodes and thoracic duct and others, the monocytes and granulocytes, being replaced by newly matured cells.

All the leucocytes have nuclei, a feature which readily differentiates them from the mature erythrocyte. The universally employed Romanowsky dyes are used for the examination of blood films and in the following discussion of the five types of leucocyte encountered in the normal blood film their appearances when fixed and stained by one of these dyes are described.

Granulocytes

These cells have distinct granules in their cytoplasm which, according to their affinity for the acidic or basic part of the Romanowsky dye, can be divided into neutrophils, eosinophils and basophils. Their nuclei can contain several lobes.

Neutrophils

The full name of this cell is the polymorphonuclear neutrophil. As its name implies its nucleus can consist of several lobes and the granules of the cytoplasm have neutral affinity for the stain. Its diameter is $10-12\,\mu m$. The purple-staining nucleus contains from 2 to 5 lobes joined together by fine filaments of chromatin. The many fine granules in the cytoplasm give it a purplish-pink appearance. It had long been considered that the number of lobes in the nucleus was an indication of its maturity. From this arose methods of performing differential counts according to the degree of lobulation of the nucleus. The maturation process would be represented with the most immature cells on the left and the most mature on the right.

From these schemes arose the expression 'shift to the left' which means that there is an increase in single or bilobed immature neutrophils, and 'shift to the right' which describes the presence of hypersegmented nuclei in the neutrophils and is usually associated with megaloblastic anaemia but which can also be seen in infections. However, although band forms (sausage-shaped nucleus) appear to be some 24 hours younger than the rest of the lobulated forms, it is believed that the so-called mature forms derive the number of their nuclear lobes from the indentations in the nucleus of the precursor stem cells.

The function of neutrophils is to capture and destroy invading organisms as soon as they enter the body. The cells move along in an amoeboid fashion, flowing easily through small spaces. They migrate *via* the blood stream, being attracted to the infecting organism by a process known as chemotaxis. The bacteria are then removed by phagocytosis. In superficial infections the bacteria are eliminated as pus. In deeper infections they are removed in faeces, urine and sputum.

Neutrophils are the most numerous of the white cells in the bloodstream, reference range $2\cdot5-7\cdot5 \times 10^9$/litre. High counts occur in many stress conditions such as burns, surgical operations, pregnancy and hard exercise. A large meal may also produce a high count.

A prolonged infection calls upon the marrow to increase its production of neutrophils and those cells which are released into the bloodstream are the previously described immature band forms. A feature often accompanying severe infections and toxic states is that known as 'toxic granulation' where corase, heavy, darkly staining granules are seen in the cytoplasm. Low neutrophil counts can be found following radiotherapy or chemotherapy for malignant conditions, in conditions where the marrow has gradually ceased to function, or sometimes towards the end of an overwhelming infection such as pneumonia when a sudden drop in the count seems to indicate exhaustion of the body's reserves of resistance.

Eosinophils

The polymorphonuclear eosinophil is generally the same shape and size as the neutrophil. Its nucleus is typically bilobed but variations do occur. Its cytoplasmic granules have an affinity for the eosin portion of the dye and appear yellowish/red. These granules are much larger than in the neutrophil; so large indeed that they often obscure the nucleus.

The normal eosinophil count is $0\cdot1-0\cdot44 \times 10^9$/litre of blood. They are found in the peripheral blood, the bone marrow, the epithelial lining of the respiratory tract, the large bowel and the skin. Eosinophilia—an increased count—is found most commonly in infestations and allergic conditions. Eosinophils have a phagocytic function which is aimed mainly at antigen/antibody complexes. They counteract the effects of histamine and assist in wound repair.

Basophils

The polymorphonuclear basophil is slightly smaller

than the neutrophil and eosinophil, being on the average $10\,\mu m$ in diameter. The nucleus is usually slightly indented or bilobed and the slightly basophilic cytoplasm contains large purple-blue granules which obscure the nucleus. The granules are water-soluble and may be dissolved during prolonged staining procedures leaving a vacuolated cytoplasm. The granules contain heparin and histamine. Basophils can be seen gathering around inflammatory lesions where they release their histamine. Their phagocytic activity is much less than the other granulocytes.

The normal basophil count rarely exceeds $0.1 \times 10^9/$litre. Some of the conditions where it may be increased are chickenpox, chronic sinus infections, ulcerative colitis and chronic myeloid leukaemia.

Monocytes

The monocyte, the largest cell normally seen in peripheral blood, is a cell with a large irregularly shaped nucleus and bluish-grey cytoplasm displaying a ground-glass appearance. Its size ranges from 16 to $20\,\mu m$ in diameter and up to $0.8 \times 10^9/$litre may be found normally in adult blood.

The monocyte is phagocytic and is capable of ingesting larger foreign particles affording protection against those bacteria with lipoid capsules such as tubercle and leprosy bacilli. An increased count, known as monocytosis, is found in conditions such as tuberculosis and chronic bronchitis.

Lymphocytes

Lymphocytes are round cells approximately $7-10\,\mu m$ in diameter with a round or slightly indented nucleus which fills most of the cell leaving a small rim of pale blue cytoplasm. Occasional azurophilic granules may be seen in the cytoplasm. Nucleoli are present in all lymphocytes but are not always demonstrated by the usual staining methods.

About 5% of the circulating lymphocytes measure $13-20\,\mu m$ in diameter. They have a less-dense irregular nucleus which is surrounded by a large volume of clear pale blue cytoplasm. These cells are known as large lymphocytes. There are also intermediate forms between the small and large lymphocyte.

The normal adult count is between 1.5 and $4.5 \times 10^9/$litre. Children have a higher count, up to $10 \times 10^9/$litre with a higher proportion of large lymphocytes. A count above the normal range is termed a lymphocytosis and

can be found in infectious diseases such as whooping cough, measles, glandular fever and infective hepatitis. The term lymphopenia is applied to a count below the normal range. Radiotherapy and drug therapy can account for this.

Lymphocytes play a major role in protecting the body from invasion by 'foreign' substances. They have long been associated with the production of antibodies because of the swollen lymph glands, packed with lymphocytes, which were observed in infections. As a result of much experimental work in recent years it is suggested that there are two populations of lymphocytes which, although similar in appearance, have different functions and are derived from different parts of the body.

In experimental work on the chicken it was found that a lymphoid organ—the Bursa of Fabricius—was responsible for the production of lymphocytes which would ultimately produce humoral antibody (antibody which circulates in the blood and tissue fluids). These lymphocytes were different from other cells which were influenced by the thymus. The 'thymus-processed' cells would eventually contain antibody-like molecules on their surface and be responsible for cell-mediated immunity. They are thought to have a very long life-span, possibly 10–20 years.

The two types of cells are called T-lymphocytes (influenced by or derived from the thymus) and B-lymphocytes (bursa-dependent).

Mammals have no single equivalent to the avian bursa. Their lymphocytes, however, are of a similar nature and recent experimental work indicates that B-lymphocytes originate in the bone marrow, with full maturation occurring in the spleen, lymph nodes and lymphoid tissue of the gut. The life-span of these cells appears to be 3–4 days, after which they disintegrate and their component material is recycled to form more lymphocytes.

On contact with an antigen B-lymphocytes are able to transform themselves into antibody-producing cells, the new cell being a plasma cell. The antibody protein produced by plasma cells acts upon bacteria by making them more easily subject to phagocytosis and by neutralising their toxins, etcetera.

T-lymphocytes recognise foreign substances and dictate to the B-lymphocytes the type of antibody which they must produce to inactivate the invader. They also hold in their 'memory' information regarding the particular antigen so that when the antigen is re-introduced the corresponding antibody can be mobilised more quickly and efficiently than the first time. This is termed the secondary response. In this way, because of the long life-span of T-lymphocytes, prolonged immunity is possible.

Referring to the thymus when discussing T-lymphocytes, and to the avian Bursa of Fabricius when discussing B-lymphocytes is a starting point in the study of these cells and it could be inferred that their pathways are distinct and separate. However, the maintenance of the body's immune mechanism is controlled by the interdependence of T and B cells and their delicate responses to each other in producing specific reactions to foreign protein.

Certain infections may be overcome without the production of antibody. Transplanted tissue is rejected in a similar manner. Large numbers of T-lymphocytes gather around the foreign substance and destroy it. This reaction is known as a cell-mediated response. Other examples are the local reactions of smallpox vaccination and the tuberculin test.

PLATELETS (THROMBOCYTES)

Platelets in the circulation vary in size from 1·5 to 4 μm. They are discoid in shape and appear as pale blue bodies containing red granules. In health the platelet count ranges from 150×10^9/litre to 400×10^9/litre. A count above the range is called a thrombocytosis; and below, a thrombocytopenia.

Platelets are fragments of the cytoplasm of very large cells, which are normally found in the bone marrow, called megakaryocytes. Megakaryocytes range in diameter from 50 to 100 μm, and have a multi-lobed nucleus and abundant cytoplasm.

The size of platelets is not now considered to be an indication of their maturity. Variation in platelet size is felt to be a reflection of the state of megakaryocyte production. The life-span of circulating platelets ranges from 8 to 12 days. Their functions are all connected with blood coagulation and will be discussed in Chapter 32.

OBSERVATION OF THE FILM

It is only by recognising the normal patterns of a blood film that abnormalities, when they occur, will be apparent. The observation of many normal blood films produces an awareness of the degree of variation which may occur in the staining and the distribution of cells without their being considered abnormal. The first approach to blood film observation, therefore, should be confined to the perusal of a large number of normal films. The approach should be systematic, following a pattern which will include red cells, white cells and platelets. The film should first be scanned using a low-power objective ($\times$10). This will give an impression of the distribution of the cells and an indication of the quality of the preparation. Subsequent examination with a high-power ($\times$50) lens will provide a more detailed appreciation of the cells. The area just before the tail of the film is where the red cells are evenly distributed without overlapping. At the head of the film the cells are too crowded and at the tail they have a flattened appearance.

When examining the film observe the size, shape and colour of the red cells and white cells. Look for precursor cells, inclusion bodies in the red cells, and rouleaux. Observe the number and size of the platelets.

Erythrocytes

Terms used to describe morphology and staining of red cells.

Anisocytosis. Variation in size to a greater degree than the normal. Present in many blood disorders.

Macrocytosis. Majority of cells larger than normal.

Microcytosis. Majority of cells smaller than normal.

Polychromasia. When reticulocytes are fixed in methanol their reticular material is evenly dispersed throughout the cell. The material stains bluish-grey.

Hypochromia. Cells stain paler than normal and are unusually thin or lack haemoglobin. The most usual cause is iron-deficiency anaemia.

Poikilocytosis. Variation in shape. Indication of abnormal erythropoiesis.

Elliptocytosis. Elliptocytes are oval or elliptical-shaped cells normally present in very small numbers.

Spherocytosis. A tendency towards a spherical shape rather than the flatter disc-like appearance of the normal red cell and therefore staining more deeply.

Schistocytes. Red-cell fragments—indicative of haemolytic anaemia.

Target cells. Abnormally thin red cells. The haemoglobin stains in a thin rim around the edge and at the centre, presenting the appearance from which its name is derived.

Leptocytes. Abnormally thin red cells. The haemoglobin stains as a thin rim around the edge. A variation of this is the target cell.

Burr cell. Red cell showing a few irregularly spaced spinous projections.

Crenated cells. Red cells with regularly spaced spines, this regularity differentiating them from burr cells. They are artifacts of a badly made film or stored blood.

Sickle cells. Holly-leaf or sickle-shaped cells.

Rouleaux. The red cells stick together one on top of another, presenting the appearance of piles of coins. The condition is caused by a high concentration of plasma proteins and is associated with diseases having a plasma protein imbalance. False rouleaux may be formed when a blood film is allowed to dry slowly leaving a high concentration of protein on the surface.

Red-cell inclusions

The presence of inclusion bodies in the red cells should be noted.

Howell-Jolly body. Eccentrically placed, well-defined purple dot about $1\,\mu m$ in diameter. It is a remnant of nuclear material. One or more bodies may be present; occurring in haemolytic and megaloblastic anaemia. They are also present after splenectomy when they are sometimes known as post-splenectomy bodies.

Punctate basophilia (basophilic stippling). Fine bluish-black granules scattered over the surface of the red cell. The cells contain ribosomes and are reticulocytes. Their presence is a sign of immaturity and is particularly associated with lead poisoning.

Heinz bodies. Although these red-cell inclusions are not observed in Romanowsky preparations they are occasionally seen in reticulocyte preparations and should be recognised. They appear as blue dots, often more than one per cell, and are complexes of denatured globin produced as a result of chemical poisoning or abnormal haemoglobin synthesis.

Leucocytes

An estimation of the relative numbers of the different leucocytes is often required, for which a differential count is performed. 100 or 200 leucocytes are examined and the number of each type is expressed as a percentage of the total. By multiplying each percentage by the total leucocyte count the count for each cell type may be obtained. A differential leucocyte count performed without great care is of doubtful value. The principal objection is that, as previously stated, the distribution of cells in a blood film is such that the larger cells, neutrophils and monocytes, congregate in the tail and at the edges. To compensate for this uneven distribution several methods of counting have been introduced which involve tracing paths of different shapes. Whichever method is used the differential count is still dependent upon a well-spread film. The interpreter of a differential leucocyte count must be aware of its inaccuracy.

The film should be perused with a low-power objective to establish that the cells are evenly distributed. If, for example, there is a conglomeration of neutrophils in the tail the film should be discarded. An area is chosen where all the cells are evenly spread without overlapping. Using a high-power objective the cells are counted following a path as indicated in Fig. 30.2.

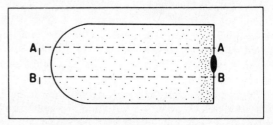

Fig. 30.2. Scheme for differential white cell counts. Count all white cells along path A–A$_1$; if insufficient cells have been counted continue along path B–B$_1$. Each path must be completed as it contains the cells spread from the original drop.

Differential leucocyte counts are expressed in absolute numbers in the same manner as the total leucocyte count. This allows direct comparison with the reference ranges below.

Differential leucocyte count: reference ranges

Neutrophils	$2 \cdot 5$–$7 \cdot 5 \times 10^9$/litre.
Lymphocytes	$1 \cdot 5$–$4 \cdot 0 \times 10^9$/litre.
Monocytes	$0 \cdot 2$–$0 \cdot 8 \times 10^9$/litre.
Eosinophils	$0 \cdot 1$–$0 \cdot 4 \times 10^9$/litre.
Basophils	0–$0 \cdot 15 \times 10^9$/litre.

The neutrophil count, for example, may be calculated thus:

Total number of leucocytes counted $= 200$
Number of neutrophils counted $\quad= 126$
Total leucocyte count $\qquad\qquad= 8\cdot0 \times 10^9$/litre

Neutrophil count $\qquad = \dfrac{126}{200} \times 8\cdot0 = 5\cdot4 \times 10^9$/litre

Neutrophil leucocytosis. An increase in the number of neutrophils may be the result of infection, pregnancy, surgical operation, vigorous exercise or emotional stress.

Lymphocytosis. An increase in lymphocytes may be caused by infectious mononucleosis (glandular fever), measles, or whooping cough.

Monocytosis. An increase in monocytes some of the causes of which are infectious mononucleosis, malaria and viral infections.

Eosinophilia. An increased eosinophil count may be the result of various allergic reactions, asthma, hay fever and intestinal parasites.

Basophilia. An increased number of basophils may be present in some virus infections, some malignant conditions and allergies. Basophilia is infrequently seen.

Neutropenia. A reduction in neutrophils may be evidenced in conditions of overwhelming infection, aplastic anaemia or treatment with drugs.

Lymphopenia. A reduced lymphocyte count may occur as a result of treatment with drugs.

There are many causes of increased or decreased counts, a few examples only have been given.

Observations on the maturity of cells should also be made and, in the case of the neutrophils, it is appropriate to use the terms 'shift to the left', 'shift to the right' and 'toxic granulation' (*see* p. 231) if applicable.

The presence of immature white cells or a gross increase in the number of a particular cell, or a combination of these and other features may lead the observer to suspect leukaemia. This is a neoplastic disease characterised by an abnormal proliferation of a specific cell type. The classification of the different leukaemias and their origins are tasks of great complexity, and are the subject of much debate which will not be covered in this book.

Platelets

With experience it is possible to conclude whether platelets are present in normal, increased or decreased numbers. Abnormalities may be checked by performing a platelet count. A reduced number of platelets may be caused by, for example, drugs, radiation treatment, chemicals, or even the presence of a small clot in the blood sample from which the film was taken. Increased platelets may be associated with haemorrhage, removal of the spleen, infections and many other conditions.

RETICULOCYTE COUNTS

The ribosomes of reticulocytes, when stained by a supravital stain, appear as filamentous strands or dots. The stain should contain an anticoagulant and, to avoid distortion of the red cells, should be isotonic. A suitable solution is:

Brilliant cresyl blue	1·00 g
Sodium chloride	0·85 g
Sodium citrate	0·45 g
Distilled water	100 ml

The reagent should be filtered before use.

Method. Place four drops of stain in a 75×10 mm tube. Add four drops of venous or capillary blood. Mix and incubate at 37°C for 20 min. Using the mixture as if it were blood make a blood film (p. 228). Examine the film under a high-power objective. Reticulocytes are those red cells which contain dark blue filamentous strands or, in the case of the more mature reticulocytes, dark blue dots. Select an area of the film where the cells are evenly dispersed without overlapping, and where the cells number approximately 100 in each field. If the film has been satisfactorily spread successive fields across its width should contain a similar number of cells. Count the number of reticulocytes in each of ten such fields and calculate the percentage. When the reticulocyte count is low it is recommended that the successive fields should be surveyed until 100 reticulocytes are counted.

If 100 reticulocytes were counted in 50 fields and each field contained approximately 80 red cells the total red cells counted would be 4000 therefore reticulocyte percentage equals

$$\frac{100}{4000} \times 100 = 2\cdot5\%$$

BONE-MARROW BIOPSY

The site usually chosen for bone-marrow biopsy in the adult is the sternum. An alternative site, the iliac crest, may be used when there is a difficulty in obtaining a specimen from the sternum. The tibia or iliac crest is used in children. The biopsy is performed by a doctor using a needle designed for the procedure which should have a well-fitting stilette and an adjustable guard which will control the depth of the puncture. Two such needles are the Salah and Klima needles illustrated in Fig. 30.3. Once the needle has penetrated the marrow cavity the stilette is removed and a syringe is fitted so that bone marrow may be withdrawn. Once the marrow aspirate has been obtained films should be made immediately, before the sample has clotted.

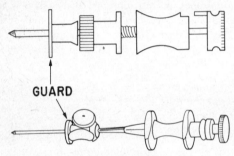

GUARD

Fig. 30.3.   Types of marrow needle
Top: Klima needle.
Bottom: Salah needle.

Six or eight slides are laid out and on to each are placed two drops of the aspirate. On each slide should be a mixture of blood and marrow particles. The blood is drawn back into the syringe leaving the particles of marrow which are then spread along the slide in the manner of a peripheral-blood film. The particles should leave a trail of cells as they are drawn along the slide. Along this trail a differential count of nucleated cells may be performed. The films are fixed in methanol for 10 min. The remainder of the contents of the syringe is expelled on to a watch glass and allowed to clot. This clot is gently rolled off into a container of formol-saline and retained for processing by the histology department.

Romanowsky preparations are essential for adequate classification of the cells but other staining procedures will provide additional information; for example a staining method for iron should always be used.

The observation of a bone-marrow film follows a similar procedure to that employed with a peripheral-blood film in that the low-power objective is used to ascertain the distribution of cells, and to look for clusters of malignant cells and the presence of mega-karyocytes. A high-power objective may then be used for the closer observation of particular cells and cell groups. While the necessity for a differential count of nucleated cells does not always arise the discipline of having to identify every cell renders it a useful exercise for the beginner. However, a detailed description of the cells to be found in bone marrow is outside the scope of this book.

Myeloid: erythroid ratio

A ratio of granular cells (at all stages of their development) to nucleated red cells. This is calculated from the results of the differential count and is an indication of the rate of proliferation of these cells. The normal range lies between 2:1 and 10:1.

Aplastic or hypoplastic marrow. Production of cells is lower than normal.

Hyperplastic. Excessive production of cells.

Dry tap. Biopsy produces very few or no marrow cells or particles—the result of poor technique or a condition of myelofibrosis or aplastic anaemia.

SUPPLEMENTARY STAINING METHODS

Several staining methods are available to supplement the information supplied by the observation of a Romanowsky-stained film.

Perls' Prussian blue reaction

Iron present in red cells is released from combination with protein by acid and combines with potassium ferrocyanide to form a blue precipitate of ferric ferrocyanide. The reaction provides useful information in the investigation of the anaemias and in haemochromatosis—a condition where there is excessive storage iron in the body tissues.

Reagents

Potassium ferrocyanide	20 g/litre (solution A)
0·2 M hydrochloric acid	(solution B)
Neutral red	10 g/litre

Method

Fix the blood film in methanol for 15 min. Mix equal volumes of solution A and solution B. Stain the slide with this mixture for 10 min at 50°C. Wash the slide in running water for 30 min and stain with neutral red for 1 min. Rinse briefly in water and allow to dry in air. The iron granules appear dark blue against a pale pink background.

Periodic acid-Schiff reaction (PAS)

Periodic acid oxidises glycogen in blood cells to form aldehydes. The aldehydes in turn react with Schiff's reagent (leuco-basic fuchsin) producing a pink colour. The dye haemotoxylin is used as a counter stain so that the pink PAS-positive material stands out against a blue background.

Reagents

(a) Periodic acid. 10 g/litre.

(b) Schiff's reagent. Bubble sulphur dioxide through a solution of basic fuchsin (5·0 g/litre) for 1 hour. If the solution is not decolorised add activated charcoal (1 g/100 ml), shake and filter. Store in the dark at 4°C.

(c) Haematoxylin. 2·0 g/litre in distilled water.

Method

Fix the film in methanol for 10 min. Allow to dry in air then place in periodic acid for 10 min. Rinse in tap water and place in Schiff's reagent for 30 min. Rinse in tap water and counterstain with haematoxylin for 1 min. Wash in tap water for 1 min.

The positivity of the PAS reaction varies a great deal and there is no strongly specific response in any disease category. However, immature granulocytes react less strongly than mature granulocytes (myeloblasts are negative) and in differentiating normal lymphocytes from those of lymphocytic leukaemia the latter are more positive.

Neutrophil alkaline phosphatase

Neutrophil alkaline phosphatase is an enzyme so called because it is present in mature neutrophils and is active at an alkaline pH (9·5–10·0). The neutrophils of chronic myeloid leukaemia show very low phosphatase activity and in the differentiation between these and non-leukaemic cells the procedure is of some assistance.

Reagents

(a) Fixative. This consists of one part formaldehyde (40 g/litre) to nine parts methanol, stored at 4°C.

(b) Substrate. This consists of:

Sodium α-naphthyl phosphate	35 mg
Fast blue RR	35 mg
0·05 M Propanediol buffer (pH 9·5)	35 ml

(c) Mayer's haemalum

Haematoxylin	1 g
Potassium alum	50 g
Sodium iodide	0·2 g
Citric acid	1 g
Chloral hydrate	50 g
Distilled water	1000 ml

Dissolve the haematoxylin in the water, gently heating if necessary. Add the potassium alum and dissolve, again using gentle heat if required. Add the sodium iodate, citric acid and finally the chloral hydrate which acts as a preservative.

Method

Prepare blood films, dry in air and fix immediately in cold (0–4°C) fixative for 30 sec. Allow to dry. Immerse in substrate at room temperature for 10 min. Rinse in tap water and counterstain with Mayer's haematoxylin for 1 min. Rinse in tap water and dry.

The phosphatase present in the neutrophils frees naphthol from the substrate which combines with the dye to form a brown precipitate in the cytoplasm. The intensity of the brown colour depends upon the amount of phosphatase activity and is graded in each cell on a scale 0–4. The total score for 100 neutrophils is established and compared with the reference range of 60–90.

Because of the variable effect of anticoagulants and unstable reagents it is usual for each laboratory to establish its own reference range.

Low scores are found in chronic myeloid leukaemia and myeloblastic leukaemia.

High scores are found in polycythaemia vera, liver disease and the neutrophil leucocytosis of infections.

31. Packed-cell volume and absolute values

PACKED-CELL VOLUME

When a test tube filled with blood is centrifuged the red cells are thrown to the bottom and after a while the space they occupy becomes a constant volume which will be only minimally decreased after further prolonged centrifugation. This 'packed-cell volume' (PCV) may serve as an indication of anaemia and, in conjunction with other measurements, may be used in the calculation of 'absolute values'.

The PCV (or haematocrit) is the volume of red cells compared with the total volume of a sample of blood and is expressed in litres/litre.

There are two methods which involve centrifugation of the blood sample: a macro-method using a Wintrobe tube and a micro-method which uses a capillary tube.

Wintrobe haematocrit

To conform with British Standard Specification 4316, 1968, the Wintrobe haematocrit tube should have an overall length of 111 ± 0.5 mm, an external diameter of 6–7 mm, an internal diameter of 2.55 ± 0.15 mm and a measuring scale of 100 ± 0.5 mm.

Blood is collected into sequestrene or heparin and mixed well. Using a long Pasteur pipette the Wintrobe tube is filled exactly to the 100 mm mark. The tube is then centrifuged using a relative centrifugal force (RCF) of 2000–2300 g. RCF is the force operating on a particle compared with the force of gravity and is dependent upon the speed of the centrifuge and the radius of the head.

$$RCF = 0.00001118 \times N^2 \times r;$$
N = revolutions per minute;
r = radius in centimetres.

An RCF in the recommended range would be achieved at 3000 r/min at a radius of 22.5 cm or 3800 r/min at a radius of 15 cm. After centrifugation the height of the column of red cells (excluding the greyish-white layer of white cells and platelets known as the buffy coat) is read as a percentage of the whole-column height.

Microhaematocrit method

To comply with the BS specification the capillary tubes used for microhaematocrit should have an overall length of 75 ± 1.00 mm, an external diameter of 1.4–1.65 mm, a minimum internal diameter of 1 mm and a wall thickness of 0.22 ± 0.04 mm.

The tubes are filled with anticoagulated blood to within 15–20 mm from the end. This end is sealed in a Bunsen flame or with a plastic sealant such as Cristaseal* and the tube is centrifuged in a microhaematocrit centrifuge. This centrifuge is a specially designed instrument which produces an RCF of 12,000 g. At this force a constant PCV is reached after 5 min. The column of red cells will be seen to have lysed but the junction of the red-cell layer and plasma is sharply defined. The height of this layer is measured and expressed as a percentage of the whole-column height. Greater accuracy is achieved if a magnifying glass is used. There are specially designed microhaematocrit readers which provide a direct reading of PCV.

The PCV is a measurement which can achieve great accuracy and reproducibility. Nevertheless, there are potential errors in both the macro and micro methods which need to be considered.

Incorrect proportions of blood to anticoagulant and delay in testing may cause an alteration in cell volume. The bore of the tubes must be constant throughout their length; a condition more easily satisfied in the macro method. There is always a small volume of plasma trapped between the red cells which, in the macro method, may account for 3% of the apparent red-cell column in normal blood.

The problem of trapped plasma has been considered by the ICSH who, in 1979, published a recommendation for a reference method for the determination by centrifugation of PCV of blood. This method involves the measurement of trapped plasma by the use of radioactively-labelled human serum albumin.

* Gelman Hawksley Ltd., 10 Harrowden Road, Blackmills, Northampton.

238

Reference range of PCV

Men	0·40–0·54 litres/litre.
Women	0·37–0·47 litres/litre.
Children	0·32–0·44 litres/litre.
Infants	0·44–0·64 litres/litre.

ABSOLUTE VALUES

Absolute values are expressions of the volume and haemoglobin content of red cells calculated from the PCV, red-cell count and haemoglobin.

Mean cell volume (MCV)

The average volume of a single red cell. This indication of cell size may be useful, for example, in establishing the red-cell macrocytosis of megaloblastic anaemia or the microcytosis of iron-deficiency anaemia.

The PCV and the RBC are used in its calculation.

Example

PCV = 0·45 litres/litre; RBC = $5·0 \times 10^{12}$/litre.

The red cells in 1 litre of blood occupy a volume of 0·45 litres, therefore one red cell will occupy:

$$\frac{0·45}{5·0 \times 10^{12}} \text{ litres} = \frac{0·09}{10^{12}} \text{ litres}$$

$$= 0·09 \times 10^{-12} = 90 \times 10^{-15} = 90 \text{ femtolitres (fl)}.$$

Simplified calculation

$$\text{MCV (fl)} = \frac{\text{PCV litres/litre} \times 1000}{\text{RBC } (\times 10^{12}/\text{litre})}.$$

Reference range of MCV

76–96 fl.

Using electronic methods of red-cell counting the reference range may be narrower (82–94 fl).

Mean cell haemoglobin (MCH)

The average weight, in picograms, of haemoglobin in one red cell. The haemoglobin (Hb) and RBC are used for this calculation.

Example

Hb = 150 g/litre; RBC = $5·0 \times 10^{12}$/litre.

In each litre there are $5·0 \times 10^{12}$ red cells and 150 g of haemoglobin, therefore each red cell will contain:

$$\frac{150}{5·0 \times 10^{12}} \text{ g} = \frac{30}{10^{12}} = 30 \times 10^{-12} \text{ g} = 30 \text{ picograms (pg)}$$

Simplified calculation

$$\text{MCH (pg)} = \frac{\text{Hb (g/litre)}}{\text{RBC } (\times 10^{12}/\text{litre})}.$$

Reference range of MCH

27–32 pg.

The MCH may be unreliable because, as stated earlier, the inherent error of the red-cell count is quite high. It may on occasions be as high as 8·8%.

Mean cell haemoglobin concentration (MCHC)

The concentration of haemoglobin in the packed red cells.

Example

Hb = 150 g/litre; PCV = 0·45 litres/litre.

One litre of blood contains 0·45 litres of packed cells and 150 g of haemoglobin, therefore 150 g Hb are contained in 0·45 litres of red cells (450 ml red cells).

Concentration of haemoglobin = (150/450) × 100 = 33·3 g/dl.

A fully saturated red cell has a haemoglobin concentration of 36 g/dl. Mean cell haemoglobin is a useful guide to the degree of hypochromia present in iron-deficiency anaemia. The haemoglobin and PCV can be estimated reasonably accurately and the derived MCHC is therefore a reliable parameter.

Simplified calculation

$$\text{MCHC (g/dl)} = \frac{\text{Hb (g/litre)}}{\text{PCV (litres/litre)}} \times 10.$$

Reference range

32–36 g/dl (or 320–360 g/litre).

The absolute values described must be considered in the light of the accuracy of the parameters from which they are derived. The PCV is the most accurate, the haemoglobin next and the RBC the least accurate (certainly by manual counting methods) although electronic methods—see Chapter 33—provide a more accurate RBC from which the MCH and MCV may be derived with more confidence.

32. Haemostasis

Haemostasis is the spontaneous arrest and control of haemorrhage following injury to the blood vessels. When injury occurs a delicately balanced process is initiated which involves platelets, the coagulation factors, the fibrinolytic system and the contraction of the vessel wall. It ends with the eventual dissolution of the clot once tissue repair has been completed. The clot which forms when blood is shed is composed of strands of fibrin within which are enmeshed red cells, white cells and platelets which together give the appearance of a solid plug of blood.

PLATELET FUNCTION

Platelets are intimately involved in the haemostatic process. As soon as any vascular injury occurs collagen fibres are exposed to the circulating platelets which immediately adhere to the wall around the site of injury and release adenosine diphosphate (ADP). ADP promotes the adhesion and aggregation of further platelets until a haemostatic plug is formed over the wound. Serotonin, which may act as a vasoconstrictor, is also released along with phospholipid (platelet factor 3) which assists in coagulation.

THE VESSEL WALL

Injury to the vessel wall results in its contraction and a consequent reduction in the flow of blood. This contraction is due to vasomotor reflexes and may also be affected by substances released from the platelets at the site.

THE COAGULATION FACTORS

To avoid the confusion arising from the several names by which each coagulation factor was known an international committee agreed on a uniform nomenclature using Roman numerals. Their commonly accepted names have also been included in the list in Table 32.1 below. It will be noticed that factor VI is missing. It is

Table 32.1   Coagulation factors

Factor	Synonyms
I	Fibrinogen
II	Prothrombin
III	Tissue extract: 'thromboplastin'
IV	Calcium
V	Accelerator globulin; proaccelerin; labile factor
VII	Proconvertin; stable factor
VIII	Antihaemophilic factor (AHF)
IX	Christmas factor; plasma thromboplastin component (PTC)
X	Stuart–Prower factor
XI	Plasma thromboplastin antecedent (PTA)
XII	Hageman factor
XIII	Fibrin-stabilising factor

no longer used. The first four factors are customarily referred to by their names rather than the Roman numerals.

Fibrinogen. A protein with a molecular weight of 340,000 which is synthesised by the liver. The action of thrombin converts fibrinogen to fibrin.

Prothrombin. A protein with a molecular weight of 72,000 which is synthesised by the liver. It is vitamin K-dependent and in the absence of this vitamin prothrombin is synthesised in an inactive form.

Thromboplastin. A complex consisting of lipoprotein and phosphatides which may be extracted from tissues and which, with the assistance of factor VII, will activate the extrinsic pathway of the coagulation system.

Calcium. In its ionic state calcium is essential for certain stages in the coagulation process.

Factor V. A very unstable factor which participates in the intrinsic and extrinsic pathways.

Factor VII. This vitamin K-dependent plasma protein, it is thought, converts factor X to factor X(a) but it may also activate factor X directly.

Factor VIII. A deficiency of this factor is observed in plasma of patients with haemophilia A. It is, however, a complex molecule with a further activity, a deficiency of which is observed in Von Willebrand's disease.

Factor IX. Molecular weight 57,000. This factor is vitamin K-dependent and participates in the extrinsic pathway. A deficiency of this factor is observed in patients with Christmas Disease.

Factor X. A vitamin K-dependent factor which is activated by both intrinsic and extrinsic pathways.

Factor XI. This is one of the contact factors and is activated by Factor XII on contact with a foreign surface.

Factor XII. This contact factor activates the intrinsic pathway.

Factor XIII. Molecular weight 320,000. This factor is essential for stabilising fibrin once it has been formed. Fibrin which has been formed without the presence of this factor lacks strength and may be dissolved in 5 M urea—a phenomenon used as a test for factor XIII deficiency.

High molecular weight (HMW) kininogen. This is required for the fibrinolytic system and assists in the activation of factor XII.

Pre-kallikrein. A precursor of plasma kallikrein which is involved with HMW kininogen and factor XII in the initial contact phase of the coagulation system.

THE COAGULATION PROCESS

The fibrin which holds the cells captive in the clot is derived from the activation of prothrombin to form thrombin, an enzyme which in its turn converts fibrinogen to fibrin. These reactions require the presence of calcium ions. There are two pathways leading to the activation of prothrombin, the 'intrinsic system' and the 'extrinsic system'.

Intrinsic system

When blood contacts a foreign surface, such as exposed collagen in a vessel wall or a water-wettable surface such as a glass test tube, a series of enzyme reactions takes place involving the coagulation factors. On contact with the foreign surface pre-kallikrein and HMW kininogen assist in the activation of factor XII to form factor XIIa ('a' indicates the activated form) which enzymatically activates factor XI to factor XIa. The process continues in this manner involving factors IX, VIII and X. Activated factor X (Xa) in the presence of calcium ions, platelet factor 3 and factor V converts prothrombin to thrombin which in turn converts fibrinogen to fibrin. Factor XIII helps to stabilise the fibrin once it has been formed. This 'waterfall' or 'cascade' system is shown in Fig. 32.1.

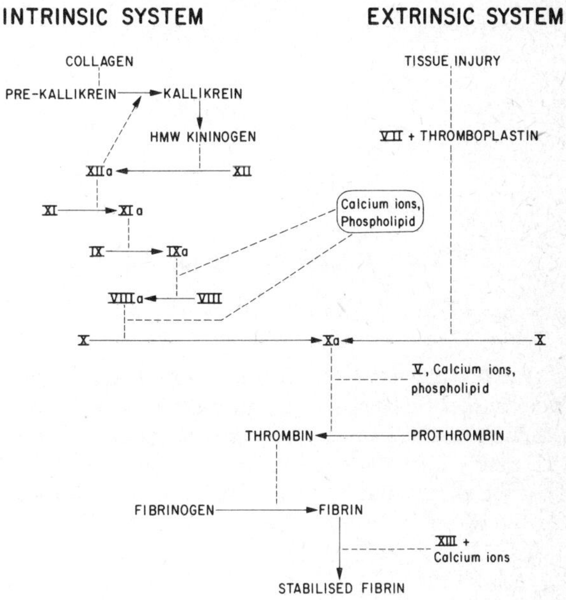

Fig. 32.1. Simplified diagram of coagulation system.

Extrinsic system

The extrinsic system is initiated when there is tissue damage. It is shorter and quicker-acting than the intrinsic system. The earlier stages of the intrinsic system are bypassed because the damaged tissue releases thromboplastin which, with the assistance of factor VII, activates factor X. From this stage it proceeds along the same pathway as the intrinsic system (Fig. 32.1).

FIBRINOLYTIC SYSTEM

The fibrinolytic system, an essential part of the haemostatic process, helps to keep the vascular system free from clots. Plasminogen present in plasma may be activated to form the proteolytic enzyme plasmin which digests fibrin and fibrinogen to form fibrin(ogen) degeneration products (FDP). The system is normally kept in balance by the presence of anti-plasmins and anti-activators (Fig. 32.2).

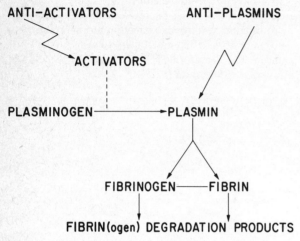

Fig. 32.2.   Simplified diagram of fibrinolytic system.

The fibrinolytic and coagulation systems are normally exquisitely balanced, as are all the factors involved in haemostasis, and in considering each mode of action separately for ease of study, it must be remembered that the checks and balances of the systems are interwoven with great complexity.

INVESTIGATION OF DISORDERED HAEMOSTASIS

A haemorrhagic disorder may be caused by:

1. A deficiency of blood coagulation factors.
2. Platelet deficiency or dysfunction.
3. Defective capillaries.
4. Excessive fibrinolysis.

Clinical history

The initial investigation of a bleeding disorder depends greatly on the patient's history. A detailed history should be taken to establish the site of bleeding and its duration. Information should be gathered on age, sex and occupation of patient; family history of bleeding tendency; drugs taken; and any previous episodes of bleeding, whether spontaneous or as the result of trauma or operation, and type of treatment given on those occasions.

The site and the type of haemorrhage may provide useful diagnostic information. The appearance of purpuric spots or bruising would suggest a platelet defect or deficiency—although these symptoms can occur in a coagulation factor deficiency. Haemorrhages from mucous membranes are also characteristic of platelet or capillary defects.

Consideration of the mode of inheritance of a possible defect is also a useful guide. A sex-linked mode of inheritance in a male could indicate a factor VIII or IX deficiency, whereas an autosomal (non-sex linked) defect could indicate Von Willebrand's disease.

Following obstetric complications or a surgical procedure such as prostatectomy the large amounts of thromboplastin which may be released not only activate the coagulation system but also stimulate the production of large quantities of plasmin. A total depletion of fibrinogen may ensue; the resultant onset of bleeding being known as the 'defibrination syndrome'. Such a history would lead to an investigation of the fibrinolytic system.

On measuring blood pressure a clinician may be aware of tiny haemorrhagic spots on the extensor surface of the patient's forearm—evidence of a vascular defect which may be inherited or due to drugs or vitamin C deficiency. The sphygmomanometer cuff, by restricting the venous return, has demonstrated a weakness of the capillary wall. This is the basis of Hess's capillary resistance test.

On the basis of such observations it may be possible to decide which part of the haemostatic process requires investigation.

Simple screening tests

The following tests are suitable for a preliminary investigation:

Full blood count.
Bleeding time.
Whole-blood clotting time.
Kaolin–cephalin clotting time.
One-stage prothrombin time.

Abnormalities in the first two tests would indicate a capillary or platelet defect, and in the last three a deficiency of one of the coagulation factors. Additionally the fibrinogen titre will be of help in the preliminary investigation of the fibrinolytic system.

Bleeding time

A prolonged bleeding time is indicative of a capillary defect, platelet dysfunction or thrombocytopenia. The ingestion of aspirin has an inhibitory effect on platelet aggregation and for this reason patients should not have taken the drug for one week prior to performing the bleeding time test.

Duke's method

Make a puncture in the tip of the patient's earlobe sufficiently deep (3 mm) to obtain a free flow of blood. Start a stop watch. Every 15 sec blot the blood with blotting paper without touching the skin, and when bleeding has ceased stop the watch and note the time.

Reference range. Up to 7 min.

Ivy method

Place a sphygmomanometer cuff around the patient's arm and inflate to a pressure of 40 mm Hg. Cleanse the forearm (extensor surface) and make three punctures at 15-sec intervals with a sterile disposable lancet. Remove the blood at 15-sec intervals with a blotting paper. Avoid touching the wound. Record the time taken for each puncture to stop bleeding and take the average of the three bleeding times.

Reference range. Up to 4 min.

Judging the depth of the stab necessary to promote a free flow of blood is difficult. In an attempt to standardise this part of the procedure templates have been introduced incorporating a blade which produces an incision of standard width and depth. These templates may be obtained commercially. However, there is a risk that these methods will produce faint scars.

Whole-blood clotting time (WBCT)

The WBCT is an insensitive test which, even when performed under strictly controlled conditions, is prolonged only when there is a marked deficiency of one of the coagulation factors. It is a test of the intrinsic system since the blood is taken directly from the vein and no tissue thromboplastin is involved. An abnormal result, therefore, indicates a deficiency of factors I, II, V, VIII, IX, X, XI or XII. Using a plastic syringe make a clean venepuncture and distribute 1 ml quantities of blood into four clean 75 × 10 mm glass test tubes which have been previously warmed to 37°C. Start a stopwatch as soon as the blood enters the syringe and place the tubes immediately into a 37°C water bath. Gently tilt the tubes in rotation at 1-min intervals until one of them can be tilted through an angle of 90° without spilling. Continue with the remaining tubes and take the average clotting time of the four tubes.

Reference range

5–10 min. Each laboratory should establish its own normal range.

Kaolin–cephalin clotting time

The reagent used for this test contains kaolin which activates the contact factors XII and XI and a phospholipid which acts as a substitute for platelets. The test is therefore sensitive to all factors in the intrinsic system. Kaolin–cephalin reagent may be obtained commercially.* It is a chloroform extract of acetone-dried brain to which light kaolin has been added.

Collect blood into trisodium citrate anticoagulant (p. 218) and obtain plasma by centrifugation. Add 0·1 ml plasma to 0·2 ml kaolin–cephalin reagent. Mix and stand in a water bath for exactly 2 min. Add 0·1 ml 0·025 M calcium chloride. Examine at 5-sec intervals and note the time taken for a clot to form. Compare the result with a normal plasma treated in the same manner.

Reference range

This is dependent on the activation time of the reagent. Figures in the range 40–55 sec can normally be expected.

Fibrinogen titre

Add 0·5 ml of saline to each of seven, 75 × 12 mm glass tubes. Add 0·5 ml of citrated plasma to the first tube, mix and carry over 0·5 ml of the mixture to the second tube. Repeat the process in each of the remaining tubes and discard 0·5 ml of the mixture from the last tube. This produces seven doubling dilutions of plasma ranging from 1 in 2 up to 1 in 128. Add 0·1 ml of thrombin* solution (20 units/ml in saline) to each tube. Incubate in a water bath at 37°C for 10 min. Examine each tube for

---

* Diagnostic Reagents Ltd., Thame, Oxon.

a clot by gently tilting it, and note the highest dilution at which fibrin clots occur. The titre is expressed as a reciprocal of the dilution.

Reference range

32–128.

As an excess of thrombin is used the action of other coagulation factors is circumvented and the test is a semi-quantitative assessment of the amount of fibrinogen present in the plasma.

One-stage prothrombin time

This test is sensitive to deficiencies of the extrinsic system. The term prothrombin time is therefore a misnomer because it not only measures factor II but also factors I, V, VIII and X; indeed the test is relatively insensitive to prothrombin deficiency. The reagent used is a tissue extract containing thromboplastin, the component produced after tissue injury which stimulates the extrinsic system. The reagent most popularly employed is a saline extract of human brain.

Reagents

Thromboplastin (saline extract of brain). Obtain a fresh human brain and remove meninges, cerebellum and blood vessels. Wash in running water, drain and remove excess water by blotting with absorbent paper. Slice the brain into small pieces and emulsify in saline using a mortar and pestle or blending machine at low revolutions. Centrifuge the emulsion at 70 g for 20 min. Use the supernatant to perform a series of prothrombin time estimations using normal plasma and dilutions of the reagent in saline (from 1 in 2 up to 1 in 10). Select the dilution which gives a clotting time of 12 sec. Dilute all the extract with phenol–saline (5·0 g phenol dissolved in 1 litre of saline) to the strength indicated, distribute in 5 ml volumes and store at 4°C. The reagent will keep for 3 months.

0·025 M calcium chloride. Dissolve 2·7 g of the salt in distilled water and make up to 1 litre.

Method. Using plastic syringes and containers obtain citrated plasma from the patient and from a normal control (p. 219). The samples should be centrifuged at 1500–2000 g for 15 min so that the plasma will be 'platelet-poor'. Into a tube in a 37°C water-bath pipette

0·1 ml of thromboplastin reagent and 0·1 ml of control plasma. Allow to warm for 2 min. Add 0·1 ml of previously warmed calcium chloride and start a stopwatch. Tilt the tube repeatedly until a clot forms and note the time. Repeat the test and take the average of the clotting time. Treat the patient's plasma similarly.

Reference range

10–14 sec.

Calculation

When reporting the prothrombin time the results may be expressed as:

$$\text{Prothrombin ratio} = \frac{\text{Patient's clotting time}}{\text{Control clotting time}}.$$

or

$$\text{Prothrombin index} = \frac{\text{Control clotting time}}{\text{Patient's clotting time}} \times 100.$$

Each report should be accompanied by a statement of the control and patient's clotting times to avoid confusion as to the method of calculating the results. The prothrombin ratio is a simple way of reporting which is readily understood.

The BCSH in 1970 recommended a scheme for the control of anticoagulant therapy which involved the use of a British comparative thromboplastin (BCT)* as a means of standardising the prothrombin time. This reagent is a standardised preparation which may be used to calibrate locally produced thromboplastin.

Using BCT five normal plasmas are tested to obtain an average normal prothrombin time. Plasma from twelve patients undergoing coumarin therapy are tested, and their ratios established. A similar procedure is followed using locally produced thromboplastin. If the results are not identical the procedure should be repeated using varying dilutions of the local thromboplastin and a dilution then selected for use which produces a mean ratio within 10% of the ratio obtained when using BCT.

Anticoagulant therapy

Anticoagulant therapy is used for the prevention of thrombosis. It interferes with the haemostatic process

* National Reference Laboratory for Anticoagulant Reagents and Control, Withington Hospital, Manchester M20 8LR.

and must, therefore, be closely controlled to prevent haemorrhage.

Coumarin–indanedione drugs

These oral anticoagulants (e.g. warfarin, dicoumarol and phenindione) act by depressing the synthesis of the vitamin K-dependent factors, II, VII, IX and X. The one-stage prothrombin time measures all these factors except IX and may be used to monitor the drugs. A level of treatment should be established which will produce prothrombin ratios between 2·0 and 4·0.

Heparin

Heparin, in conjunction with a co-factor, acts on the haemostatic mechanism by neutralising thrombin. It also has an effect on the activation of factor X. The drug is used in the treatment of deep-vein thrombosis and pulmonary embolism.

The laboratory control of this drug is the subject of much discussion. A recommended test is the kaolin–cephalin clotting time which gives an overall reflection of heparin activity. The reagent, however, should be strictly standardised by reference to a national quality control scheme.* A level of 1·5–2·5 times the normal control value would indicate adequate heparin treatment.

* National Reference Laboratory for Anticoagulant Reagents and Control, Withington Hospital, Manchester M20 8LR.

33. Automation in haematology

The high capital outlay involved in introducing automation into the haematology laboratory must be contrasted with the increased accuracy and reproducibility achieved by the equipment, its convenience in use, the amount of time saved and its effect on staffing levels.

Automated and semi-automated equipment is available for many of the routine procedures in haematology. Their commonest application has been in the electronic measurement of red-cell and white-cell counts. The principles on which electronic methods are based may be exemplified by the Coulter Counter and Technicon Autoanalyser.

THE ELECTRICAL RESISTANCE METHOD—Coulter counter*

This system depends on the measurement of the difference in electric resistance between a cell (low conductivity) and the fluid in which it is suspended (high conductivity).

A mechanical pump controlling a mercury manometer draws a known volume of diluted blood through an aperture in a glass tube (Fig. 33.1). The diluting fluid is particle-free isotonic saline. There are electrodes situated inside and outside the tube and as the diluent is an electrolyte a current will pass through the fluid from one electrode to the other. A sensing zone is created around the aperture through which each cell passes displacing its own volume of electrolyte and, because of its lower conductivity, the resistance between the two electrodes is momentarily altered. Provided the current remains steady the voltage will be proportional to the resistance. The tiny pulses produced by these changes in voltage, when amplified and counted, are equal to the number of cells.

Thresholds

Each particle passing through the aperture creates one pulse of an amplitude proportional to its volume. To obtain an accurate count of cells all pulses which represent smaller particles and background electrical noise must be eliminated. This is achieved by means of

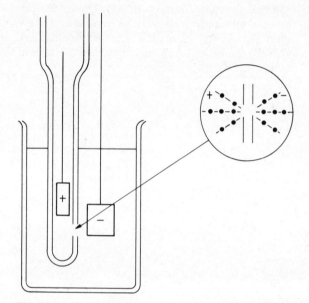

Fig. 33.1. Aperture tube of the Coulter Counter (Coulter Electronics Ltd.)

an electronic filter which can be adjusted so that pulses smaller than the cells being measured may be excluded. This setting is known as the threshold setting.

Red-cell and white-cell counts

The diluent, which may have a preservative added, is isotonic saline. For a red-cell count a dilution of 1 in 50,000 is obtained by adding $20 \mu l$ of well-mixed blood to 10 ml of saline (1 in 500). This is further diluted by taking $100 \mu l$ of the dilution and adding it to 10 ml of saline (1 in 50,000). The count may be performed, at the appropriate settings, immediately after mixing.

Before a white-cell count can be performed it is necessary to eliminate the red cells. This is achieved by the addition of a lysing agent which destroys the red cells whilst leaving the white cells intact. 20 g/litre saponin may be used for this purpose, or a commercial preparation such as Zaponin.* It is added to a dilution of 1 in 500 ($20 \mu l$ of blood added to 10 ml of saline).

* Coulter Electronics Ltd., Northwell Drive, Luton, Beds.

After allowing 5 min for red-cell lysis to be complete the cells may be counted. If the lysing agent is allowed to act for longer than 30 min the white cells may also start to disintegrate.

Counts are repeated until two results correspond. For red-cell and white-cell counts a 100 µm orifice tube is used.

Platelet counts

To distinguish platelets from red cells and white cells a count is performed at two threshold settings; a lower threshold setting which will include red cells, white cells and platelets, and an upper threshold which will be set to exclude platelets. Prior to this a preliminary separation is effected by allowing the whole blood to settle leaving the platelets suspended in plasma along with small numbers of red cells and white cells (Fig. 33.2).

cells due to over-exposure to lysing agent, presence of air bubbles and particulate matter in the cleansing fluid, dirty glassware in the instrument, and variations in pressure due to leaking taps and changes in atmospheric pressure.

All these faults may be easily avoided or remedied. Particular attention should be paid to the daily cleansing of the orifice tube in the manner recommended by the manufacturers.

Coulter Model S

Based on the principle that a cell passing through the sensing zone will produce a pulse proportional to its volume, the model S counter is able to measure the red-cell count (RBC), white-cell count (WBC) and mean cell volume (MCV). The haemoglobin is also measured and by a calculation involving RBC, MCV

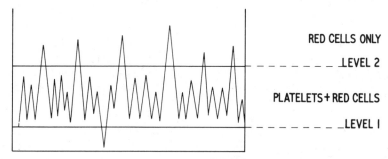

Fig. 33.2.   Coulter counter: counting platelets using two threshold levels.

Separation by sedimentation

Reagent. Methyl cellulose 2% aqueous sp.gr. 1·005; 1·6 ml.
Triosol 440 (Nyegaard, Oslo) sp.gr. 1·2; 1·2 ml.
This mixture should have a sp.gr. of 1·08.

Layer 1 ml of EDTA blood into 1 ml of the sedimentation reagent in a narrow test tube. Allow to stand for 15 min when a layer of erythrocyte-free plasma will be visible. Make a dilution (1 in 5000) of this platelet-rich plasma and count at two threshold settings using a 70 µm orifice tube.

Calculation. Subtract high threshold count (red cells and white cells) from the low threshold count (red cells + white cells + platelets) to arrive at the platelet count. Multiply by the dilution factor.

The sources of error using the electrical resistance method of counting cells include: inaccurate machine calibration, inaccurate dilution, destruction of white

and haemoglobin a further three parameters—haematocrit, mean cell haemoglobin and mean cell haemoglobin concentration, are computed.

The instrument aspirates, dilutes, mixes and counts the sample and in 20 sec produces the seven parameters in a print-out format. Separate baths are used for counting the red cells and white cells, and each bath has three orifices producing three results from which an average is taken. A facility is also provided for testing small samples whereby a preliminary dilution may be prepared manually and presented to the instrument.

Several steps are taken by the instrument to avoid errors. To reduce carry-over blood is aspirated in a long column, effectively washing out the previous sample. If one of the three counts differs significantly from the other two a red light indicates the error and the count is rejected. If more than one reading is rejected the whole count is not recorded and must be repeated. An automatic wash procedure is included in the process.

There are, however, some errors which the operator must guard against.

(a) In leukaemia the WBC may be reduced because the strong lytic agent used may lyse the weak white cells.

(b) The high white-cell count in leukaemia may significantly affect the WBC of the following sample. This high count would also affect the haemoglobin because of the increased turbidity. High concentrations of lipids produce the same effect.

(c) The presence of cold agglutinins may give erroneously low counts.

Most of these errors will be easily discovered by the observation of a stained blood film and an examination of printed results.

A further modification of these machines is the model S Plus, which additionally measures the number and size of platelets and produces a size distribution curve.

THE ELECTRO-OPTICAL
METHOD—Technicon AutoAnalyser

The electro-optical method counts cells by sensing the scattering of light that occurs when cells suspended in a column of fluid pass through an illuminated optical chamber (Fig. 33.3).

from the light source will pass straight through and be blocked by the dark-field disc. However, if a suspension of cells flows through, the cells will be illuminated by the light source and will scatter the light forward towards the objective lens where it will be focused onto the photomultiplier through an aperture. The aperture excludes stray light so that only the light scattered by the cells is measured. The tiny current produced in response to the flashes of light is amplified and printed out on to a chart recorder.

This principle is incorporated in the Technicon Haemalog 8/90,* a fully automated machine which processes whole blood at a rate of 90 samples per hour. The parameters measured are haemoglobin, RBC, WBC, PCV and platelets. On the basis of the measured parameters three others are calculated: MCV, MCH and MCHC.

A well-mixed sample of whole blood in EDTA is aspirated through a probe (Fig. 33.4). The sample is propelled along tubing by means of a pump. It is then split into several streams as it progresses along the system where it is diluted to optimum concentrations for measurement of the various parameters. Reagents are also added: urea for the lysis of the red cells prior to platelet counting, cetrimide–acetic acid for the lysis of

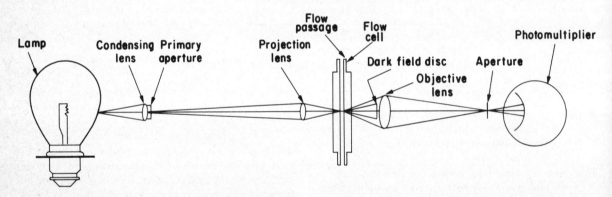

Fig. 33.3.   Optical system—Technicon Autocounter (Technicon Instruments Co. Ltd.)

Light from a lamp passes through a condensing lens on to the primary aperture which has a small rectangular opening at its centre. The projection lens forms a reduced image of this aperture in the centre of the flow cell, thus a very small sensing zone is created through which the sample stream will flow. The light passing through the cell is blocked by a dark-field disc. A photomultiplier is situated at the end of the system. The dark-field disc prevents any light falling on the photomultiplier tube.

If a clear solution passes through the flow cell light

red cells prior to white-cell counting, saline for dilution of the red cells for red-cell counting and cyanide reagent for the conversion of haemoglobin to cyan-methaemoglobin. One of the streams is directed to a centrifuge system which measures the packed-cell volume (PCV).

The machine has built-in procedures to guard against carry-over and a series of electronic alarms which monitor functions. They could, for example, indicate low reagents or a pump tube leak.

* Technicon Instruments Co. Ltd., Basingstoke.

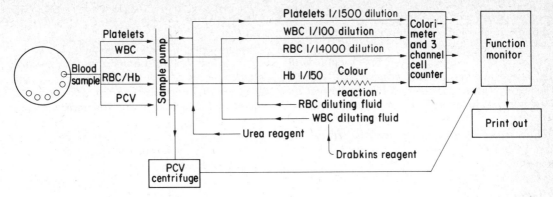

Fig. 33.4.   Simplified diagram of progress of a blood sample in the Haemalog 8 (Technicon Instruments Co. Ltd.)

It will be seen that the electro-optical system measures the PCV and calculates the MCV in contrast to the electro-resistance method which calculates the PCV from a measured MCV and RBC.

AUTOMATIC DIFFERENTIAL COUNTERS

The differential white-cell count as performed in many laboratories is laborious, time-consuming and relatively inaccurate. The introduction of automated differential leucocyte counters is an attempt to eliminate these disadvantages. The systems may be generally divided into two groups:

(a) Continuous flow cytochemistry
This is as employed in the Haemalog D,* in which the white cells are stained supravitally, the amount of colour produced by the different staining reactions being measured by light absorption, and their different sizes measured by the light-scattering method described on p. 248.

(b) Digital image processing systems
This system is employed in the Diff 3 (Coulter Electronics), Abbott ADG 500 and Haematrac (Geometric Data Corporation), in which a Romanowsky-stained film is scanned by a microscope driven by a computer. Although the systems vary in detail they are all essentially pattern-recognition methods.

* Technicon Instruments Co. Ltd.

COAGULOMETERS

These instruments are automated or semi-automated clot-sensing devices which are used in coagulation experiments; the simplest being a semi-automated machine consisting of coupled clot-sensing and timing devices, and a thermostatically controlled heating block. The operator starts the clock as the reagents are added and when the reaction is complete the clock is automatically stopped. Instruments vary in their sophistication, incorporating automatic timing, magnetic stirring or pre-warming facilities.

Fully automated instruments incorporate facilities for adding sample and reagents automatically, a sample tray which maintains plasmas of 4°C and brings them to a temperature of 37°C immediately before sampling, and a print-out facility which will calculate concentration of a coagulation factor after the end-point has been measured.

Clot-sensing devices are designed to detect the formation of fibrin which is the end-product of most routine coagulation experiments. Two methods of detection are in general use:

(a) A photoelectric cell triggers the timing mechanism when the amount of light passing through the test solution is altered by the formation of fibrin.

(b) Two probes are immersed in the test solution; one is immobile while the other agitates the solution and picks up strands of fibrin as they are formed. In this electromechanical method the resultant alteration in current stops the timer.

The use of coagulometers for measuring the one-stage prothrombin time is increasing. Instruments vary, some detecting the first signs of fibrin formation; others the presence of a fibrin clot. Automated methods in general appear to give shorter prothrombin times, a difference which may be reduced to some extent by reporting prothrombin times as ratios. Direct comparison between the manual and automated techniques is therefore inadvisable and instruments should be calibrated by reference to a national quality control scheme.

AGGREGOMETERS

These instruments are used to study platelet aggregation. The light passing through a suspension of platelets is measured by a photoelectric cell. As the platelets aggregate more light is transmitted to the cell. These alterations in light intensity are traced on a moving chart, the final result being a record of the rate of platelet aggregation. The instruments are useful in the further investigation of haemorrhagic disorders involving platelet function.

34. Further considerations of haemoglobin

HAEMOGLOBINS A, A₂ AND F

The haemoglobin molecule as described in Chapter 29 consists of a globin portion composed of two identical pairs of closely linked polypeptide chains labelled α and β, in each of which is inserted a haem group (Fig. 29.1).

This is the type of haemoglobin normally present in the adult and is designated haemoglobin A (HbA). If the amino acids in the globin portion are arranged in a different sequence they will affect the properties of the haemoglobin. This is evidenced by fetal haemoglobin (HbF) which is more resistant to alkali denaturation than HbA because of the altered amino acid sequence on its non-α chains. These chains are designated γ chains and HbF is therefore composed of two α chains and two γ chains ($\alpha_2\gamma_2$). HbF is present at birth in concentrations up to 90% and is gradually replaced by HbA during the first 4 months of life.

A further constituent of normal haemoglobin is HbA₂ which is present at a concentration of approximately 3%. HbA₂ contains two α chains and two δ chains. These three haemoglobins may be represented:

$$HbA = \alpha_2\beta_2 \qquad HbF = \alpha_2\gamma_2 \qquad HbA_2 = \alpha_2\delta_2.$$

The synthesis of haemoglobin is genetically controlled and certain conditions exist which are the result of inherited defects in the formation of the α and β chains. These defects may range from a simple substitution of one amino acid residue to the suppression of a whole polypeptide chain. Thalassaemia, for example, is a disease in which there is failure to produce one type of chain, decreased synthesis of the α chain being designated α-thalassaemia and decreased β chain synthesis β-thalassaemia. The seriousness of any condition associated with abnormal haemoglobin depends on whether it is inherited from both parents (homozygous), in which case the symptoms are more severe than when inherited from one parent (heterozygous) where there may be no detectable symptoms.

The haemoglobinopathies are conditions in which the substitution of an amino acid residue has taken place in either the α or β chains.

Haemoglobin F

Beta-thalassaemia, where the suppressed β chains are replaced by γ and δ chains, shows an increase in HbF. The demonstration of this increase is a useful aid to diagnosis of the disorder.

Estimation of haemoglobin F

The method is based on the resistance of HbF to denaturation at an alkaline pH.

Reagents. 1·2 M NaOH.
Drabkin's solution (*see* p. 224).
Saturated ammonium sulphate.

Method. Prepare a red-cell lysate by diluting an EDTA sample with distilled water until the solution of haemoglobin approximates to 10·0g/dl. Add 0·6 ml of this lysate to 10·0 ml of Drabkin's solution. Place 2·8 ml of this cyanmethaemoglobin solution in a separate tube and add 0·2 ml of 1·2 M NaOH. Stopper the tube and place it on a roller-mixer for 2 min. Add 2·0 ml of saturated ammonium sulphate, shake and allow to stand for 5 min. Filter through a double layer of Whatman No. 6 filter paper.

Prepare a standard by adding 1·4 ml of original cyanmethaemoglobin solution to 3·6 ml of distilled water. Dilute this standard 1 in 10 and compare test and standard in a colorimeter at 415 nm.

Calculation.

$$\% \text{ HbF} = \frac{\text{Absorbance of test}}{\text{Absorbance of standard} \times 20} \times 100.$$

Reference range. Adults 0·5–0·8%.

HbA₂

Another important diagnostic aid in β-thalassaemia is the estimation of HbA₂. The suppressed β chain synthesis allows the formation of increased amounts of

HbA$_2$. This pigment may be estimated by means of a chromatographic process on DEA cellulose, a procedure beyond the scope of this volume.

HAEMOGLOBINS S AND C

HbS

This abnormal haemoglobin is the result of a substitution of an amino acid in the β chains. The haemoglobin readily crystallises under reduced oxygen tension and as a result the red cells become distorted into sickle or holly leaf shapes. The term sickle-cell anaemia is derived from this appearance of the red cells. The disease has its highest incidence among African Negroes and to a lesser extent American Negroes.

The heterozygous condition—only one HbS gene being inherited—is known as the sickle-cell trait. Here there are no symptoms or red-cell distortion apparent until the stress of reduced oxygen tension is imposed. Such a situation can occur, for example, when under an anaesthetic. The homozygous condition is called sickle-cell anaemia and here symptoms of haemolytic anaemia are evident. Occlusions of small blood vessels caused by the sickling of red cells gives rise to painful crises. Attacks of thrombosis often occur as well as infections.

Demonstration of sickle cells

Sickling of the red cells may be promoted under conditions of reduced oxygen tension.

Reagents.

(a) Sodium dithionite 2·0 g/100 ml.
(b) Disodium hydrogen phosphate 1·62 g/100 ml.
For use mix 2 volumes of (a) with 3 volumes of (b).

Method. On to a clean microscope slide place a drop of the prepared reagent. Add a very small drop of blood (10 μl), sufficient to make a very thin suspension of red cells, mix and cover with a coverslip. Seal the edges of the coverslip with Vaseline. Incubate at 37°C. Examine the preparation under the microscope at intervals up to 2 hours. Treat positive and negative controls in like manner. In sickle-cell anaemia marked sickling occurs almost immediately but up to 1 hour is necessary for changes to occur in sickle-cell trait, the appearances in the latter condition being much less marked. When positive this test merely demonstrates the sickling

phenomenon. Further tests are necessary to differentiate between sickle-cell anaemia and sickle-cell traits.

Solubility test for HbS

Blood is added to a buffered reducing agent containing a lysing agent, Saponin.

Buffer. Potassium dihydrogen phosphate　135·12 g
　　　　　Dipotassium hydrogen phosphate　237·32 g
　　　　　White saponin　　　　　　　　　10·0 g
　　　　　Distilled water　　　　　Up to 1 litre

Working solution. Dissolve 1·0 g sodium dithionite in 100 ml of buffer.

Method. Add 20 μl of blood to 2·0 ml of working solution in a test-tube, 75 × 12 mm. Mix and allow to stand for 5 min. Place the tube against a white card on which thick black lines have been drawn. View the black lines through the solution. A positive test is indicated by an opaque solution through which the black lines may not be seen. Cells containing HbS resist lysis, leaving the solution cloudy and giving the positive reaction described above. Red cells containing HbA lyse and the haemoglobin dissolves. A mixture of HbA and HbS produces a reaction intermediate between the two. Positive and negative controls should be included in the test. Centrifugation of the tubes at 1200 g for 5 min will help to clarify doubtful results. Positive reactions now appear as a clear almost colourless solution with a layer of HbS-containing red cells at the surface.

Compared with the other haemoglobinopathies HbS and HbC have a relatively high incidence. There are no simple tests similar to those described for HbS which would be applicable to HbC. The diagnosis of all haemoglobinopathies is confirmed by haemoglobin electrophoresis.

METHAEMOGLOBIN, SULPHAEMOGLOBIN AND CARBOXYHAEMOGLOBIN

Methaemoglobin

All but a tiny portion of the iron in haemoglobin is normally present in the ferrous state. Approximately 2% of the iron, however, exists in the oxidised, trivalent state, and forms methaemoglobin. The pigment is inert and is therefore incapable of transporting oxygen or carbon monoxide. An increase in the concentration of methaemoglobin in the blood may occur for three reasons:

(a) The action of certain drugs such as nitrites which act as oxidising agents;

(b) a congenital defect in which there is a lack of the red-cell enzyme which normally reduces methaemoglobin; and

(c) an inherited defect of the haemoglobin molecule producing a variant known as haemoglobin M.

The molecular abnormality is such that the ferrous atom of the haem group loses an electron and methaemoglobin is formed. The pigment is formed, therefore, when the iron in the haem portion of the haemoglobin molecule is oxidised to the ferric state. The condition produces cyanosis. The reducing agents methylene blue and ascorbic acid may be used in treatment to revert the pigment to haemoglobin. They are not effective in the hereditary haemoglobin M disease.

Sulphaemoglobin

Sulphaemoglobin is a compound of haemoglobin and sulphur and is not normally present in the red cells. It is formed by the action of certain drugs and may be found in association with methaemoglobin; unlike methaemoglobin it cannot be reverted by reducing agents. Once formed in the red cell it remains throughout the whole of the cell's lifespan.

Carboxyhaemoglobin

The combination of carbon monoxide and haemoglobin produces a cherry-red pigment called carboxyhaemoglobin. Because of its high affinity for haemoglobin (200 times greater than oxygen) carbon monoxide will form carboxyhaemoglobin at relatively low concentrations of the gas. The absorption of large amounts of carbon monoxide from sources such as car exhaust fumes may lead to anoxia and death. However, the pigment is readily dissociated at high concentrations of oxygen.

For the differentiation of the pigments carboxyhaemoglobin, methaemoglobin and sulphaemoglobin a spectroscope may be used. This instrument contains prisms or a diffraction grating arranged in such a way that light entering one end is split up into its component colours, the spectrum being viewed through an eyepiece at the other end. The three pigments absorb light of different wavelengths and when viewed through a spectroscope the absorbed light appears as dark bands in the spectrum. These absorption bands are specific for each compound and are known as its absorption spectrum, the wavelength at which absorption occurs being measured in nanometres (nm).

A 1 in 5 to 1 in 10 dilution of blood is made in distilled water. This lyses the sample, which must be centrifuged to remove cellular debris and obtain a clear solution. The solution should be of such a strength that the band may be clearly defined. Too low a dilution will result in overlapping of bands, and at too high a dilution they will be indistinct. The diluted blood is

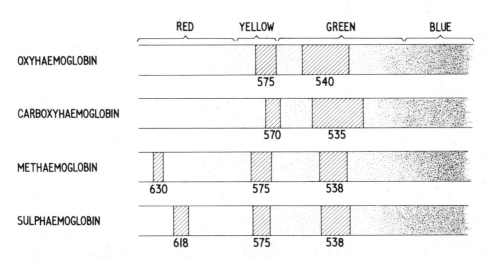

Fig. 34.1. Absorption spectra produced by haemoglobins.

viewed through a spectroscope. Absorption bands will appear in the red or green part of the spectrum according to the pigment present (*see* Fig. 34.1). The absorption bands for oxyhaemoglobin occur at 540 and 578 nm and those of carboxyhaemoglobin at 535 and 572 nm. This difference is difficult to detect with a simple spectroscope but there is a more sophisticated instrument—a reversion spectroscope—with which the wavelength of the bands may be measured.

The direct visual observation of a 1 in 500 dilution of blood in a test tube is a useful indication of the presence of carboxyhaemoglobin. The pigment will have a purplish tint whilst an equivalent dilution of oxyhaemoglobin will be yellowish-red; also, a drop of blood may be placed on a slide and two drops of sodium hydroxide (250 g/litre) added. Normal blood turns brownish and blood containing carboxyhaemoglobin remains red. These results are only well marked when the carbon monoxide saturation is above 20%.

The bands of methaemoglobin occur at 538, 575 and 630 nm, those of sulphaemoglobin at 538, 575 and 618 nm (Fig. 34.1). These pigments therefore have an extra absorption band at the red end of the spectrum in addition to the two bands in the yellow and green which are present in each of the two pigments. The addition of 2 or 3 drops of a solution of sodium cyanide (50 g/litre) will convert methaemoglobin to cyanmethaemoglobin. On re-examination the band in the red will have disappeared. Sulphaemoglobin will be unaffected by the cyanide and its band will remain.

35. Miscellaneous investigations

HAEMOLYTIC DISORDERS

A haemolytic disorder occurs when the life-span of the red cells is shortened by premature destruction. When the rate of red-cell destruction exceeds the rate of replacement by the bone marrow haemolytic anaemia ensues. In severe cases the normal life-span of 120 days may be reduced to a few days. Haemolytic disorders may be divided into two groups: (1) those which are due to a defect of the red cell, (2) those which are due to an external haemolytic mechanism acting upon the red cell.

The corpuscular defects. These may be the result of an abnormality of the haemoglobin molecule, the cell membrane or an enzyme controlling cellular metabolism, e.g.

(a) Conditions associated with abnormal haemoglobin synthesis, e.g. sickle-cell disease.

(b) Deficiency of an enzyme causing the red-cell membrane to be sensitive to the action of certain drugs resulting in haemolysis, e.g. glucose-6-phosphate-dehydrogenase deficiency.

(c) Hereditary spherocytosis, a defect of the cell membrane which results in the cell taking the shape of a sphere.

The extra-corpuscular defects. These are acquired defects which may be due to numerous causes, e.g.:

(a) Haemolytic disease of the newborn where antibodies formed in the mother's circulation cross the placenta and subsequently destroy the baby's red cells.

(b) Septicaemia—certain bacteria may destroy red cells, e.g. *Clostridium welchii*.

(c) Malaria infections.

(d) The action of certain drugs and chemicals.

Intravascular haemolysis

This term describes the haemolysis which occurs when red cells are ruptured in the circulation. The loss may be chronic—the loss of small numbers of cells taking place over a long period, or acute, with a consequent destruction of a large number of cells in a short time.

Extravascular haemolysis

In many of the haemolytic disorders red-cell destruction takes place in the reticuloendothelial system, particularly in the spleen and to a small extent in the liver. The term extravascular haemolysis therefore describes an acceleration of the normal process of red-cell destruction.

An increased reticulocyte count, polychromasia, anisocytosis, and occasionally the presence of normoblasts, evidence the increased marrow activity present in haemolytic anaemia. Once a haemolytic disorder has been established by these and other observations, involving the breakdown products of haemoglobin, tests may be performed to establish the type and cause of the disorder.

Red-cell osmotic fragility

Spherocytes are found in many haemolytic disorders. Cells of this shape are more easily lysed than others. The red-cell osmotic fragility test is designed to measure the amount of spherocytosis present in a blood sample by observing the amount of haemolysis produced in hypotonic solutions of varying salt concentration. Target cells, because of their shape, are more resistant to this treatment than normal red cells. The red-cell membrane is semipermeable and therefore allows the passage of water but not dissolved substances. In an attempt to balance the concentration of salts on each side of the membrane water will flow into the chamber containing the highest concentration of salt. The process is called *osmosis* and the pressure exerted is the *osmotic pressure*. Solutions which exert the same osmotic pressure are said to be isotonic. In the case of physiological solutions the tonicity is usually compared with the osmotic pressure of blood; hypertonic solutions having a higher, hypotonic solutions a lower, and isotonic solutions the same, osmotic pressure as blood.

Reagents

(a) Stock sodium chloride solution osmotically equivalent to 100 g/litre NaCl:

NaCl   90·00 g
NaHPO$_4$ 13·65 g
NaH$_2$PO$_4$ · 2H$_2$O   2·43 g
Distilled water up to 1 litre

(b) Working solution equivalent to 10 g/litre NaCl diluted from the stock solution.

Method

Prepare a series of dilutions as below:

Tube No.	1	2	3	4	5	6	7	8	9(Std)	10(Blank)
Working solution (ml)	3·0	3·5	4·0	4·5	5·0	5·5	6·0	6·5	—	10·0
Distilled water (ml)	7·0	6·5	6·0	5·5	5·0	4·5	4·0	3·5	10·0	—
Concn. of NaCl (g/litre)	3·0	3·5	4·0	4·5	5·0	5·5	6·0	6·5		

Mix and transfer 5 ml of each solution to another tube. There are now two rows of tubes containing the range of dilutions. One row will be used for the test and one row for a control (normal) sample. Add 50 μl of fresh heparinised test blood to each tube of the test row, mix, and allow to stand at room temperature for 30 min. Treat the control blood similarly. After 30 min centrifuge all the tubes at 1500 g for 5 min. Read the absorbance of each test supernatant at 540 nm (Ilford 625 filter) against the 'test blank'. The 'test blank' is tube No. 10 containing 10 g/litre NaCl and 50 μl of *test* blood. It should show no haemolysis. Read the control supernatants against the 'control blank' which is tube No. 10 containing 10 g/litre NaCl and 50 μl of *control* blood.

Calculation

Test readings. The standard tube containing test cells in distilled water (tube number 9), represents 100% lysis. The percentage lysis in each tube is calculated as follows:

$$\text{Percentage haemolysis} = \frac{\text{absorbance of test}}{\text{absorbance of standard}} \times 100.$$

Control reading. The haemolysis in these tubes is calculated in the same manner as above using the standard tube containing control blood. A graph for normal and control bloods is prepared by plotting the percentage haemolysis against the concentration of salt solution (Fig. 35.1).

Notes on the method

(a) Fresh blood should be used. Heparin is the preferred anticoagulant.

(b) The amount of blood added to the salt solution affects the results. A ratio of 1:100 is used; if the haemolysis in the standard tube is too great (an absorbance greater than 0·5) it should be diluted.

(c) The pH of the buffered salt solution is pH 7·4, the optimum for the test.

(d) The control blood should be sampled and treated in every way the same as the test.

(e) The reference range of osmotic fragility should

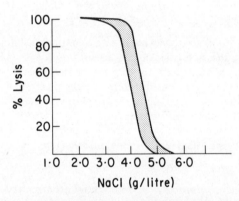

Fig. 35.1.   Osmotic fragility. The shaded area between the two curves indicates the limits of the reference range.

be established as a shaded area on the graph after performing many 'normal' tests. The shaded area may then be reproduced on subsequent graphs for comparison with the test. The median corpuscular fragility (MCF) which is the concentration of saline causing 50% haemolysis is sometimes used as a numerical expression of osmotic facility. The reference range for MCF is 4·0–4·5 g/litre NaCl.

(f) Osmotic fragility is increased in hereditary spherocytosis and decreased in thalassaemia, sickle-cell disease, iron-deficiency anaemia and liver disease.

SYSTEMIC LUPUS ERYTHEMATOSUS (SLE)

Renal insufficiency, liver enlargement, rash, fever, weight loss and hypertension are some of the symptoms manifested by this relatively rare disease. The haematological changes which may be demonstrated are thrombocytopenia, anaemia, raised erythrocyte sedimentation rate and, characteristically, an anti-nuclear factor which is active against the nuclei of lymphocytes and neutrophils.

LE cells

The anti-nuclear factor in SLE lyses the nuclei of leucocytes rendering them susceptible to phagocytosis by neutrophils, a phenomenon which occurs outside the body. It is only effective on the nuclei of dead leucocytes and after a certain amount of trauma. The leucocytes in a defibrinated sample of blood have undergone the necessary degree of trauma to make them susceptible to the action of anti-nuclear factor and if such a sample is incubated some of the leucocyte nuclei will be lysed and subsequently engulfed by neutrophils. The appearance is that of a round, homogeneous, structureless body surrounded by the nuclei of one or more netrophils (Fig. 35.2). LE cells can also be demonstrated if the patient's serum is allowed to act upon normal cells under the same conditions.

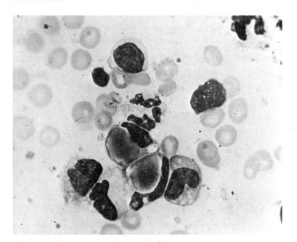

Fig. 35.2   LE cells in a 'buffy coat' preparation.

Method

The final stage of nuclear engulfment requires comple-

ment and calcium ions. Anticoagulants should, therefore, be avoided although satisfactory preparations may be made from heparinised blood. This method uses defibrinated blood.

Add 10–15 ml of blood to a universal bottle containing several paper clips, or a small amount of anti-bumping granules or glass beads. Mix vigorously until the blood is defibrinated. Rotate on a mixer for 30 min and incubate at 37°C for 1 hour. Transfer the liquid blood to two 75×12 mm test-tubes and centrifuge at $1500\,g$ for 5 min. Transfer the top layer of cells to two Wintrobe haematocrit tubes. Centrifuge these at $1500\,g$ for 10 min. With a Pasteur pipette discard most of the supernatant plasma and prepare blood films from the buffy coat. Stain the films by a Romanowsky method.

The LE body stains pale purple, the nuclei of the engulfing neutrophils dark purple in the usual manner.

ERYTHROCYTE SEDIMENTATION RATE (ESR)

The erythrocyte sedimentation rate is a measure of the rate of fall of red cells in plasma. The rate is influenced by a number of factors, the greatest being the rate at which the cells will aggregate to form rouleaux; the increased weight of the aggregates causes them to sink faster than single cells. The formation of rouleaux depends upon the concentration of globulins and fibrinogen in the plasma; when these are increased the ESR is raised. Other influences on the sedimentation rate are:

(a) Anaemic conditions where a reduction in red cells will alter the ratio of red cells to plasma and encourage the formation of rouleaux.

(b) The size and the shape of red cells which will affect their ability to aggregate.

(c) Viscosity of the plasma.

(d) Technical and environmental factors such as temperature, dimension of sedimentation tube, anticoagulant and the position of the tube which should be vertical.

Sedimentation takes place in three phases—a period of several minutes during which aggregates form, a period when the aggregates fall freely at a constant rate, and a final period of approximately 15–20 min when there is a retardation due to packing of cells at the bottom of the tube.

A raised ESR is found in a wide range of disorders such as chronic or acute infections, renal disease and neoplastic and degenerative disorders; all of which involve changes in the plasma proteins. The ESR, therefore, is a non-specific test. However, it is a useful screening test for organic disease and a guide to the progress of conditions such as rheumatism and tuberculosis.

Method

In 1973 the ICSH recommended the Westergren method for the estimation of the ESR.

Materials

Anticoagulant: 0·105 M trisodium citrate dihydrate (30·88 g/litre).
Westergren tube: To conform with BS 2554: 1968 the tube must have the following dimensions:

(a) Overall length: $300 \pm 1·5$ mm.
(b) Tube bore: $2·55 \pm 0·15$ mm.
(c) Uniformity of bore: $\pm 0·05$ mm.

The scale should be graduated and numbered from 200 at the bottom to 0 at the top in steps of 10 or less, the maximum tolerated error between two subsequent markings being 0·2 mm.

Test

(a) Take blood into trisodium citrate solution in the proportions 4 volumes of blood to 1 volume of citrate.
(b) Using a syringe or rubber teat draw the blood into a Westergren tube up to the 0 mark.
(c) Place in a Westergren rack which has been adjusted so that the tube will be vertical. The rack should be placed in a position which is free from vibration and draughts and under room temperature conditions (18–25°C).
(d) Allow the tube to stand for 1 hour and record in millimetres the distance the red cells have fallen.

The ESR should be reported as follows:

ESR (Westergren 1 hr) = x mm

Reference range

Men 0–5 mm; women 0–7 mm.

INFECTIOUS MONONUCLEOSIS

Infectious mononucleosis (IM) is a disease characterised by sore throat, fever, enlarged glands and an enlarged spleen. It occurs in older children and young adults and infrequently in the very young and adults over 40 years. The causative agent is considered to be a virus called the Epstein–Barr (EB) virus.

The presence of antibodies in the sera of patients with IM which will agglutinate sheep red cells was described by Paul and Bunnell in 1932. These antibodies, which are active against other antigens (e.g. those present in sheep cells) as well as the antigen against which they were originally formed (the causative organism of IM), are called heterophile antibodies. The reaction with sheep red cells is not specific for IM; at least two other types of anti-sheep-cell haemagglutinins occur in human serum. However, these may be absorbed by guinea-pig kidney. IM antibody is only slightly affected by guinea-pig kidney but is completely absorbed by ox cells. These reactions are used to advantage in the diagnosis of IM.

Paul–Bunnell–Davidsohn test

The test measures titres of agglutinins for sheep erythrocytes before and after absorption with guinea-pig kidney and ox cells. The test uses patient's serum which has been inactivated by heating at 56°C for 30 min.

Reagents

(a) Guinea-pig-kidney suspension: strip two pairs of guinea-pig-kidneys of fat and capsules. Homogenise in physiological saline and autoclave. Centrifuge and discard the supernatant, resuspend in saline and centrifuge once more. Again discard the supernatant and resuspend in saline. Centrifuge once more (this process is known as washing). Discard the saline and make a 1 in 6 suspension of the deposit in phenol–saline (5 g phenol in 1 litre of saline).
(b) Ox-cell suspension: wash ox cells in saline. Make a 30% suspension in saline and autoclave. Allow to cool and remove coarse particles by sieving through muslin. Make a 10% suspension in phenol–saline.
(c) 0·4% suspension of washed sheep cells.

Method

Take three tubes (75 × 12 mm), A, B and C:

into tube A pipette	0·25 ml serum
	1·00 ml saline
into tube B pipette	0·25 ml serum
	0·75 ml saline
	0·30 ml guinea-pig-kidney

into tube C pipette
0·25 ml serum
0·75 ml saline
0·25 ml ox cells

Mix all three tubes and stand at 4°C for 2 hours. Centrifuge and retain the supernatant.

Supernatant A is now a 1 in 5 dilution of unabsorbed serum.

Supernatant B is a 1 in 5 dilution of serum absorbed with guinea-pig-kidney.

Supernatant C is a 1 in 5 dilution of serum absorbed with ox cells.

Make doubling dilutions of these supernatants from 1 in 5 up to 1 in 640 using 0·25 ml volumes. Add 0·25 ml of sheep-cell suspension to every tube in each row. Incubate at 37°C for 2 hours. A known positive control serum should be treated similarly.

After incubation note which tube shows agglutination. The observation of the end-point is improved by gently resuspending the cells and viewing them through a concave mirror placed beneath the tube. The titre is expressed as the reciprocal of the highest dilution in which agglutination is observed.

Examples of results:

(a) Row A: 320   Row B: 160   Row C: 20   POSITIVE
(b) Row A: 40   Row B: 40   Row C: NIL   POSITIVE
(c) Row A: 320   Row B: 20   Row C: 160   NEGATIVE

Very little absorption by guinea-pig-kidney and significant absorption by ox cells is therefore indicative of infectious mononucleosis.

Screen test for IM

It is known that horse cells are more readily agglutin-ated by IM sera than are sheep cells. Horse cells are, therefore, a more sensitive indicator of IM. However, this sensitivity is such that a small number of non-IM sera give positive results. If the horse cells are used in conjunction with the guinea-pig-kidney and ox-cell absorption procedure, the false-positive results will be eliminated and a sensitive screening test may be established.

Reagents

(a) Guinea-pig-kidney prepared as above but at a final dilution of 1:10.

(b) Ox-cells, 2% suspension in phenol–saline.

(c) Horse cells, 2% suspension in saline.

On one end of a glass slide place one drop of ox-cell suspension and on the other end one drop of guinea-pig-kidney. To each of these drops add one drop of patient's serum, mix thoroughly and add one drop of horse cells. Rock the slide gently. A positive reaction should be evident within 2 min.

READING LIST

Dacie, J.W. and Lewis, S.M. (1975). *Practical Haematology*, 5th Edition. London: Churchill.

Thompson, R.B. (1978). *Disorders of the Blood*. London: Churchill.

Thomson, J.M. (Ed.) (1980). *Blood Coagulation and Haemostasis*, 2nd Edition. London: Churchill.

PART FIVE

Blood group serology

36. Introduction to blood group serology

Man has always recognised the connection between blood and life. Primitive man was aware that excessive loss of blood meant loss of life and it is not surprising that, over many centuries, he attributed to it mystical and divine properties. Sacrificial blood was used to appease his gods, promote the growth of his crops and was bathed in and drunk to cleanse his soul. The blood of dying warriors was imbibed by their slayers to acquire the victims' heroic qualities and prophets derived inspiration from sucking the blood of sacrificed animals.

The transfusion of animal blood into humans was advocated by scientists in the 17th and 18th centuries. Cases have been described which produced symptoms including pyrexia, rapid pulse, backache, vomiting and death; symptoms now associated with haemolytic transfusion reaction. In the 19th century experiments in transfusing human blood met with variable success and it became clear that while, under certain conditions human blood could be transfused successfully, blood from another species could not be tolerated.

The demonstration of Karl Landsteiner, in 1900, of three different groups of human blood, and the subsequent discovery of a fourth in 1902, helped to explain some of the early transfusion failures. Human blood was divided according to whether the cells contained A or B antigens. The groups were A, B, AB and O (containing neither antigen). He also demonstrated the presence of naturally occurring antibodies which were active against the A or B antigens. These were present in the serum of individuals whose cells did not contain the antigen. Group A contained anti-B and group B contained anti-A.

In 1914 sodium citrate, in small quantities, was recommended as a low-toxicity anticoagulant and direct transfusion was superseded by the transfusion of stored blood. Two major wars in the 20th century have, not surprisingly, advanced the state of transfusion therapy, and with this increased use came the realisation that diseases such as hepatitis, syphilis and malaria could be transmitted. It was also noticed that occasionally a patient who had been successfully transfused with ABO-compatible blood on one or two previous occasions would suffer a reaction on a further transfusion.

Landsteiner and Wiener, in 1940, produced an antibody against the blood of rhesus monkeys which agglutinated the red cells of 85% of the human blood samples they tested. The antibody which gave this reaction was called anti-Rh and the cells which were agglutinated by it were called Rh-positive. Those which did not react were called Rh-negative.

It was subsequently shown that the sera from the unexplained transfusion reactions above gave a parallel reaction to the anti-Rh sera. It was therefore deduced that Rh-positive blood, when transfused, could stimulate the production of antibodies in a Rh-negative patient.

In 1939 Levine and Stetson described an antibody in the serum of the mother of a still-born fetus which they postulated had been the result of immunisation by the fetus. The antibody subsequently appeared to have the same specificity as the Rh antibody of Landsteiner and Wiener. The fetus had died as a result of haemolytic disease of the newborn (HDNB) caused by the action of the maternal antibody on its cells.

Today transfusion therapy has advanced to such a degree that specific blood components may be transfused according to need, so that more than one patient may benefit from the same unit of blood.

ANTIGENS AND ANTIBODIES

Why did the transfusion of blood from a different species have such catastrophic results?

When the body is invaded by an infectious organism information about the infection is recorded and the body prepares its defences so that a subsequent infection will be met by a specific response. In this manner the childhood diseases of whooping cough and mumps are rarely experienced twice. This recognition of substances which are 'non-self' is the basis of immunity. In those early experiments the transfused blood cells from a different species, being 'non-self', were destroyed producing the severe symptoms which, in some cases, resulted in death.

The components of blood which are capable of recognising foreign substances and building up a memory are the T-lymphocytes (p. 232) which instruct the B-lymphocytes to form antibodies. The substances which stimulate the production of antibodies are called antigens.

The introduction of an antigen into a subject produces a 'primary response' in which the antibody level reaches a peak and falls. Exposure to a further dose of antigen elicits a stronger response with greater rapidity. In this 'secondary response' the antibody level remains high for a longer period.

Antigens

Antigens are usually proteins of large molecular size. Certain sites on the molecule determine its antigenicity (ability to stimulate antibodies) and specificity. The antibodies formed by B-lymphocytes are manufactured to fit the sites exactly. An antigen has been defined as a substance which, when introduced into a subject which lacks that substance, will stimulate the production of a specific antibody.

Antibodies

Antibodies are proteins and are known as immunoglobulins. In the human there are five major types of immunoglobulin.

Immunoglobulin G (IgG). Molecular weight approximately 150,000. IgG comprises approximately 80% of the immunoglobulin normally present in serum. It is the most important immunoglobulin produced during the secondary response to antigenic stimulus. It can cross the placenta and is responsible for protecting the baby from infection during the first few weeks of life. It can also cause HDNB.

Immunoglobulin M (IgM). Molecular weight 900,000. It comprises approximately 8% of normal human immunoglobulin. IgM is produced in the primary response to antigenic stimulus. This large-molecular weight protein does not cross the placenta or diffuse through the tissues. It has many combining sites and characteristically behaves as an agglutinin.

Immunoglobulin A (IgA). Molecular weight 160,000. IgA comprises 13% of normal human immunoglobulin and may be found in colostrum, tears, saliva, sweat and nasal fluid where it protects the exposed external surfaces. It does not cross the placenta.

Immunoglobulin D (IgD). This immunoglobulin has a molecular weight of 185,000 and comprises only 1% of human immunoglobulins.

Immunoglobulin E (IgE). Molecular weight 200,000. Serum IgE levels are raised in patients with diseases such as hay fever, eczema and asthma. The immunoglobulin is associated with the release of histamine from the mast cells in these conditions.

Antibody production

The information required for the synthesis of antibodies is genetically controlled and is already present on the antibody-producing cells. When the antigen is in contact with the cell the correct combination of amino acids is synthesised and the chains are folded to make specific antigen-combining sites which will fit the antigen. The currently held view is that each B-lymphocyte possesses the material to make a particular antibody and the molecules of this antibody act as receptors on the cell-surface membrane. As each cell contains a different antibody there is a potential in the body for the formation of many antibodies. When an antigen combines with a lymphocyte it provides a stimulus for reproduction which results in a clone with a large number of offspring each having the capacity to produce antibodies to the same antigen. A clone is a group of cells which have the same characteristics because they are derived from a common precursor cell.

DEMONSTRATION OF ANTIGEN–ANTIBODY REACTIONS

Naturally occurring antibodies

These are antibodies present in serum of which there is no known antigenic stimulus although there is a widely held view that they are formed in response to substances such as bacteria, food and dust particles which are widespread in nature. They are present in several blood group systems, notably the ABO system which, as stated above, contain anti-A and anti-B antibodies. They are mainly IgM and are usually demonstrated by their ability to agglutinate saline suspensions of red cells at 4°C, although they do have a wide thermal range (2–40°C). Their large molecular size prevents them from crossing the placenta and causing haemolytic disease of the newborn.

Immune antibodies

Antibodies produced in response to the stimulus of a known antigen are immune antibodies and are most commonly IgG. They are able to cross the placenta and may cause damage to the fetus *in utero*. In contrast to naturally occurring antibodies they generally have a narrow thermal range for detection *in vitro* (optimum 37°C) and do not directly agglutinate red cells in saline. They do, however, sensitise red cells and with the assistance of a further stage in the reaction agglutination is complete. For this reason they are also known as 'incomplete antibodies'.

Three ways in which antigen–antibody reactions may be demonstrated in the laboratory are precipitation, haemolysis and agglutination.

Precipitation

When an antigen is mixed in the correct proportions with serum containing an antibody a precipitate is formed. This precipitin reaction may be used as a basis for the quantitative assessment of an antibody.

Haemolysis

Some antibodies react by causing lysis of the cells carrying the corresponding antigen. When they react in this manner with erythrocytes they are termed haemolysins. They require 'complement' to complete the reaction.

Complement is a complex system of factors consisting of eleven proteins, which reacts with antibodies in the immune reaction and causes lysis by punching out small holes in the cellular membrane of the cells sensitised with antibodies. If serum is heated at 56°C for 30 min its complement activity is destroyed.

Agglutination

This reaction, where the combination of antigens on cells and antibodies in serum results in the clumping or agglutination of the cells, is the most commonly used method of observing the antigen–antibody reaction in blood group serology.

Red cells possess negative electric charges on their surfaces which are due to the carboxyl groups of sialic acid. The electric potential (zeta-potential) which keeps the cells apart is dependent upon these surface charges and upon the ionic cloud formed by the sodium and chloride ions of the saline which surrounds the cells.

The ease with which naturally occurring antibodies agglutinate saline suspensions of red cells is explained by the fact that IgM molecules, of which the antibodies are usually composed, because of their large molecular size are able to bridge the gaps between cells bringing them together to form agglutinates. Immune or incomplete antibodies, on the other hand, are mainly of the IgG type and are small molecules which can coat the cells but cannot bridge the gaps between. For this reason they will not agglutinate cells in saline and methods have been devised which will reduce the zeta-potential and bring the red cells into closer proximity or detect the IgG antibody coating the cells. These are:

(*a*) The use of colloidal suspensions such as 20% bovine albumin or human serum added to the tube after the cells and antiserum have had sufficient time to react together. The colloidal suspension should be used at a sufficient strength to reduce the zeta-potential to an optimum for the immunoglobulin to bridge the gap.

(*b*) The use of the enzymes papain, bromelin or ficin. One explanation of their action is that they act upon the sialic acids and reduce the surface charge on the red cells. In some cases this treatment may also increase the number of available antigen sites on the cell surface.

(*c*) The use of anti-human globulin (AHG). The antibody which coats the red cells is a γ-globulin and a suitable serum may be prepared which will react with this γ-globulin. When purified human globulin is injected into a rabbit, AHG antibodies are produced. This rabbit serum, when placed in contact with the sensitised red cells, will bridge the gap sufficiently to cause agglutination (Fig. 36.1).

THE INHERITANCE OF BLOOD GROUPS

Within the nucleus of a cell is found darkly staining material which appears as irregularly shaped masses without any organised pattern. However, when the cell divides to reproduce itself this material begins to condense and forms a number of rod-shaped bodies. These bodies are called chromosomes and in each cell, except the sex cells, there are 46.

Chromosomes contain molecules of desoxyribonucleic acid (DNA) arranged in such a manner as to form units along the chromosomes called genes which determine the characteristics of each cell and the whole organism. The many ways in which the DNA molecule can be arranged in a chromosome ensures that every

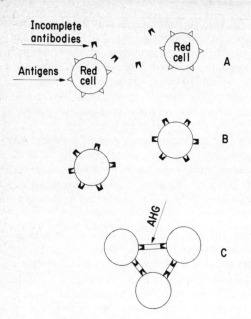

Fig. 36.1. Diagrammatic representation of the anti-human globulin test
A Incomplete antibodies and red cells with antigen sites indicated.
B Red cells coated with antibody (sensitised).
C After the sensitised red cells have been washed and resuspended in saline AHG is added and completes the linkage between the cells to form agglutinates.

animal is unique. In order to pass on the coded instructions (genetic information) contained in the molecule of DNA the chromosomes must be able to reproduce themselves. They achieve this by dividing longitudinally, forming two identical chromatids each passing to a separate daughter cell. The process of cell division by which these daughter cells are formed from a parent cell is called mitosis. Mitosis may be broadly divided into four phases (Fig. 36.2):

1. Prophase. In the first stage of cell division the chromosomes become visible as elongated strands which gradually shorten and become thicker as the stage proceeds. The chromatids are discernible, each pair being joined at a centromere.

2. Metaphase. The chromatids arrange themselves along one plane at the equator of the cell.

3. Anaphase. The centromere connecting the chromatids splits and they separate, rapidly moving to opposite poles of the cell.

4. Telophase. In this last stage of mitosis the cytoplasm divides, two daughter cells are formed and their chromosomes reform into nuclei.

Sexual reproduction involves the union of sperm and ovum. If each of these contained 46 chromosomes, as in the other cells of the body, this union would result in the formation of a cell with 92 chromosomes. The maturation of the sex cells therefore proceeds in a different manner; a process of reduction division takes place called meiosis whereby each sex cell eventually contains 23 chromosomes.

Some terms used in genetics

Allelomorph (or allele). Two or more genes occurring at the same position on both chromosomes and conferring the same characteristics.

Autosome. Any chromosome other than the sex chromosomes.

Heterozygous. Having different allelic genes inherited from each parent.

Homozygous. Having the same allelic genes inherited from each parent.

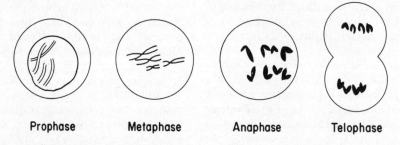

Prophase   Metaphase   Anaphase   Telophase

Fig. 36.2. Diagram of mitosis.

Locus. Position of a gene on a chromosome. Genes are always arranged in the same sequence on a chromosome.

Dominant. A dominant gene is one which expresses itself over its allelomorph; it therefore expresses itself in the homozygous or heterozygous state.

Recessive. Recessive genes are only expressed in the absence of a dominant allelomorph, i.e. only in the homozygous state.

Genotype. The genetic make-up of an individual or cell.

Phenotype. The observable characteristics of an individual or cell, e.g. the observable characteristics of an individual of group AO genotype would be A because the O gene is recessive.

THE ABO BLOOD GROUP SYSTEM

The ABO group of a child is determined by the inheritance of three genes which are situated on the same locus of the two parental chromosomes which carry them. These genes are A, B and O. Only one of these genes may be inherited from each chromosome and the possible gene combinations (genotypes) are demonstrated in Table 36.1. It will be seen also that the genotypes AO and BO are expressed as A and B respectively. This is because the O gene is recessive to both A and B.

Table 36.1. The ABO systems

Genotype	Group	Naturally occurring antibodies	Frequency (%) in United Kingdom
AO⎫ AA⎭	A	anti-B	42
BO⎫ BB⎭	B	anti-A	9
AB	AB	—	3
O	O	anti-A+ anti-B	46

The original classification of the ABO groups was made by Landsteiner in 1900 when he mixed the cells and serum of different individuals and from the resultant pattern of agglutinations was able to recognise three groups. The fourth and rarest group, AB, was discovered in 1902 by Descastello and Sturli.

The naturally occurring antibodies present in the sera he tested were always compatible with the individual's own blood and were, therefore, only present when the corresponding antigen was lacking (Table 36.1). These naturally occurring antibodies do not fully develop until the age of 3–6 months.

Although it is a feature of all cells in the body the ABO system is primarily concerned with red cells because of their importance in blood transfusion and their availability as test material.

As a result of the discovery that certain group A red cells react more weakly than others the A group was further sub-divided into two sub-groups, A_1 and A_2. There were then six groups in the ABO system: A_1, A_2, B, A_1B, A_2B, and O; and the naturally occurring antibodies in Group B individuals agglutinated A_1 and A_2 cells.

By absorbing the serum in Group B individuals with A_2 cells the A_2 agglutinins may be removed, leaving a pure anti-A_1 agglutinating serum. The reactions of the several groups against antisera are shown in Table 36.2.

Table 36.2. The ABO system: reaction of cells with known test sera

Group	Anti-A	Anti-B	Anti-A + B (Group O serum)
A	+	−	+
B	−	+	+
AB	+	+	+
O	−	−	−

Approximately 20% of group A persons belong to the sub-group A_2, the same distribution occurs in the AB group. Another manifestation of the A sub-group is the presence of naturally occurring anti-A_1 in a proportion of A_2 and A_2B individuals. Two per cent of A_2 and 25% of A_2B sera contain the antibody. From this it is evident that the A_2 sub-group is not merely a weaker form of the group A_1.

ABO GROUPING METHODS

Determination of a patient's ABO group is a necessary preliminary to blood transfusion and for this reason requires a meticulous attention to details of technique and identification of blood samples. The group may be determined by detecting the antigens on the red cells or the agglutinins in the serum. In practice both procedures are combined in one technique; each serving as a check on the other.

Two methods are available; a tile technique, which is suitable for providing a rapid result, and a tube technique which is the standard method and is more reliable.

Tile technique

(1) Obtain a clotted sample of blood and after centrifugation remove the serum to a tube and label it with the patient's identity and origin. From the same sample prepare a 10% suspension in physiological saline of the free red cells in the tube.

(2) Mark a clean white tile in sections with a grease pencil as indicated in Fig. 36.3.

For the interpretation of the reaction between cells and antisera see Table 36.2.

Tube method

(1) Wash the patient's cells by placing a few drops of cells in a centrifuge tube, diluting with saline, mixing and centrifuging. Replace the supernatant with fresh saline. Mix and repeat the process twice more. Make a final 2–5% suspension of cells in saline. In this manner the patient's serum is removed from the cells and the possibility of rouleaux formation due to an excess of globulin is circumvented.

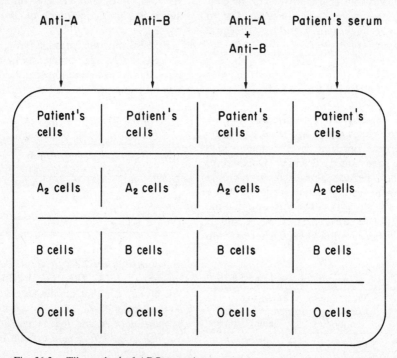

Fig. 36.3.   Tile method of ABO grouping.

(3) Place one drop of relevant antisera and test serum in each square of the vertical rows as indicated.

(4) Place one drop of 10% suspension of the relevant cells in each square as indicated.

(5) Mix the cells and serum gently with a wooden applicator stick, using a fresh stick for each mixture.

(6) Allow to stand for 5 min at room temperature.

(7) Rock the tile gently. Read the controls and if they have reacted satisfactorily read the tests. Take care to wash out the Pasteur pipette thoroughly several times in saline between each serum and cell sample.

(2) Set up precipitin tubes ($50 \times 5 \cdot 5$ mm) in a rack as shown in Fig. 36.4.

(3) Using a Pasteur pipette add cells and sera in one-drop volumes as indicated. Rinse the pipette thoroughly in saline between each addition.

(4) Mix by tapping the tubes gently and allow to stand for $1\frac{1}{2}$ hours at room temperature.

(5) Read by gently tapping the tubes and examining for agglutination. Doubtful results must be checked by spreading the cells gently on a slide and viewing them under a microscope (low-power objective). Examina-

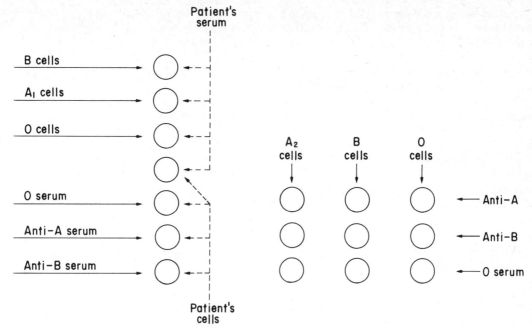

Fig. 36.4.   Tube method of ABO grouping.

tion of the controls must precede the reading of the tests.

Whichever method of grouping is used it is essential to include controls to check on the integrity of the reagents and the satisfactory performance of each stage of the test.

Positive controls. Weak-reacting A_2 cells are used against anti-A serum to prove its sensitivity. They are also used against O serum (anti-A + B) for the same reason.

Negative controls. These are included to check the specificity of the antisera. Known A and B cells should only be agglutinated by their specific antisera, and O cells not at all.

Auto control. This mixture of patient's cells in his own serum is to exclude the possibility of his having autoagglutinins which will react with his own cells, a rare occurrence but one in which the agglutinin is often active against all red cells. If autoagglutinins are present the grouping should be repeated on a fresh sample which has had the serum separated from the cells before the sample has had time to cool to room temperature. Obvious agglutination observed in a sample prior to processing may often be dispersed by washing the red cells with warm saline.

Sub-groups of the ABO system

The previously discussed sub-groups of the ABO system vary in their strengths of reaction with anti-A serum in descending order, A_1, A_1B, A_2, A_2B. There are also some very weak-reacting sub-groups of A which may not be detected by standard anti-A serum. They do, however, react with group O serum which is the reason for its inclusion in the routine ABO protocol.

As anti-A_2 serum does not exist the A_2 and A_2B antigens are established by a process of elimination. Anti-A_1 serum is used against the cells and those which do not react are assumed to belong to one of the sub-groups (Table 36.3).

Table 36.3.   *The ABO system: subgroups*

Group	Anti-A	Anti-A_1	Anti-B
A_1	+	+	−
A_2	+	−	−
A_1B	+	+	+
A_2B	+	−	+

Anomalous results

Reactions are occasionally encountered which, even when the controls are satisfactory, do not correspond to the usual pattern.

Weak reactions. Weak reactions with anti-A grouping serum should be re-tested with a different sample of anti-A and a potent group O serum.

Absence of agglutinins. Infants do not start to develop anti-A and anti-B until they are about 3 months old. The infant's group cannot, therefore, be checked by the agglutinins in its serum. The antigens may also be weakly reacting.

Haemolysis. The patient's serum may haemolyse the standard A, B or O cells. In this case the test should be repeated after heating the serum at 56°C for 30 min to destroy the complement.

Rouleaux. A high concentration of globulins in a patient's serum may cause the formation of rouleaux. This is difficult to distinguish from true agglutination. If the serum is diluted with an equal volume of saline, thereby lowering the concentration of protein, the test may be repeated but with a consequent weakening of the reaction due to the dilution of antibody.

Autoagglutination. This has been discussed above.

SELECTION AND PREPARATION OF ABO GROUPING SERA

Only 2% of human sera are suitable for use as ABO grouping sera. A satisfactory serum should have high avidity, a high titre and must be specific. It should be free from fat and any tendency to form rouleaux.

Occasionally some high-titre sera may cause haemolysis, a property which may be removed by heating at 56°C for 30 min.

Screening test

To assist in the selection of grouping sera a screening test may be used in which a small sample of the donor serum is diluted 1 in 4 with saline, one volume of this being added to one volume of a 2·5% suspension of the relevant A_1 or B cells. After standing for 1 hour at room temperature suitable sera will show complete agglutination.

An alternative procedure is to collect a small amount of blood by finger-prick into an equal volume of sodium citrate anticoagulant. This is mixed and centrifuged. One drop of this supernatant plasma is mixed on a tile with one drop of a 5% suspension of the relevant A_1 or B cells. A suitable antiserum will show agglutination within 30 sec.

Collection of serum

Blood is collected from the donor into a dry sterile glass bottle without anticoagulant and allowed to clot at 37°C for 2 hours. It is then allowed to stand at 4°C overnight to allow the red cells to absorb any cold agglutinins. The serum is then removed into a sterile bottle using an aspirator set. An air trap bottle is used to prevent water being sucked back into the bottle and contaminating the serum (Fig. 36.5). Any red cells still remaining in the serum may be removed by centrifugation. A few ml of the serum is retained for testing and the rest

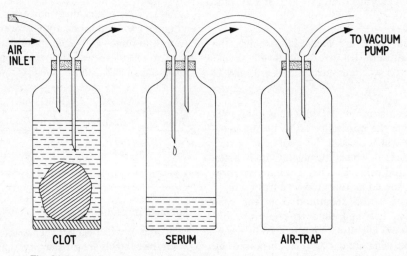

AIR INLET

TO VACUUM PUMP

CLOT   SERUM   AIR-TRAP

Fig. 36.5.   Separating serum from donor blood.

distributed in small amounts, labelled and stored at −20°C. When serum is thawed and refrozen several times it loses potency. The storage of small quantities of serum ensures that each sample is only thawed once. Aseptic precautions should be used throughout the whole process; indeed some workers recommend as a final stage the sterilisation of the serum by Seitz filtration using a grade HPEK pad.

Avidity

Avidity is a measure of the ability of an antiserum to agglutinate cells quickly and completely. It is most conveniently assessed by placing equal volumes of a 5% suspension of appropriate cells and serum on a tile, mixing and noting the time taken to produce complete agglutinations. The avidity of a grouping serum should be established before it is used in a tile grouping method. Suitable sera produce complete agglutination in 30 sec. It is possible to find sera which have a high titre but low avidity.

Titration of antisera

Set up a row of ten 75 × 12 mm test tubes and into each pipette 0·5 ml saline. Into the first tube pipette 0·5 ml of the antiserum under test, mix and transfer 0·5 ml to the second tube. Repeat the process until a row of doubling dilutions from 1 in 2 to 1 in 1024 is achieved.

Set up a row of 10 precipitin tubes corresponding to the row of dilutions and transfer 0·1 ml of each dilution to a precipitin tube. Add 0·1 ml of a 5% suspension of appropriate cells. Mix and allow to stand at room temperature for 2 hours. Read the results microscopically. The titre is expressed as the reciprocal of the highest dilution causing agglutination when viewed under the microscope.

Anti-A sera should be selected which agglutinates A_1 cells at a titre of 512 and A_2B cells at 64. Anti-B sera should have a titre of 256 and group O sera a titre of 8 against A_x cells.

Specificity

The specificity of an antiserum may be established by testing equal volumes of neat serum against a 5% suspension of cells of all ABO groups. Agglutination should only occur with the appropriate cells.

Lectins

Extracts of the seeds of certain plants have been shown to have red-cell agglutinating activity. These seed agglutinins (lectins) may be extracted and diluted until they show a required specificity. An extract of *Dolichos biflorus*, for example, will react very strongly with group A_1, much less strongly with A_2 and not at all with the other sub-groups of A. It may, therefore, be diluted until it reacts only with the sub-group A_1.

Anti-A_1 from Dolichos biflorus

Soak the seeds in a large volume of distilled water overnight at room temperature. Pour off the distilled water and grind the seeds in a mortar. Add three volumes of saline, transfer to a flask and agitate for 60 min. Centrifuge and, if necessary, filter the supernatant through Whatman No. 1 filter paper. Store the filtrate in small amounts at −20°C. The extract should be titrated against A_1 and A_2 cells and used at a dilution which will only agglutinate A_1 cells.

Human anti-A_1 serum

Anti-A_1 serum may be prepared by absorbing high-titre anti-A serum with washed, packed A_2 cells at 4°C for 2 hours. The supernatant serum from the centrifuged mixture should give no reaction with A_2 cells and agglutinate A_1 cells at a titre of 64.

Naturally occurring anti-A_1

The naturally occurring anti-A_1 which is present in a small percentage of A_2 and A_2B individuals may be used as typing serum provided the titre is sufficiently high (16 or more).

THE Rh BLOOD GROUP SYSTEM

The original Rh factor of Landsteiner and Wiener is now considered to be a single complex locus of six genes, C, D, E, c, d and e which are inherited as three closely linked allelomorphs. The eight possible combinations of these are shown in Table 36.4 along with their shorthand symbols. These gene combinations, being carried on homologous chromosomes can give rise to 64 different combinations. The most frequently occurring combinations are shown in Table 36.5. In the Rh system the D antigen (what was thought to be the original Rh antigen) is the most strongly antigenic and readily stimulates the production of anti-D when introduced into D-negative individuals. The other antigens form antibodies infrequently (anti-d has yet to be

Table 36.4.   The eight possible combinations of the Rh genes

	Shorthand
CDe	R_1
cDE	R_2
CDE	R_z
cDe	R_0
Cde	r'
cdE	r''
CdE	r_y
cde	r

Table 36.5   The most frequently occurring Rh combinations

R_1R_1	CDe/CDe
R_1r	CDe/cde
R_1R_2	CDe/cDE
R_2R_2	cDE/cDE
R_2r	cDE/cde
R_0r	cDe/cde
$r'r$	Cde/cde
$r''r$	cdE/cde
rr	cde/cde

demonstrated) and in Rh grouping the emphasis is therefore placed upon the identification of the D antigen. Anti-D is formed as the result of immunisation by the transfusion of incompatible blood or during pregnancy when a fetus with D antigen on its cells stimulates the production of anti-D in the mother's serum. As it is an immune antibody it is most usually of the incomplete (IgG) type and when used as a grouping serum requires special techniques to demonstrate the agglutination of the cells. However 'complete' anti-D is available as well as 'incomplete' anti-D. Techniques for Rh grouping using both types of antisera will be described.

Saline method using complete anti-D

Prepare a 5% suspension of the cells to be tested in saline. In a precipitin tube place one drop of complete anti-D and add one drop of the cell suspension. Mix by tapping the tube and incubate at 37°C for 90 min. After incubation remove some of the button of cells at the bottom of the tube by means of a wide-bore Pasteur pipette and transfer to a glass slide. Examine microscopically for agglutinates.

Albumin displacement method using incomplete anti-D

The principles of several methods of bringing about the association of IgG antibodies with their corresponding antigens have been outlined above. The usual method for Rh grouping uses the colloidal suspension, bovine albumin.

Add one drop of incomplete anti-D and one drop of 5% cell suspension to a precipitin tube. Mix by tapping and incubate for 60 min. Run one drop of 20% bovine albumin down the side of the tube on to the cells. This displaces the saline/serum mixture and layers itself on top of the cells. Incubate for a further 30 min and read microscopically as described above.

Stratton sandwich method

When the occasion arises for a rapid Rh grouping prior to cross-matching blood for urgent blood transfusion this method may be used. The operator should be well versed in its interpretation and it is essential that the result be checked by the tube method. It is a method evolved for use with incomplete anti-D and the antiserum should be one which is known to work satisfactorily under the conditions outlined below, and should have a titre of at least 64.

On a clean microscope slide place one drop of anti-D, one drop of packed, washed red cells and one drop of 30% bovine albumin. Mix well with an applicator stick and place a second clean microscope slide on top. Incubate this 'sandwich' at 37°C for 10 min and examine microscopically. Treat known D-positive and D-negative controls similarly.

Enzyme technique (see also p. 275)

The enzyme, bromelin, may be used for a rapid Rh group. In a precipitin tube place one drop each of anti-D, 2% suspension of cells and bromelin working solution (p. 275). Mix and incubate at 37°C for 15 min, centrifuge at 1000 r.p.m. for 1 min and read. Treat positive and negative controls similarly.

Controls for rhesus grouping

Positive control. Weak-reacting D-positive cells should be used. Suitable cells are group R_1r (CDe/cde).

Negative controls. Ideally Cde/ceE cells should be used in order to check that the anti-D is not contaminated with anti-C or anti-E.

Group AB Rh-negative cells should also be included

as a check that anti-A or anti-B is not present in the grouping serum. An equal volume of AB serum must be used instead of the anti-D serum to check for false positives which may be due to the presence of rouleaux or atypical autoantibodies.

SELECTION AND PREPARATION OF Rh GROUPING SERA

When a D-negative woman has a D-positive baby the chances of her forming anti-D antibodies are quite high. Subsequent pregnancies with D-positive infants will increase the strength of the antibodies and at the second or third pregnancy the mother's serum will contain antibodies of sufficient strength to be used as a grouping serum. This, until recently, was one of the main sources of Rh antisera.

These immunoglobulins are able to cross the placenta and on entering the baby's circulation destroy its red cells—the original antigenic stimulus—producing a condition known as haemolytic disease of the newborn (HDNB) which in its severest form is fatal. It has become current practice to inject mothers who have been delivered of a D-positive baby with anti-D. The antiserum destroys any of the baby's D-positive cells which may have entered the mother's circulation and prevents the formation of antibodies in future pregnancies with D-positive babies. This practice has reduced the amount of anti-D grouping serum available from this source and increasing use is being made of volunteers in whom the antibody may be stimulated by the injection of D-positive cells. These cells contain other antigens and the antiserum produced may contain, most commonly, anti-C in addition to the ABO antibodies generally found.

Collection of serum

Serum is collected in the manner described for ABO grouping sera. Complement is destroyed by heating the serum at 56°C for 30 min.

Removal of unwanted antibodies

The inadvertent use of sera containing a mixture of antibodies may have dangerous consequences. If, for example, a grouping serum containing a mixture of anti-C + D were assumed to be pure anti-D, patients who were D-negative but C-positive would be erroneously grouped as D-positive.

The unwanted antibodies may be removed by absorption with cells containing the relevant antigens. ABO antibodies may be absorbed most satisfactorily using A_1B cells. Unwanted Rh antibodies may be absorbed using a mixture of cells containing the correct combination of antigens other than D.

The chosen mixture of cells is washed three times in saline. An equal volume of serum is added to the packed cells and after mixing is left at 4°C overnight. The mixture is centrifuged and the supernatant serum absorbed again in the same manner with fresh washed cells.

Specificity

To establish that all unwanted antibodies have been absorbed the anti-D serum is tested against the cells of group A_1B containing the Rh antigens CcddEe using the procedure in which the serum is to be employed, e.g. albumin, enzyme and/or indirect antiglobulin techniques. The results should be negative.

Titre

The anti-D serum should be titrated against group O CDe/cde and O cDE/cde cells prepared as in the manner described for the titration of ABO grouping sera.

Set up a row of six precipitin tubes corresponding to the row of dilutions and transfer one drop of each dilution to a precipitin tube, using a Pasteur pipette. By starting at the 1 in 64 dilution carry-over from lower dilutions will be eliminated. Add one drop of a 5% suspension of washed O D-positive cells to each tube. Mix and incubate at 37°C for 60 min. Displace with 20% albumin. Incubate for 30 min and examine under a microscope. When titrated with O CDe/cde cells a titre of 64 is acceptable.

OTHER BLOOD GROUP SYSTEMS

The ABO and Rh systems are of major practical importance in blood group serology. There are, however, other blood group systems which, although they do not form antibodies as frequently, are of clinical importance in that they are capable of causing transfusion reactions and HDNB. These systems include MNSs, P, Lutheran, Kell, Lewis, Duffy, and Kidd. Standard cross-matching techniques (Chapter 37) will detect atypical antibodies from the systems and specific antibody tests may then be performed.

A very complex system known as the HLA system (human lymphocytic system A) is of great importance in transplant surgery and can produce reaction to transfused blood. It is present in leucocytes and platelets and has a profound influence on the satisfactory establishment of grafted tissue. Differences in HLA types between graft and host will result in the rejection of the graft, and if the grafted tissue contains immunologically competent cells (as in bone-marrow transplants) a condition may arise in which those cells will attack the host tissue. This is known as graft versus host disease.

37. Blood transfusion techniques

COMPATIBILITY TESTS

For blood to be transfused safely it must be established that there is compatibility between the recipient's and donor's blood. An antibody circulating in the recipient's plasma which was active against the donor's cells would destroy them causing a severe, dangerous haemolytic reaction. Antibodies in the donor's plasma, on the other hand, would be diluted in the relatively large volume of recipient's plasma and partially neutralised by antigenic substances there. Attention is therefore concentrated on the detection of antibodies in the recipient's plasma using a technique called the major cross-match. The minor cross-match is not normally performed in the UK because the National Blood Transfusion Service screens all donor blood for antibodies before issue. The major cross-match involves a combination of the methods discussed in the previous chapter—enzyme, albumin and indirect antiglobulin techniques at 37°C, and saline tests at 37°C and room temperature. These techniques, of course, may be used to detect antigens as well as antibodies; known sera being used to demonstrate antigens and known cells to demonstrate antibodies.

Enzyme techniques

The enzymes which may be used to detect antibodies are papain, trypsin, bromelin or ficin. Incubation times are critical and over-exposure of the cells to the enzyme may give false-positive results. However, when adequately controlled and standardised these methods are extremely sensitive and the incidence of false-positives is very low. They are useful in the detection of Rh antibodies.

Papain method

Reagent: The solutions required for the preparation of the reagent are:

 buffered saline which consists of 85 g sodium chloride dissolved in 1 litre of 0·1 M phosphate buffer (Sörensens) pH 5·4;

1·0 M cysteine hydrochloride (157 g/litre)—used as an activator to overcome inhibitory effects of serum;
1·0 M sodium hydroxide (40 g/litre).

(1) In a mortar grind 1·0 g papain with 50 ml of buffered saline. Clear the solution by filtration or centrifugation.
(2) Add 5 ml of 1·0 M NaOH to 5 ml of 1·0 M cysteine hydrochloride to produce a neutral solution.
(3) Add 5 ml of the neutralised cysteine hydrochloride solution to the clarified papain solution and make up to 100 ml with buffered saline.
(4) Incubate at 37°C for 60 min.
(5) Store in small quantities at −20°C.

One-stage method

In a precipitin tube place one volume of patient's serum, one volume of a 5% suspension of donor's cells and one volume of activated papain solution. Incubate at 37°C for 60 min. Read microscopically.

Two-stage method

In a 75 × 12 mm tube place equal volumes of papain reagent and a 50% suspension of washed donor cells. Incubate for 15 min. Wash the cells twice and prepare a 2% suspension in saline. Place one volume of serum in a precipitin tube at 37°C. Allow to warm and add an equal volume of pre-warmed papain-treated cells. Mix and incubate for 60 min at 37°C. Read microscopically.

Bromelin method

Reagents

 (i) Stock solution: in a mortar grind 5·0 g of bromelin with small quantities of phosphate buffer pH 5·4. Make up to 100 ml with buffer and store at 4°C. At this temperature the solution will keep for 2 months.
 (ii) Working solution: dilute the stock solution 1 in 10 with saline.

Method. In a precipitin tube place one drop each of serum, 2% suspension of red cells and bromelin working solution. Incubate for 60 min at 37°C and examine microscopically.

Albumin technique

The method is the same as described under Rh grouping.

Indirect antiglobulin techniques (IAGT or Coombs' technique)

The principle of the IAGT is described on p. 265.

Tile test

All tubes should be scrupulously clean and the opalescent tile used in the final stage washed with soap and water then dried and polished with a clean cloth.

(1) In a 75×12 mm test tube place one drop of washed 50% donor cells and four drops of patient's serum.

(2) For a positive control place one drop of D-positive cells and two drops of weak anti-D serum in a test tube and for a negative control use D-negative cells and weak anti-D serum.

(3) Mix the contents in each tube and incubate all tubes at 37°C for 90 min.

(4) Using a Pasteur pipette carefully remove the serum/saline mixture from each tube and discard. Resuspend the cells and wash three times in saline. Resuspend the cells in three drops of saline.

(5) Place one drop of each cell suspension on a tile and add saline and AHG as shown in Fig. 37.1.

(1) Using a 2% suspension of washed red cells place one drop of test and control cells in relevant tubes. Add two drops of test serum.

(2) In a precipitin tube place one drop of a 2% suspension of washed donor's cells and two drops of patient's serum. Mix and incubate at 37°C for 90 minutes.

(3) Treat positive and negative controls similarly.

(4) Remove the supernatant serum/saline mixture from each tube with a Pasteur pipette and wash cells three times in saline. After the final wash remove all the supernatant saline and add one drop of fresh saline.

(5) Add an equal volume of AHG reagent.

(6) Mix the cells and reagent and allow to stand for 2 min.

(7) Centrifuge lightly (2000 rpm for 2 min).

(8) Examine for macroscopic agglutination. A concave mirror may be used to advantage. Doubtful reactions may be checked microscopically.

The antiglobulin test is very sensitive and may give false-positive results in the presence of dust particles and plasma clots. Colloidal silica may also cause false agglutination and for this reason it is recommended that anti-human globulin (AHG) and cells are mixed with wooden applicator sticks rather than the corner of a glass slide. The presence of serum proteins may inactivate the reagent and produce a negative result. Careful attention to cell washing procedures is therefore essential.

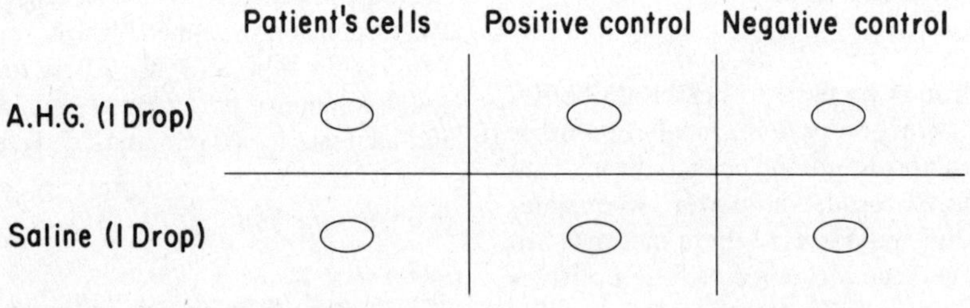

	Patient's cells	Positive control	Negative control
A.H.G. (I Drop)	⬭	⬭	⬭
Saline (I Drop)	⬭	⬭	⬭

Fig. 37.1.　Layout of tile for IAGT.

Mix with an orange stick, allow to stand for 1–2 min, then gently rock the slide for 3 min. Tests which do not show agglutination after 5 min are negative.

Spin test

This test is more sensitive than the tile test and more convenient to use.

PREPARATION OF ANTI-HUMAN GLOBULIN REAGENT

A satisfactory AHG reagent should be capable of detecting all antibodies when used at a single dilution. As well as the immunoglobulins already described there are antibodies which require complement for their reaction to be completed. An AHG which contains an anti-complement component will, therefore, be able to detect these complement-binding antibodies on the red cell. Such a reagent, which is capable of detecting the full range of antibodies, is called a 'broad-spectrum' reagent and requires much skill in its preparation. The animals commonly used for its production are the rabbit and goat, and as a single animal may not produce a serum with a sufficiently broad spectrum of antibodies the pooled sera from several animals of the same species is often required. The antigen is a gamma-globulin from human group O serum. Sera from group A, B or AB individuals are undesirable because of the risk of stimulating anti-A or anti-B in the animal. After an immunisation regime has been completed serum is collected from the animal and heated at 56°C for 30 min to destroy complement.

All animal sera contain 'anti-human species' antibody which must be removed before the serum can be used against human red cells. If the titre of the antibody is very high the amount of absorption necessary to remove it may reduce the titre of the AHG reagent to such a degree as to make it not worth while processing. A preliminary titration may be performed.

Prepare sensitised cells by incubating a mixture of O D-positive cells and anti-D serum at 37°C for 90 min. Wash the cells four times. Prepare doubling dilutions of AHG in saline ranging from 1 in 2 up to 1 in 512. Transfer one drop of each dilution into each of two positions on a tile as indicated by Table 37.1. To each drop on the top row add one drop of a 5% suspension

Table 37.1. AHG preparation: preliminary titration

AHG dilution	1/2	1/4	1/8	1/16	1/32	1/64	1/128	1/256	1/512
Sensitised cells	+	+	+	+	+	+	+	−	−
Unsensitised cells	+	+	−	−	−	−	−	−	−

of the sensitised O D-positive cells. Proceed in a similar manner along the bottom row using a 5% suspension of washed unsensitised group O D-positive cells. Mix and allow to stand for 1–2 min then rock gently while examining for agglutination. If the titre against the sensitised cells is less than 20 times the titre against unsensitised cells the AHG should be discarded.

Removal of unwanted antibodies

Once it has been established that the AHG titre is sufficiently high the next procedure is to remove the anti-human-species antibodies and any anti-A or anti-B agglutinins. This is achieved by absorption with group O cells and then group AB cells.

(1) Thoroughly wash the cells at least six times in large volumes of saline.
(2) Mix equal volumes of packed group O cells and AHG serum and allow to absorb at 4°C for 2 hr.
(3) Centrifuge and collect the supernatant serum.
(4) Repeat the absorption using packed AB cells.
(5) Collect the supernatant.

Further tests are necessary to establish the potency of the reagent but these are beyond the scope of this volume.

Saline cross-match at 37°C and room temperature

Equal volumes of a 2% saline suspension of donor cells and patient's serum are incubated at 37°C to detect immune 'complete' antibodies, and at room temperature to detect cold agglutinins such as anti-A or anti-B.

Of the several methods described above for the detection of antibodies in recipient's plasma it is essential that the saline and indirect antiglobulin tests be performed along with an albumin or enzyme technique. As plasma antibodies detectable by albumin will not fail to react with the antiglobulin technique the omission of albumin would be justifiable. However, as many workers prefer to use all four a protocol is described which includes them.

Protocol for cross-match

(1) Group the patient's blood as described in chapter 36; retain serum and select suitable donor blood.
(2) For each unit of donor's blood set up five precipitin tubes.
(3) Wash the donor's cells in saline and prepare a 5% suspension in saline.
(4) Place one drop of patient's serum in tubes 1, 2, 3 and 4 and four drops in tube 5 (Fig. 37.2).
(5) Add one drop of 5% cell suspension to each tube.
(6) Add one drop of papain reagent to tube 3.
(7) Mix all tubes by tapping and remove tube 1 to a rack at room temperature.
(8) Incubate all other tubes at 37°C.
(9) At 60 min read tube 3 (enzyme) and add 20% albumin to tube 4.
(10) At 90 min read tubes 1, 2 and 4.

(11) Wash cells in tube 5 and perform antiglobulin test.

(12) Positive controls using weak anti-D serum against group O CDe/cde cells are included to confirm the potency of the albumin, enzyme and antiglobulin reagent.

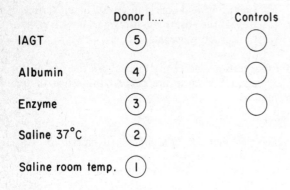

Fig. 37.2.   Protocol for cross-match.

Emergency cross-match

Clinicians who request blood urgently should have balanced the need for the immediate replacement of lost blood against the inherent dangers in transfusing inadequately cross-matched blood. The primary danger from haemorrhage is not the loss of cells but the reduction in blood volume, and while other volume-expanding fluids are being infused a cross-match may be performed. Whatever the circumstances it must be remembered that, using standard methods (the use of low-ionic strength saline will be discussed later), incubation periods of less than 20 min reduce the likelihood of detecting antibodies.

A tile ABO group and a Stratton sandwich or other rapid Rh group may be performed, but must be accompanied by a full complement of controls.

For the cross-match saline, albumin, enzyme and indirect antiglobulin techniques may be performed with an incubation period of at least 20 min and read after the tubes have been given a light spin. Again a full complement of controls must be employed. The incubation time should be as long as circumstances permit.

In parallel with the emergency procedures a full group and cross-match must be performed which may be read after the blood has been issued. All units of blood issued under these conditions should bear the label 'Emergency Cross-Match Only'. The stress of emergency cross-matches, especially at night, increases the risk of faulty patient identification and there must be no relaxation of the discipline requiring inadequately labelled blood samples to be discarded.

LOW-IONIC-STRENGTH SALINE (LISS)

It has been stated previously that the association of antigen and antibody molecules is greatly affected by the charges they carry and the degree of ionisation of the sodium chloride solution in which the cells are suspended. It has been found that if the strength of the sodium chloride is reduced from 0·15 mol/litre (the strength of physiological saline) to 0·033 mol/litre the resultant LISS produces a remarkable increase in the antigen-antibody association.

The use of LISS has had a marked influence on the methods used for the detection of antibodies, and incubation times may be drastically reduced without detracting from the increased sensitivity of tests performed in this medium. It may be used to great advantage in an emergency cross-match when a spin IAGT using cells suspended in LISS may be incubated for 20 min without fear of missing important antibodies. When using LISS there is a necessity for strict attention to the details of reagent preparation, temperature, time of incubation and the ratio of serum to cells (which will affect the ionic strength of the medium).

LISS (0·033 mol/litre salt)

Preparation

(1) Dissolve 18 g glycine in 500 ml distilled water.

(2) Add 1·0 mol/litre NaOH dropwise until pH 6·7 is achieved.

(3) Prepare 0·15 mol/litre phosphate buffer by adding 0·15 mol/litre $NaH_2PO_4 \cdot 2H_2O$ to 25 ml of 0·15 mol/litre Na_2HPO_4 until pH 6·7 is achieved. Add 20 ml of this buffer to the glycine solution.

(4) Add 1·7 g NaCl dissolved in 100 ml distilled water to the solution and make up to 1 litre with distilled water. Distribute in 100 ml amounts and sterilise by autoclaving at 100°C for 20 min.

In the cross-match the red cells are washed with saline and finally resuspended in LISS.

INVESTIGATION OF A TRANSFUSION REACTION

Transfusion reactions can range from a mild pyrexia to sudden total collapse and the causes are various. The reaction may be due to an allergy; too rapid transfusion of the blood; incompatibility of red cells, white cells or platelets because of a faulty cross-match or clerical error; infected blood; haemolysed blood; or the patient's aversion to the idea of blood transfusion being physically expressed.

When a transfusion reaction is reported the following steps should be taken.

(1) Obtain the remains of the transfused blood and check the identity on the label and group the blood to see that it is as stated. Centrifuge a small amount and examine the plasma for haemolysis. Send a sample to the microbiology department for culture.

(2) Obtain a fresh sample of EDTA blood and perform a blood count for comparison with the pre-transfusion sample.

(3) Obtain a fresh sample of clotted blood and repeat the group and cross-match.

(4) Repeat the group and cross-match with the original sample of patient's blood.

(5) Obtain a sample of urine and examine for haemoglobin and haemosiderin.

(6) Obtain a clotted sample from the patient after 7–10 days when antibodies may be detectable which were not obvious earlier because of their absorption on to the donor's cells.

(7) Test the pre- and post-transfusion samples against a panel of standard cells using all techniques for antibody detection.

HAEMOLYTIC DISEASE OF THE NEWBORN (HDNB)

The fetus has many antigens inherited from its father which are foreign to its mother. Any of these antigens could theoretically stimulate antibodies in the maternal circulation. If, for example, a baby is group D-positive and a few cells manage to cross the placenta into the circulation of its group D-negative mother, anti-D antibodies will begin to form in the maternal circulation. In a first pregnancy only a small quantity of antibody is produced, but later pregnancies with D-positive children will increase the strength of the anti-body and as it is the smaller IgG molecule it is capable of crossing the placenta into the fetal circulation and destroying its red cells.

Haemolytic disease of the newborn is therefore a condition in which the lifespan of an infant's cells is shortened by the action of antibodies derived from the mother by placental transfer. The antigen responsible for the highest percentage (about 95%) of cases of HDNB is the D antigen of the Rh system. This is followed by the other Rh antigens, the ABO antigens and antigens of other blood group systems.

The opportunity for fetal cells to enter the maternal circulation is at its greatest when the placenta is detached from the wall of the uterus during delivery. The prophylactic treatment with potent anti-D discussed previously is designed to destroy this sudden influx of D-positive red cells.

Ante-natal screening

Early in her pregnancy each woman should have her ABO and Rh blood groups typed, and her serum tested against known group O CDe/cDE cells by suitable antibody testing techniques. Any antibody present should be identified and its strength ascertained by titration. Titrations should be repeated regularly until delivery, when preparation will be made to treat the baby should it be severely affected with HDNB. Women whose first tests do not demonstrate any antibodies need to be tested only at the 32nd week and at delivery.

Detection of fetal cells. Acid-elution test (AET)

The AET is used to assess the need for prophylactic treatment with anti-D immunoglobulin of D-negative mothers who have been delivered of a D-positive infant. It is based on the principle that adult haemoglobin may be eluted from red cells in an acid medium (pH 1·5) leaving the cells as pale ghosts while the cells containing resistant fetal haemoglobin stain bright pink.

Reagents

Fixative: 80% ethanol.

Solution A: 0·75% haematoxylin in 96% ethanol.

Solution B: 2·5 g ferric chloride.
2·0 ml of 25% hydrochloric acid.
Distilled water to 100 ml.

Elution solution. Two volumes of A mixed with two volumes of B and one volume of 80% ethanol. This gives a mixture of pH 1·5.

Counterstain. 0·5% aqueous eosin.

Method

Dilute a small quantity of EDTA blood with an equal volume of saline. Make blood films from the mixture in the usual manner and fix in 80% ethanol for 5 min. Dry thoroughly and place in the elution solution for 20 sec, rinse in distilled water and counterstain for 2 min. Examine, microscopically, at least 50 fields for fetal cells using ×40 objective.

Current practice is to treat with immunoglobulin regardless of the presence or absence of fetal cells. The test is used as a guide to the size of dose required.

Treatment of infants suffering from HDNB

On occasions samples of amniotic fluid may be obtained to ascertain the severity of the disease. The fluid may be examined for the presence of bilirubin which would indicate the breakdown of haemoglobin from the red cells—the level of bilirubin indicating the severity of the disease. Intrauterine transfusion may be considered when this examination has indicated a severely affected fetus but it is a procedure which is not commonly practised. For this approximately 100 ml of fresh group O Rh-negative blood is transfused into the fetal peritoneal cavity from where the cells find their way into the circulation.

At birth the infant may require an exchange transfusion. This is effected by withdrawing a small quantity of baby's blood and replacing it with an equal volume of fresh, concentrated Rh-negative cells. The process is continued, using 20–30 ml quantities until approximately 500 ml of blood has been exchanged.

Tests on the infant's blood

A sample of cord blood should be obtained for haemoglobin, direct antiglobulin test, serum bilirubin level and ABO and Rh groups.

The results of these tests will serve as a guide to the need for exchange transfusion. A moderately affected infant would have a haemoglobin level of 10·0 g/dl or below and show evidence of jaundice. The direct antiglobulin test would be positive, although the test is not a useful guide to the severity since a mildly affected infant may have a strong positive reaction.

Direct antiglobulin test

Place one drop of a well-washed 5% suspension of baby's blood in a precipitin tube. Add one drop of AHG reagent. Mix and allow to stand for 2 min. Spin lightly in a centrifuge and examine for agglutination.

Positive control. Use CDe/cde cells sensitised with anti-D.

Negative control. Use the baby's cells and substitute saline for AHG reagent. This will eliminate false-positives due to Wharton's jelly, a sticky substance sometimes found in cord specimens.

AUTOMATION IN BLOOD GROUP SEROLOGY

Automated blood group systems

The processing of large numbers of blood groups and antibody screen tests may be facilitated by the use of automated machinery. The machinery most commonly used in the UK is that supplied by Technicon Instruments Limited, based on their continuous-flow system first used for biochemical analysis.

To bring about agglutination in a minimum time the system employs substances such as polyvinylpyrrolidone (PVP) or methyl cellulose which will encourage rouleaux formation. Sensitivity is increased by pretreatment of the red cells with an enzyme, i.e. bromelin. The rouleaux formed by unsensitised cells is easily dispersed on the addition of saline.

EDTA blood samples are placed in small test tubes and centrifuged to separate the cells and plasma into two layers. A double probe samples cells and plasma and sends them along separate pathways. Red cells are automatically diluted with enzyme and the channel

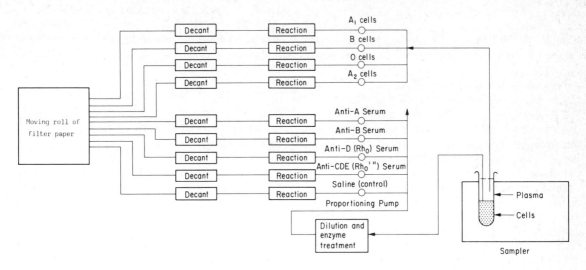

Fig. 37.3. Automated blood group (Courtesy of Technicon Instrument Co Ltd)
(a) Diagrammatic representation of the Technicon system.

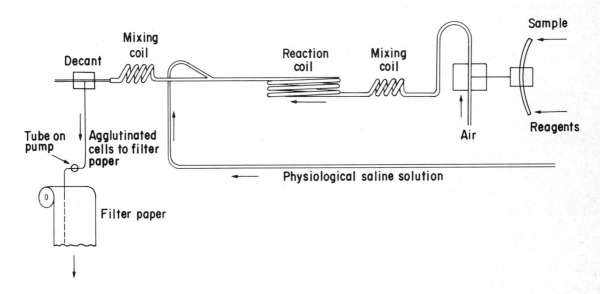

Fig. 37.3. (b) Detail of one channel.

divided into streams for ABO and Rh grouping. The appropriate antisera are pumped into the channels along with PVP. After passing through a large reaction coil, at which stage agglutinates form, rouleaux is dispersed by the addition of saline and the true agglutinates are collected on to a continuous-filter paper strip. The group may then be determined from the appearance of the agglutinates on the filter paper which may be kept as a permanent record (Fig. 37.3).

The plasma sample is separated into four channels and standard A, B, O and A_2 cells automatically join their relevant channels. After treatment with bromelin and PVP they proceed in a similar manner to the red cell sample.

The same principle is used in the detection of antibodies.

These machines show an increased sensitivity in the detection of antibodies, and provided an adequate range of standard cells are used they produce reliable results. In the earlier machines some workers had reservations about their use because of the possible errors introduced during manual transcription of data and misreading of results. The current model, the Autogrouper-16C system, provides 16 channels with a fully computerised print-out and a positive sample identification by means of a label scanner.

Automated Coombs systems

Automated systems exist for the performance of the antiglobulin test from the first washing of the sensitised cells through to the final light spin after the automatic addition of antiglobulin reagent. An audible warning device indicates completion of the cycle and the operator removes the tube and examines the button of red cells for agglutination. They are useful in a department which performs large numbers of antiglobulin tests. Each batch of tests must include weak positive, strong positive and negative controls. Two such instruments are the Dade C-7M and the Becton Dickinson Spectra 111.

QUALITY CONTROL IN BLOOD SEROLOGY

In blood serology departments relaxation of vigilance in the correct identification of patient and sample may have dramatic and dangerous consequences. Frequent checks of identity must therefore be built into every procedure.

Positive-reacting cells and sera of varying strengths should be included with each batch of tests to confirm the sensitivity of the method, along with negative controls to exclude the possibility of false-positive reactions.

All antisera should be used in the manner advocated by the supplier. If used incorrectly, unwanted antibodies may become active and would result in an incorrect typing.

Many Regional Transfusion Centres run a quality control programme, supplying panels of cells of different groups either as one pooled sample or several samples from different donors. Participation in these schemes is voluntary. Cells may be also supplied to enable a laboratory to run its own quality control scheme. Quality control programmes are also available commercially.

38. Blood bank procedures

THE BLOOD DONOR

The success of the National Blood Transfusion Service is dependent upon the voluntary blood donor. Professional blood donors have never been used in the UK and while an enthusiastic regular campaign is carried out in local communities by a voluntary donor organisation along with national publicity campaigns the rate of voluntary donations will still, hopefully, keep pace with consumption and the need for professional blood donors will not arise.

Blood donors must be healthy adults between the ages of 18 and 65 and should not have suffered from any transmissible diseases such as malaria or syphilis. Conditions such as anaemia, heart disease, kidney disease, high blood pressure, tuberculosis and epilepsy would lead to rejection as a donor. Transfusion Centres will usually require potential donors to complete questionnaires on these points before their acceptance on the panel. Donors in the UK do not normally give blood more than twice a year. Women are not bled during pregnancy nor if they have been pregnant within the previous year.

The donor session

Screening test for anaemia

Taking blood from an anaemic donor is dangerous to the donor, and anaemic blood is of little use to the recipient. The National Blood Transfusion Service will not take blood from males with a haemoglobin level below 13·5g/dl or females with a level below 12·5g/dl. A simple screening test used at donor sessions is to allow one drop of the donor's blood, taken by finger-prick, to fall on the surface of a copper sulphate solution of known specific gravity. If the drop of blood sinks immediately the level of haemoglobin is acceptable. If the blood rises to the surface before sinking the haemoglobin is too low. The specific gravity of the two copper sulphate solutions used is 1·055 and 1·053, indicating haemoglobin levels of not less than 13·5g/dl and 12·5g/dl respectively.

This screening test is necessarily simple because blood donor sessions are usually run by mobile teams who visit village halls, factories and offices and elaborate procedures would be difficult to perform under these conditions.

Blood donation

The term 'venesection' is applied to the procedure of obtaining a large quantity of blood from a vein. The blood is collected into a specially designed plastic bag which contains 67·5 ml of acid-citrate-dextrose anticoagulant (see below). The amount of blood taken, 420–450 ml, is assessed by weight using a small spring balance designed for the purpose. Glass bottles may also be used but have been largely superseded. If used they must be vented by means of a needle through the cap to allow air to escape when the blood enters the bottle. If the air vent is blocked pressure will build up inside the bottle and may cause air to pass back into the circulation. This will occur when the tourniquet, which was placed on the arm during the donation, is removed allowing the venous pressure to drop below the pressure which has built up inside the bottle. The result could be fatal. The problem does not arise with plastic bags.

During the procedure the bags or bottles are agitated frequently to mix the blood with the anticoagulant to prevent clotting. On completion of the donation a small dressing is applied and after a further few minutes lying on the couch the donor is allowed to get up and is given a cup of tea. Some donors are liable to faint after rising suddenly from a lying position. All donors should therefore be advised to get up slowly. Mild symptoms of fainting such as sweating, nausea or dizziness may be expected in about 5% of subjects.

Regeneration of haemoglobin and iron after venesection

Haemoglobin reaches its pre-donation level approximately 3–4 weeks after venesection. Iron stores take longer to build up and for this reason the interval between donations should be 6 months.

Plasmapheresis

An individual who wishes to donate his plasma, for example, as a grouping serum, may do so without losing his red cells. This may be achieved by a procedure known as plasmapheresis. A donation of 450 ml is taken into ACD or CPD in a plastic bag. This blood is centrifuged and the plasma removed. The red cells are then returned to the patient's circulation through the vein which has been kept open by a saline drip. This saline drip also serves to compensate for the reduction in plasma volume. The process may be repeated using a double amount of plasma after which the donor is no more affected than he would be after a normal blood donation. This double plasmapheresis may take up to an hour to complete but machines have been developed which will complete the process automatically. These cell separators will collect 500 ml of plasma from a donor in 20 min.

STORAGE OF BLOOD

Red cells must be suitably stored so that when transfused they are not destroyed immediately they enter the patient's circulation. This may be expected in a small proportion which are approaching the end of their natural lifespan but the majority should remain viable long enough to be of benefit to the patient. Red-cell viability is decreased on prolonged storage.

During storage there is a progressive fall in pH and a loss of the organic phosphates, adenosine triphosphate (ATP) and diphosphoglycerate (DPG). These changes are reduced at 4°C. Red cells stored at this temperature lose potassium into the plasma.

Anticoagulants

Heparin may be used for storing blood but has many disadvantages: potassium diffuses from the cells relatively quickly, the blood clots after 12 hr unless a large amount is used, and red-cell viability is low. It may be used at a concentration of 15–30 mg for 500 ml of blood. Trisodium citrate is unsatisfactory, again because of low red-cell viability, but with the addition of dextrose, which helps in the synthesis of ATP and DPG, the life of red cells is prolonged. Disodium citrate (acid-citrate) along with dextrose prolongs red-cell life even further. Citrates when transfused in large amounts produce toxic effects.

Citrate dextrose (ACD) anticoagulant

Dissolve 2 g disodium citrate and 3 g dextrose in 120 ml of pyrogen-free distilled water. At 4°C blood stored in ACD is at pH 7·4–7·5 and although the red cell volume is increased by about one-fifth their viability is not affected. This anticoagulant was used in the past with glass bottles, 120 ml being sufficient for 420 ml of blood.

A modified ACD solution known as ACD-A is now widely used with plastic bags:

Trisodium citrate (dehydrated)	2·2 g
Citric acid (monohydrate)	0·8 g
Dextrose	2·5 g
Water (pyrogen-free)	to 100 ml

67·5 ml of this solution is sufficient for 450 ml of blood.

Citrate-phosphate dextrose solution (CPD)

A solution containing less acid than ACD has been evolved which shows less haemolysis and slightly better post-transfusion survival. The solution may be prepared as follows:

Trisodium citrate (dihydrate)	26·30 g
Citric acid (monohydrate)	3·27 g
Sodium dihydrogen phosphate (monohydrate)	2·22 g
Dextrose	25·50 g
Water (pyrogen-free)	to 1 litre

63 ml of this solution is sufficient for 450 ml of blood.

Pyrogen-free distilled water

Pyrogens are substances which when injected cause a pyrexia. They are generally of bacterial origin. If the distilled water used for making intravenous solutions is not sterilised as soon as possible after manufacture the residual bacteria left from the cleaning of the bottles will have time to form pyrogenic material and although killed in subsequent sterilisation the pyrogenic effect will still be observed. Fluids may be tested for pyrogens by injecting them into rabbits. The fluid under test is injected into three rabbits and after 3 hr if the total rise in temperature of all three exceeds 2·65°C the fluid is pyrogenic and is discarded.

Blood-bank refrigerators

The temperature at which blood is stored is 4–6°C. At this temperature the changes in the organic phosphates discussed above are reduced, as is the multiplication of any bacteria which may have been introduced into the containers. The temperature in a blood-bank refrigerator must be strictly controlled within the stated range and a temperature-recording device should be installed. An audible warning, indicating when the temperature strays outside the range, should be run off a battery system independent of the main electrical supply so that it may function during a power failure. It is usual to have the warning signal showing at the main telephone switchboard in the building or at a station that is manned throughout the night. The alarm system should be tested daily to check that the batteries are not run down. Various commercial firms produce refrigerators specifically designed as blood banks. These should conform to BS 4376.

Blood should never be stored in a ward refrigerator. The temperature varies too greatly; on occasions dropping to freezing point. If blood is allowed to freeze under these conditions on subsequent thawing the red cells will haemolyse, releasing haemoglobin into the plasma. During this slow freezing process pure ice is formed leaving a liquid with a high salt concentration. When the blood thaws the red cells become exposed to varying concentrations of salt and the change from hypertonic to isotonic conditions damages the cells.

Frozen blood

If red cells are frozen rapidly there is little separation of ice and the red cells remain intact. Methods have been evolved for the storage of blood in the frozen state and, while there is some destruction of the cells (about 5%), after washing, the remaining red cells show a high post-transfusion survival rate.

Glycerol may be added to packed cells from a unit of CPD or ACD blood and the mixture transferred to a special plastic pack which may then be plunged into a bath of liquid nitrogen ($-196°C$). After 3 min the blood will be frozen and may be stored in liquid nitrogen vapour. The cells may be recovered, when required, by thawing at 40°C after which they are washed several times and resuspended in CPD. The loss of red cells may be as little as 4%.

Red cells may be stored in this manner for months or years. The system has the advantage that stocks of red cells containing rare antigens may be accumulated. It is not unknown for a patient with a rare antibody to have units of his own blood stored in this manner prior to surgery for use if needed, a so-called autologous trans-

fusion. Frozen blood may also be used to transfuse to patients with white-cell antibodies.

BLOOD PRODUCTS

The processing of blood has advanced so far that many components are available to provide for the individual needs of patients. One unit of blood, therefore, has a wide potential and blood donors may be assured that their blood will not be wasted.

Concentrated red cells

These cells, from which the supernatant plasma has been removed, may be used in cases of anaemia where the volume of transfused blood must be kept to a minimum to prevent cardiac failure.

Preparation

The red cells in a unit of blood are centrifuged or allowed to sediment by standing in a refrigerator. The plasma from the plastic bag is collected into another bag by means of a transfer pack. The sterile needle at the end of this pack is inserted and the supernatant plasma is removed by squeezing the bag. The connecting tubing may then be severed and sealed with a clip. Small units are available (Fig. 38.1) which apply even pressure to the bag so that the cells are not disturbed. The removal of too much plasma will result in a viscous product which would be difficult to transfuse. A preparation with a haematocrit of 0·6–0·7 litres/litre would meet the need for a high concentration of red cells and yet have a viscosity low enough to be transfused conveniently.

Leucocyte-poor blood

It is sometimes neccessary to transfuse blood to patients who have developed antibodies to leucocytes. To reduce the risk of a transfusion reaction from this cause the leucocytes in each unit of blood should be removed prior to use. This may be achieved by dextran sedimentation, in which dextran is used to promote rouleaux formation and the rapid sedimentation of the red cells; or by filtration through a sterile cotton wool or nylon filter. Frozen red cells may also be used as leucocytes are destroyed during the thawing process. Platelet-free blood may be prepared by similar methods.

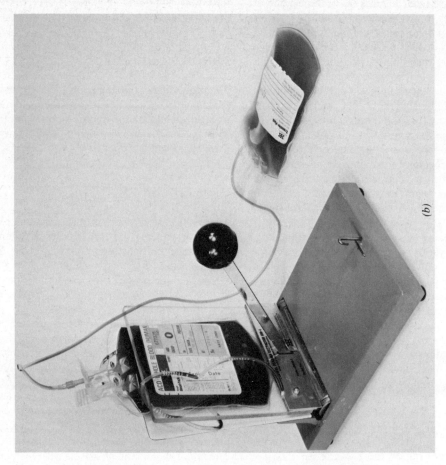

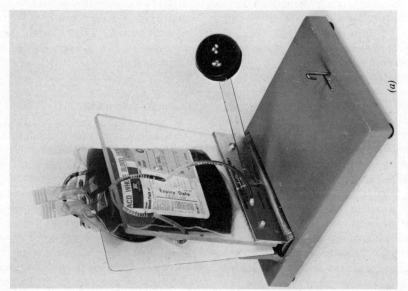

Fig. 38.1. Fenwall plasma Extractor
(a) Commencement of procedure; (b) concentrated cells prepared with plasma removed to satellite bag.

Platelet concentrate

The transfusion of platelets has been recommended in the presence of a platelet count of 50×10^9/litre when there is overt bleeding such as epistaxis, haematuria, etc., or when there is a fall in platelet count to 10×10^9/litre with a consequent high risk of bleeding.

Thrombocytopenia may be the result of marrow failure, drugs, an enlarged spleen removing platelets from the circulation at an increased rate or cytotoxic therapy for the treatment of a malignant condition. In all of these conditions a platelet transfusion will help to arrest the spontaneous bleeding which may occur when the platelet count drops to too low a level. Another condition with an abnormally low platelet count is idiopathic thrombocytopenia. This condition is not helped by platelet transfusion because platelets are rapidly destroyed in the patient's circulation.

Platelet preparations should be used as soon as possible after collection. If stored for longer than 24 hr their viability decreases. Preparations which are stored at 4°C show a high coagulant activity but disappear from the patient's circulation within 36 hr. When stored at 22°C platelets have a longer life-span but do not reach a peak of activity until 24 hr after transfusion. The usual method of storage is at 22°C with constant agitation. The best indication of the efficacy of platelet transfusion is not the rise in platelet count but whether bleeding has been arrested.

Preparation

Blood is collected in plastic bags containing ACD anticoagulant and centrifuged at $275\,g$ for 20 min. The platelet-rich plasma is transferred to a plastic bag and centrifuged at $1300\,g$ for 25 min. The preparation is allowed to stand for $1\frac{1}{2}$ hr by which time the platelets will disaggregate. They are then resuspended in 20–30 ml of plasma and stored at 22°C with gentle agitation. The single units may be pooled immediately before use. Concentrates prepared in this manner will yield up to 86% of the platelets in the original unit of whole blood.

Fresh whole blood may sometimes be requested when a patient is anaemic as well as thrombocytopenic. Blood is taken in the usual manner and transfused as soon as a cross-match has been completed. Blood transfused as quickly as this (within 2 hr) will contain up to 90% viable platelets.

Fresh-frozen plasma (FFP)

Fresh-frozen plasma is useful as a blood-volume expander by virtue of its albumin content, and as a source of coagulation factors. Generally, when coagulation factors are required the specific factor is given as a concentrated fraction; indeed the amount of FFP needed to supply a demand for an individual factor may, on occasions, lead to a circulatory overload. However, in a situation where there has been a general depletion of coagulation factors FFP may be indicated. FFP contains blood group agglutinins and must, therefore, be given to patients of the correct blood group. Its preparation involves the removal of plasma by centrifugation and freezing it within 6 hr of the donor being bled. The plasma is stored at −20°C or lower.

Cryoprecipitate

We have seen from chapter 32 that of the inherited coagulation disorders haemophilia is the one most frequently encountered. This is a condition in which there is a shortage of factor VIII, the anti-haemophilia factor. FFP contains about 60% of the factor VIII present in the original material and might, therefore, be considered a worthwhile product for the treatment of this condition; but the product takes 40 min to thaw, requires a large volume to raise the factor VIII level by a small amount, and frequently induces allergic reactions to the protein present. It is nowadays rarely used in the treatment of bleeding episodes caused by the lack of factor VIII.

If FFP is allowed to thaw slowly at 4–8°C a precipitate is formed which contains factor VIII and fibrinogen. This cryoprecipitate may be concentrated by centrifugation and removal of the supernatant plasma so that only 10–15 ml of the product remains. Cryoprecipitate does not cause a burden on the circulation because a large amount of factor VIII may be injected in a relatively small volume of fluid. A further advantage is that it has a low tendency to cause allergic reactions.

Preparation of cryoprecipitate

Blood taken into CPD anticoagulant gives a measurably higher yield of factor VIII than blood taken into ACD anticoagulant. A plastic bag system is used and immediately after collection the blood is centrifuged and the plasma expressed into a satellite bag. The plasma is frozen to −70°C by immersing in alcohol and solid carbon dioxide mixture for 30 min. The bag is then suspended in a cabinet at 4–8°C when it will slowly thaw and a cryoprecipitate will form; this is then centrifuged. The supernatant plasma is then expressed, leaving about 10–20 ml of plasma and cryoprecipitate. The cryoprecipitate is stored at −30°C. The ABO and Rh group should be stated on the label.

This method of preparation may be expected to yield about 70 units of factor VIII per bag. Cryoprecipitate may also be prepared in the same manner using FFP already in stock.

To prepare the cryoprecipitate for injection first select the number of packs required and thaw in a 37°C water bath for no longer than 5 min. Dry the bags, which are now pliable; flatten them and hang them on a hook. Examine them for leaks. Draw the cryoprecipitate into 50 ml syringes using a No. 1 needle. The injection may be performed using a 'butterfly' cannula or directly through a No. 1 needle.

The amount of factor VIII required may be calculated as follows:

Number of units required =

$$\frac{\% \text{ rise required} \times \text{weight of patient}}{1.5}.$$

Each bag may be assumed to contain 70 units.

The advent of cryoprecipitate and its convenience in use has led to the adoption of a policy of home treatment for haemophiliacs. Patients are taught how to treat themselves and are given a supply of cryoprecipitate for storage at home. The policy results in a greater independence, more rapid treatment and less hospitalisation for the patient.

Freeze-dried plasma

The plasma from 10 units of blood is aseptically removed and pooled. So that the antibodies present may be neutralised by antigenic substances a mixture of groups is used in the proportion 4 group A, 4 group O and 2 group B or AB. The pooled 10 units are distributed in glass bottles in 400 ml amounts. The bottles are rotated in a vacuum at 4°C in which manner the plasma is freeze-dried.

Freeze-dried plasma is commonly prepared from time-expired blood and in consequence has a high concentration of potassium due to leakage from ageing red cells. Stored at room temperature in the dark it has a shelf life of 8 years. Reconstitution is with 400 ml of pyrogen-free distilled water.

Freeze-dried plasma was originally prepared from large pools of plasma. The knowledge that blood transfusion could transmit hepatitis brought the realisation that one unit from an infected donor could contaminate the whole pool. The risk is now reduced by the use of small pools as described above. In addition to this, blood donors are nowadays routinely tested for the presence of hepatitis B antigen.

The use of freeze-dried plasma is nowadays restricted to conditions which require a restoration of plasma volume as in acute haemorrhage or severe burns cases.

Plasma protein fraction (PPF)

Plasma protein fraction has a higher albumin content than plasma but the overall protein content is lower. Its advantage lies in the fact that because of a lower globulin content it may be heated at 60°C for 10 hr with little aggregation of the protein; this treatment destroys hepatitis virus. The risk of transmitting hepatitis is therefore removed.

The product, having the same osmotic pressure as plasma, is used as a plasma volume expander without the risk of increased levels of potassium which may be found in freeze-dried plasma.

The solution contains 45 g/litre of protein, 90% of which is albumin and the rest α and β globulins. 130–160 mmol/litre of sodium chloride are added to make the solution isotonic. The potassium content is 0.2 mmol/litre or less and there is no fibrinogen.

Fibrinogen

Fibrinogen is presented as a freeze-dried powder prepared in the fractionation process of plasma. It may be used in treating the defibrination syndrome which may occur as a complication of labour or any other fibrinolytic condition.

The product is available in bottles containing 2–3 g of dried powder which is reconstituted by the addition of pyrogen-free distilled water.

Plasma substitutes

Blood transfusion in severe haemorrhage is aimed at sustaining the blood volume. As stated previously this may be achieved by the use of plasma until red cell transfusion is eventually needed to maintain oxygen-carrying power. A substitute for plasma must exert the same osmotic pressure as blood, should not leave the circulation rapidly after transfusion and should not be stored in the tissues.

Dextran

This is a polysaccharide of glucose which may be manufactured in a range of molecular sizes. The average molecular weight of the dextran is an important consideration when it is to be used as a volume expander. Molecules with a molecular weight less than 70,000 are rapidly excreted by the kidneys and solutions with a high molecular weight will cause 'sludging' of the red cells in the circulation. The choice of dextran will be dictated by the need to balance the degree of rouleaux formation against the length of time the substance will remain in the circulation maintaining plasma volume expansion. The serum from patients treated with dextran may create difficulties in cross-matching blood because of the tendency to form rouleaux, and for this reason it is a wise policy to obtain, if possible, a sample of serum prior to treatment which may be stored for cross-matching purposes.

PVP

Polyvinylpyrrolidone (PVP) is a high molecular-weight colloid which is used in the same manner as dextran but is excreted more rapidly. It is not generally used in the UK.

BLOOD BANK ORGANISATION

The Regional Blood Transfusion Centre will supply to hospital blood banks: whole blood, blood products, grouping sera and standardised cells. It will usually conduct a quality control scheme for the region and assist in programmes of training. It will maintain lists of donors with rare blood types and will act as a reference centre for antibody testing. Before issuing blood it performs the following investigations:

1. ABO and Rh group

The Rh group is performed using anti-D, anti-C and anti-E and only blood of genotype cde/cde is issued as 'Rh-negative'. These Rh-negative bloods are further tested by the antiglobulin reaction for the 'D^u' antigen, a weakly reacting variant of the D antigen. If this antigen were missed the donor blood would be erroneously grouped as Rh-negative and when trans-

fused into a D-negative patient the D^u antigen could stimulate the production of anti-D.

2. Screening for the presence of high titre anti-A and anti-B agglutinins in group O blood

Approximately 10% of group O blood contains anti-A or anti-B agglutinins of a sufficiently high titre to cause a reaction if transfused to group A or B patients. As group O Rh-negative blood may be transfused in an emergency before a cross-match can be completed it is advisable to screen the donations for these high titre agglutinins and if found the bottle should be suitably labelled.

3. Tests for syphilis

Screening tests for syphilis are performed on every blood donation and any with positive results are rejected.

4. Tests for hepatitis

The introduction of tests for hepatitis B surface antigen (HBS) has made a large contribution towards reducing the risk of transmitting hepatitis by transfusion. Once a positive result has been established the donation is incinerated, the donor is informed and his name is removed from the panel.

Hepatitis B antigen—safety precautions

Any worker who handles large numbers of blood samples is open to the risk of contracting serum hepatitis and all suspect material should be treated circumspectly. When testing for the antigen HBS the risk is even greater and the following precautions are recommended:

(1) All suspect samples should be labelled 'hepatitis risk'. Their accompanying forms should be similarly labelled.

(2) Disposable gloves, plastic aprons and masks should be used when handling the material.

(3) The tests should be performed in an area specially designed for the purpose, access being restricted to authorised personnel only.

(4) Samples should be opened and processed in an exhaust protective cabinet conforming to BS 5726, 1979.

(5) Oral pipetting must be forbidden.

(6) Where possible all disposable items should be incinerated after use. Articles which cannot be incinerated should be soaked in 2·5% hypochlorite solution (2500 ppm available chlorine). A stronger solution (10,000 ppm) should be used for blood spillages.

(7) All working surfaces should be disinfected with 2·5% glutaraldehyde.

For further reference to safety procedures see Chapter 1.

Blood bank documentation

Conscientious attention to the details of documentation is essential for the safe supervision and control of material passing through a blood bank. Patient's well-being and economy of products will result from a well-planned system which controls the issue of blood and blood products and includes identity checks at

BLOOD TRANSFUSION

AFFIX IDENTIFICATION LABEL HERE AND ON DUPLICATES OR HERE ↓

UNIT No.	UNIT GROUP	EXPIRY DATE	GIVEN BY DATE	TIME	INITIALS
1					
2					
3					
4					
5					
6					

SURNAME   Other names
Address: Date of Birth

Record Number

General Practitioner | Hospital | Ward/Clinic | Consultant

FOR USE
DATE
TIME   REQUIREMENTS:-   UNITS

IF OTHER THAN WHOLE BLOOD PLEASE STATE

GROUP AND SAVE SERUM ONLY   PLEASE TICK

BLOOD NOT USED WITHIN 48 HRS. OF STATED TIME WILL BE RETURNED TO STOCK UNLESS THE LABORATORY IS OTHERWISE INFORMED.

FOR LABORATORY USE

BLOOD GROUP_____ RH(D)_____

ANTIBODY SCREEN   DIRECT ANTIGLOBULIN TEST

DATE   LABORATORY No.

TRANSFUSION   ISSUE OF BLOOD - THIS SLIP IS REQUIRED TO CHECK & OBTAIN BLOOD FROM THE BANK WHEN THE TRANSFUSION HAS BEEN COMPLETED. PLEASE FIX THIS SLIP IN THE CASE NOTES.

REASON FOR TRANSFUSION_____

BLOOD GROUP (IF KNOWN)_____

PREVIOUS TRANSFUSIONS YES/NO (IF YES, PLEASE GIVE DETAILS)

PREGNANCIES, ABORTIONS, MISCARRIAGES (GIVE FULL DETAILS)

SIGNATURE OF DOCTOR   DATE

Fig. 38.2. Cross-match form.

									GROUP	CROSS MATCH	

RACK No. (R.T.) _____ 37°C _____ TIME:-

PATIENT | HOSP. INDEX No.
| WARD AND HOSP.

	ANTI SERA			AUTO	CELLS				ANTI D	A/B SCREEN		GP Rh
A	A₁	B	A I B		A₁	A₂	B	O		ENZ	IAG	

CROSS - MATCH

EXPIRY DATE	DONOR		ABO	Rh	SALINE		ALB. 37°	A.H.G.	A.H.G. No.	TIME (Incub. mins.)	FOR ISSUE
	SERIAL Nos. As on front of card		A.B.O.	Rh	Room Temp.	37°					
	1										
	2										
	3										
	4										
	5										
	6										

SET UP BY
READ BY _____ INITIALS _____ DATE _____ TIME _____

Fig. 38.3. Cross-match form. The top of this back copy serves as a file card.

several stages in the process of cross-matching and issuing of blood. Blood group, cross-match, and blood products books may be kept as separate documents.

The blood group book should contain patient's identity, age and origin, and the name of the clinician. In columns ruled for the purpose the reactions in each tube of the ABO and Rh grouping should be entered and in the final column the ABO and Rh group.

The cross-match book should also contain patient information along with a note on the clinical condition. The serial number of each unit of blood is entered, as well as expiry date, and columns should be provided for the time and date of issue and the signature of the individual collecting it from the bank. Space should also be left for information on the fate of the blood, whether used or not.

The blood products book may be kept as a record of transactions other than whole blood. Here, again, full patient information is required along with ABO and Rh groups.

Columns should be provided for a description of the product, its serial number, expiry date and where applicable, as in the case of FFP, its ABO group.

The form illustrated in Fig. 38.2 may serve as a request for grouping or cross-matching. It consists of a top copy which on completion of laboratory tests may be sent to the ward with the results entered, and a bottom card which serves as a laboratory record. The back of this card (Fig. 38.3) is used to detail the reactions of the various antisera and, in the case of a cross-match, the reactions of each unit of donor blood against the recipient's serum.

Among other records which may be kept are a despatch book with details of specimens sent to other centres, and a record of stored patient's sera.

RECOMMENDED FURTHER READING

1. Mollison, P.L. (1979). *Blood Transfusion in Clinical Medicine.* 6th Edition. London: Blackwell.
2. Boorman, K.E., Dodd, B.E. and Lincoln, P.J. (1977). *Blood Group Serology.* 5th Edition. London: Churchill.

PART SIX

Clinical chemistry

39. Quality control in clinical chemistry

Clinical chemistry is that part of pathology which deals with the detection and measurement of the chemical constituents of body fluids and excretions. Its limits are, of course, ill-defined. Other names for the same type of laboratory include chemical pathology, biochemistry, and diagnostic chemistry.

Quality control is a term used to indicate the procedures used by a laboratory to ensure that the answers which it reports are correct.

Quality control may be thought of in three parts:
Pre-analytical
Analytical
Post-analytical

PRE-ANALYTICAL QUALITY CONTROL

This subject includes patient status and the collection of specimens.

Patient status

For some results to be useful the patient must be fasting (plasma triglyceride) or resting (plasma lactate). Time is often important (plasma glucose, cortisol) and posture may be relevant (urine protein).

Collection of specimens

Blood specimens

If the patient is difficult to bleed or the venesectionist is inexperienced, the cuff used to enlarge the vein may be in position for a considerable period. In this event some constituents (protein, calcium) have been reported to become raised.

Some constituents are metabolised in shed blood. When this happens the values obtained do not reflect the status of the patient. These changes will be discussed when discussing the constituents, but a brief general guide is given. Specimens originating as whole blood are used in the laboratory as:

(a) Serum. When blood is shed it clots, and if the clotted blood is filtered, or more usually centrifuged, the supernatant fluid is serum. This means that serum is the same as circulating blood plasma, except for the substrates of blood clotting. This type of specimen is satisfactory for almost all analyses, and is preferred for protein and enzyme measurements.

(b) Plasma. Anticoagulants are used to prevent clotting, because the yield of plasma from a given volume of blood is greater, the specimen can be processed immediately, and some constituents (fibrinogen, bicarbonate) change from their physiological level when blood is allowed to clot. Glucose is a special case (*see* Chapter 40).

(c) Erythrocytes. These are rarely used for clinical chemistry. Erythrocyte transketolase is measured as an indicator of Vitamin B1 deficiency.

Urine specimens

Urine collections can be:
Timed.
Early morning.
Random.

(a) Timed. Most timed specimens are collected by the ward staff or by the patient, but the laboratory worker must be able to explain the correct way of collecting such a specimen since it is surprising how often this simple procedure is carried out incorrectly. Instructions for the collection of a 24-hr urine are as follows; they can of course be adjusted to any other time period. The patient empties the bladder and the time is noted. This specimen is *discarded*. All the urine passed until the same time on the following day is collected. The patient should then empty the bladder and this sample is *included*. Care should be taken during defaecation to prevent either loss or contamination of the urine. If the full collection period cannot for some reason be completed the time of the last collection included should be noted. It is much better to have a collection that is known to have been for 22 hr 50 min than to believe it

to be a true 24-hr collection. Collections for periods other than 24 hr are sometimes required, but it must be remembered that there is great variation in excretion rates of many substances throughout the day.

(b) Early morning urine. The first urine voided on waking in the morning is sometimes used. Usually it is more concentrated than others passed later and therefore some abnormalities are more easily detected.

(c) Random. Urines can also be examined specially for substances not normally found, for example, blood or bilirubin, where the presence is indicative of an abnormality and the concentration less important.

Preservation of urine

A number of changes take place in urine on keeping. Some of these will be mentioned in later chapters when specific tests are described. Many of these changes are due to bacterial action. If the specimen is collected into clean containers and stored in a cool place some of these changes will be delayed. If the urine cannot be examined soon after the collection a preservative will be required.

For many purposes acidification is a satisfactory means of preservation and about 10 ml of concentrated HCl should be used in a 24-hr urine. Nurses and patients should be warned of what the bottles contain to prevent accidents. In cases where acidification is undesirable or unsatisfactory a number of other substances have been employed. These include thymol, chloroform, toluene and formalin. Probably the most satisfactory for general purposes is a few millilitres of a 10% solution of thymol in propan-2-ol for a 24-hr urine, or 15 g of boric acid.

Naturally the storage of large volumes of urine presents a problem, and since most investigations require very little sample volume it is more convenient to keep a small representative portion rather than the whole collection. To do this the urine should be mixed thoroughly and carefully measured. The mixing is very important, particularly if any precipitate is present. A small volume is placed in a suitable container, a universal (30 ml) bottle being most convenient, and this bottle is carefully labelled with the patient's details, the time and date of collection, and the total volume.

Faeces

Random, timed or marked specimens are used depending upon the requirements. For qualitative investiga-

tions such as occult blood, a number of random samples should be tested. In these cases a portion of the stool is usually sent to the laboratory in a waxed carton or plastic container.

For investigations such as faecal fat where a quantitative result is required the entire stools are sent to the laboratory, usually for a period of about 5 days. The most convenient and least unpleasant way of dealing with these specimens is for them to be collected onto polythene sheeting in a bedpan; the ends of the polythene can then be gathered together and secured with an elastic band or wire closure. The whole specimen should then be placed is a deep-freeze cabinet. For analysis the polythene is peeled from the sample; if this is done whilst the specimen is still deep-frozen it will be found to come away almost completely, and whatever remains on the polythene can be easily washed off with water into the container to be used for the analysis. It should be noted that the above instructions apply only to faecal specimens to be used for chemical analysis, those requiring microbiological investigation should be treated in accordance with the instructions given in the relevant part of this book.

Cerebrospinal fluid (CSF)

Cerebrospinal fluid is frequently received in the chemical laboratory for the estimation of glucose and protein, and occasionally for other investigations. It is important to co-operate with the Microbiology Department since most CSFs require culture and cell count as well as the chemistry, and there is usually a limited quantity available.

The investigations should be carried out as soon as possible after receipt, or the specimen refrigerated. It is advisable to place some of the specimen into a container with the same preservative as is used for blood glucose. Remember that the collection of CSF is somewhat unpleasant for the patient so great care must be taken of the specimen.

Finally, two things must be remembered about all types of specimen. First, they all come from patients whose welfare is in some degree in your hands. Secondly, the fact that they are not in a microbiology laboratory does not mean that they are any less likely to be infective, so the necessary precautions must still be taken.

Identification

This subject is not as simple as it seems. The author has

been to a ward to collect blood and identified the bed indicated by the nursing staff as belonging to Mrs. Jones. When asked, the elderly patient sitting on the bed agreed by nodding and smiling that she was indeed Mrs. Jones. It was only as he was about to leave that Mrs. Jones returned from a bath to 'evict' Mrs. Brown from the bed, and the correct identification was made. Wrist name-tags have decreased the chance of this type of error, but not eliminated it. Local rules to ensure correct labelling exist, and should be followed. Identification must follow the specimen throughout its time in the laboratory.

Transport

Some constituents of blood may change very quickly even in the presence of anticoagulant. Blood pH, and oxygen and carbon dioxide levels are examples. The change may be minimised by cooling the specimen (anticoagulated) to 0°C by immersing in an ice/water mixture. Samples kept like this are suitable for analysis for up to 2 hr.

Storage

Every constituent of blood where the cellular level is different from the plasma or serum level will change if the shed blood is not centrifuged and the cells separated from the supernatant fluid. Samples which are not separated within a very few hours of venesection will be unsuitable for measurement of, for example, some enzymes, potassium and phosphate. Some analyses (e.g. renin) require that the plasma is frozen solid during storage.

Let us suppose, then, that the specimen has been taken, identified, transported, and stored properly. There are many potential errors still waiting to be made.

ANALYTICAL QUALITY CONTROL

Training

Probably the most effective means to ensure correct results is thorough training. A useful question to be borne in mind is 'Why is there never time to do it properly, but always time to do it again?' If a laboratory worker is not given time to learn the techniques, then that worker will constantly make mistakes and

require close supervision to achieve a satisfactory standard of work. Training is complementary to and different from education, and consists of equipping an individual with the skills required to complete properly the tasks allocated to him within the laboratory.

Instrument maintenance

In some laboratories the most neglected aspect of quality control is instrument maintenance. Spectrophotometers are often supplied with the means to check optical alignment, and this is certainly done for those instruments which are regularly maintained by the manufacturer. Filters are available which have a very closely defined absorption curve, such as didymium filters—these can be used to ensure that the wavelength indicated is the wavelength measured. Another means of doing this is to use a solution such as Holnicob,* which also has a well-characterised absorbance spectrum. There have been recent attempts to alert laboratories to errors caused by badly aligned and calibrated spectrophotometers. Specimens of absorbing solutions have been distributed to laboratories, which have reported to a central organiser on the wavelength and absorbance values. The results showed that there is room for improvement. In general it may be said that clean, well-maintained instruments may go wrong; dirty, badly maintained ones *will* go wrong. Most equipment manufacturers give detailed information in the handbook concerning the upkeep of their instruments. It is amazing how breakdowns are virtually eliminated, if the handbook is not lost and the instructions are followed!

Choice of method

This will be made by more senior members of the laboratory staff, but the aspects of methods taken into consideration for quality control purposes include:

(a) *Specificity*. Does the method measure only the substance under investigation, or does it measure other, chemically similar, substances as well? Lack of specificity does not automatically bar a method— non-specific glucose methods were used for several decades—but it is a drawback.

(b) *Simplicity*. A simple method is more likely to be

* From Scientific Hospital Supplies Ltd., 38 Queensland St., Liverpool, L7 3JG.

robust—that is to maintain its accuracy and precision in relatively inexperienced hands. It can also be faster than a complex method, allowing a greater work-flow.

(c) Precision. If reagents are unstable, or if an insensitive part of the spectrum of a spectrophotometer is used, or if the method is not specific or if one of many other criteria is not met, the precision will suffer.

(d) Sensitivity. If a method has been devised for another purpose, for example, testing drinking water or controlling an industrial process, it is likely that the range of concentrations commonly met will be different from those found in body fluids. Care must be taken when adapting a chemical reaction which works well from one concentration to another.

Other considerations in the choice of a method include cost, including that of new instruments and of reagents; safety of reagents and procedures; and availability of reagents or special glassware.

Again let us assume we have the right specimen and a suitable method—how do we know if the answers are correct? The errors which are made fall into two groups—random errors and systematic errors.

Random errors include the errors which are made by an operator—for example, bad pipetting or inconsistent reading of an end-point in titrations.

Systematic errors include some of the points we have considered—instrument, standard and reagent errors, incomplete reaction or interference from other substances.

To minimise random errors the best policy is to ensure good technique; other errors may be monitored by 'quality control' techniques, and steps taken to eliminate them as far as possible. It must be emphasised that no method is ideal, and no laboratory is perfect. Mistakes will occur. All we can do is to try to minimise them.

Definitions of terms used in quality control

Accuracy

Accuracy is the nearness of a result to the true value.

Precision

Precision means reproducibility. Thus a method is precise but not accurate if a true value is 100 units, and the values obtained from 5 repeat analyses are 110, 111, 109, 110, 110 units.

Standard deviation (SD)

Standard deviation is a statistical value which may be used to measure precision. It assumes that the values used for the statistical procedure will be 'normally' or symmetrically distributed. One way in which it may be determined is to repeatedly analyse a single sample and to apply the formula:

$$SD = \sqrt{\frac{\Sigma (x - \bar{x})^2}{n - 1}}$$

When $\Sigma (x - \bar{x})$ is the sum of the differences of each individual test from the mean, and n is the number of observations, which should be greater than 30 for an adequate measure.

Coefficient of variation (CV or % CV)

The standard deviation is difficult to interpret, because it will vary with the value of the mean. An SD of 0·7 with a mean value of 30 shows the same precision as SD of 1·4 with a mean of 60. The coefficient of variation overcomes this difficulty by expressing the SD as a percentage of the mean, thus in the cases cited above,

$$CV = \frac{0·7}{30} \times 100 = 2·3\% \quad \text{or} \quad \frac{1·4}{60} \times 100 = 2·3\%$$

The general applicability of CV does not mean that the value can be measured for only one level of analyte. The CV must be obtained for several levels, in the normal and abnormal ranges, and the mean value should be quoted when using any CV.

Control sample

A control sample simulates the chemical and physical characteristics of the unknown samples being analysed, and is taken through all the steps of the analytical procedure. A value for the analyte is assigned to it, either by special analysis, or because the analyte is weighed in.

Quality control techniques

Intra-laboratory control consists of the internal arrangements being made by a laboratory to measure performance with respect to accuracy and precision.

(a) Drift control. A large pool of material (usually serum) is divided into suitable volumes and frozen. Only the amount of serum required for immediate use

is thawed. An assayed value gradually becomes available as more tests from a single batch are done. In automated systems a control is placed at intervals throughout the run to check on the consistency of results within the batch.

(b) Commercial control samples. These consist of samples (usually freeze-dried) of serum which may have human or animal origin. They are made in large batches and bottled, so that any bottle from a given batch will contain serum with the same constituent values as that of any other bottle. Values are assigned to the constituents by a number of reference laboratories.

(c) Interbatch controls. One or more samples from a previous batch are reassayed with a new batch of analyses to check on the consistency of results from day to day.

(d) Daily means. If sufficient analyses of one type are done in a batch (more than about 40), then it is possible to assume that the population of results is likely to stay constant from day to day. If the mean of the results, excluding grossly abnormal ones, is calculated, it may detect an error of standardisation, which would affect all the answers.

(e) Quality control programmes. In this type of control, a central laboratory sends a sample to each of several hundred participating laboratories. Each laboratory measures a predetermined set of analytes, and sends the results back to the organiser. The results are analysed statistically and the processed information is returned to each participant. That laboratory can see how the results which it is reporting compare with the results from other laboratories using the same method, and with results from other methods. The standard deviations of results from each method gives useful information to a laboratory worker who is thinking of changing a method.

Quality control charts

A simple check on the precision of results can be obtained by the production of control charts, and there are a number of ways in which this can be done. A useful example can be seen in Fig. 39.1. The mean value obtained from a series of analyses (at least 30) and the acceptable limits (usually two standard deviations on either side of the mean) are shown, and the results obtained are plotted daily. In the example shown it can be seen that during the first 18 days the method was 'in control' but from day 9 onwards we see a trend occurring, in this case downwards. This could be caused by the deterioration of reagents or an increase in standard concentration by evaporation or

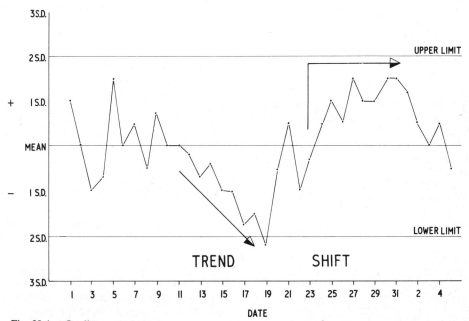

Fig. 39.1. Quality control chart.

contamination. An upward trend may be caused by a decrease in standard concentration, by incomplete protein precipitation or by a deterioration of reagents.

In our example we have corrected this fault, but from about day 25 a shift becomes apparent. This shift could be due to one of a number of factors including: change of worker to one less experienced, a new standard or reagent incorrectly prepared, loss of control of incubation due to a faulty timer, alteration in incubation temperature or any similar type of fault. It will be seen that in our example only one value has fallen outside of the acceptable range but that a great deal of valuable information has been obtained by careful inspection for trends and shifts. A log book for each method showing when reagents, standards or personnel are changed should be kept as this helps in the diagnosis and treatment of faults revealed by the control chart.

To make charting more flexible it is possible to draw a similar chart for a number of different control values. In this case instead of standard deviations, percentage changes from the various means are plotted. This type of chart is used in the same way as the previous example and has the added advantage that the various unknowns can be presented to the analyst in random sequence thus preventing bias, either conscious or subconscious, towards an expected result. A further advantage is that with carefully chosen control values the performance of the test over a wide range of concentrations can be determined.

'Cusum' technique

Cusum is an abbreviation of cumulative sum and is a running total of the difference between each measurement and its reference value, taking into account the + and − signs. A graph is made which plots the cusum value for each result obtained from the control sample. From the sample in Table 39.1 it will be seen that the

cusum quickly indicates a developing error. While the system was in control during the first six measurements the differences above and below the mean cancelled each other and the graph (Fig. 39.2) oscillated around the zero line. In the last four measurements an upward trend of 0·2 was indicated by a sharp upward turn of the graph.

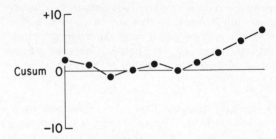

Fig. 39.2. 'Cusum' chart.

If, in a routine batch, a control sample is measured after every ten tests and the cusum curve indicates that the system is in control, it can be assumed that the tests between the control samples have been accurately assayed. If the system is out of control it can be readily seen from the graph which batch will need to be repeated.

A good quality control programme can only come about in a laboratory that is keen to improve the standard of its work. To be successful the programme should be continuously reviewed. Consideration should be given, for example, to narrowing the range of acceptability as work improves, and to the use of charts in training programmes for technical staff and to show the clinicians what degree of confidence can be placed on an individual result. It must be remembered that quality control is the responsibility of every member of the laboratory staff.

Table 39.1

Control reference value	Control estimated value	Difference	Cusum
120	122	+2	+2
120	119	−1	+1
120	118	−2	−1
120	121	+1	0
120	121	+1	+1
120	119	−1	0
120	122	+2	+2
120	122	+2	+4
120	122	+2	+6
120	122	+2	+8

POST-ANALYTICAL QUALITY CONTROL

A neglected area of quality control is that which covers clerical errors. All the technical and scientific resources of a laboratory, and the considerable cost of maintaining those resources, are wasted if an accurate answer is assigned to the wrong patient. Constant vigilance is required to ensure that the tedious task of giving each of perhaps several hundred specimens a day its correct documentation is performed accurately. The author deplores the practice of allowing untrained, non-professional workers to perform such tasks without adequate supervision.

All laboratories have checking procedures which make 'howlers' less likely. Such checking is usually done by a pathologist or a biochemist. Each result is compared with previous results, with the diagnosis, and with the treatment if this information is given. This task is made much more difficult without the co-operation of the clinical staff.

40. Tests of carbohydrate metabolism

GLUCOSE

The level of glucose in the blood is maintained within fairly narrow limits by the homeostatic mechanisms shown in Fig. 40.1. When these mechanisms fail the blood glucose may either be high (hyperglycaemia) or low (hypoglycaemia). A level over about 10 mmol/litre will cause the amount of glucose in the glomerular filtrate to be greater than the capacity of the renal tubules to reabsorb all of it, and glucose will appear in the urine. This finding is characteristic of diabetes mellitus—which means 'lots of urine tasting of honey'. Glucose is an example of a threshold substance, and the lowest blood level at which it appears in the urine is called the renal threshold.

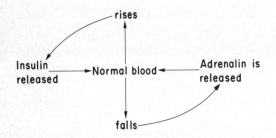

Fig. 40.1.   Glucose homeostasis (simplified).

Formerly blood glucose methods depended on the reducing properties of the sugar. Other sugars and some other metabolites share this property, however, and so most of the methods were not very specific. It is obviously better to have a method which measures only glucose and the enzyme system incorporating glucose oxidase confers a high degree of specificity on techniques for the measurement of blood and urine glucose.

Specimens

When blood is shed the cells do not die immediately. They continue to metabolise and use glucose as an energy source. This means that the blood glucose concentration would decrease with time if an enzyme inhibitor were not added. Fluoride is such an inhibitor, and is used to preserve specimens with oxalate or sequestrene as an anticoagulant. Fluoride inhibits the enzyme enolase, which occurs in the metabolic pathways of glucose, but has little effect on glucose oxidase and peroxidase.

Blood glucose has classically been measured on a protein-free filtrate of whole blood, which gives a value lower than that of plasma because of the presence of RBCs. Recent modifications in methods have removed any reason to treat glucose differently from the other constituents of plasma, which is now generally preferred.

Estimation of blood glucose (Royle C.M. and Hardwell T.R. Unpublished method)

(1) Principle

The aminophenazone–phenol reaction of Trinder is used to measure the oxygen evolved from the following coupled enzyme reactions:

$$C_6H_{12}O_6 + H_2O + O_2 \xrightarrow{\text{Glucose oxidase}} C_6H_{12}O_7 + H_2O_2$$

Glucose + water   Gluconic acid + hydrogen peroxide

$$H_2O_2 \xrightarrow{\text{Peroxidase}} H_2O + O$$

Hydrogen peroxide   water + oxygen*

It will be seen that oxygen appears at the beginning and at the end of the reaction sequence. The oxygen marked * is nascent (newly formed) and is much more able to enter into reactions.

(2) Reagents

(a) *Phosphate buffer pH 7·0.* 8·52 g of disodium hydrogen phosphate and 5·44 g potassium dihydrogen phosphate are dissolved in 500 ml distilled water, the pH is adjusted if necessary, and the volume is made up to 1 litre.

(b) Colour reagent.

Fermcozyme 952 DM*	5 ml
(Glucose oxidase + peroxidase)	
Phenol (analytical grade)	0·30 g
Sodium azide	0·30 g
4-aminophenazone	0·10 g
Phosphate buffer to	300 ml

Adjust the pH to 6·8 if necessary. Stable for 8 weeks at 4°C and away from light.

(3) Standards

(a) 10 mmol/litre. 1·80 g glucose are dissolved in saturated benzoic acid and made up to 1 litre.

(b) 20 mmol/litre. 3·60 g glucose are dissolved in saturated benzoic acid and made up to 1 litre.

These standards must be made up at least 24 hr before use. Glucose achieves the final proportion of alpha and beta form in solution very slowly, and glucose oxidase is specific for the beta configuration.

(4) Method

(a) Set up four test tubes as follows:

Blank   Test   Standard 10   Standard 20.

Add 3·0 ml working reagent to each tube. Add 20 μl isotonic saline to the blank tube and 20 μl of the test plasma and appropriate standards to the other tubes.

(b) Mix well on a vortex mixer and incubate at 37°C for 10 min.

(c) Read the absorbance of the test and standards against the blank at 515 nm.

(5) Calculation

The blood glucose concentration is given by:

$$\frac{\text{Abs. test}}{\text{Abs. standard}} \times \text{Standard value (mmol/litre)}$$

Use the standard absorbance which is closer to the test absorbance for the calculation.

(6) Note

For values greater than 30 mmol/litre use 6·0 ml colour reagent + 20 μl test plasma and multiply the result by 2.

* Hughes and Hughes, Ltd., Romford, Essex.

(7) Reference range

3·5–7·6 mmol/litre (fasting).

Commercial stick tests

These tests have been developed to give a rapid answer for blood glucose when full laboratory facilities are not immediately available. They depend on a test area which is impregnated with glucose oxidase and peroxidase in a buffer together with an indicator which changes colour in the presence of nascent oxygen.

Attempts to reduce the subjective nature of the strips, and to improve the accuracy and precision, have been made. They consist of:

(1) including a second complementary test area, and

(2) reading the colour of the test strip with a reflectance photometer (*see* Chapter 47).

REDUCING SUBSTANCES IN URINE

The detection, identification and quantification of reducing substances in urine has long been of interest in clinical chemistry. Recent advances in techniques have greatly simplified the task. The three questions that most commonly need answering are:

1. Is glycosuria present?

2. To what degree is glycosuria present?

3. If the reducing substance detected is not glucose, what is it?

1. Is glycosuria present? The question is asked, for example, during the diagnosis of suspected diabetes or during its treatment.

2. To what degree is glycosuria present? This information is frequently required to help in the regulation of the treatment of a diabetic.

3. If the reducing substance detected is not glucose what is it? A number of other reducing substances can occur in urine. These include other sugars; lactose (especially in pregnancy and lactation), galactose, fructose and pentoses, these last three occurring either after excessive intake or as the result of a congenital abnormality. Apart from sugars other reducing substances can occur, for example, salicyluric acid (after taking salicylate drugs, e.g. Aspirin); uric acid and creatinine (both normally present they can, in highly concentrated urines, give a positive reaction for reducing substances); and glucuronates in which form certain drugs are excreted in the urine.

Of the reducing substances of interest glucose is the

most common, and positive tests (Benedict's or Clinitest) should be checked in cases of doubt by a specific test for glucose.

Tests for reducing substances

1. Benedict's qualitative test

This is based on the reduction to red cuprous oxide (Cu_2O) of blue cupric sulphate ($CuSO_4$) in alkaline solution.

Reagent

173 g sodium citrate and 100 g anhydrous sodium carbonate are placed in a beaker with about 600 ml of water and dissolved with the aid of heat. 100 ml of 17·3% cupric sulphate ($CuSO_4 . 5H_2O$) is added slowly with constant stirring. After cooling, transfer to a 1-litre volumetric flask and make up to volume with distilled water.

Method

0·5 ml of urine and 5 ml of reagent are mixed in a test tube and heated in a boiling water-bath for 3 min. Observe for coloured precipitate formation. White precipitates are due to phosphates and are ignored. If the solution remains blue or slightly green with no precipitate the test is negative. Positive results go from a green solution with yellow precipitate (approximately 0·25%) through yellow and brown to orange or red (2% or more).

Commercial tests are available and are described in Chapter 45.

Identification of reducing sugars

There has been described in the past a multitude of tests for the identification of reducing sugars occurring in urine. These have now been superseded, for all practical purposes, by chromatography.

CHROMATOGRAPHY

Chromatography in its many and various forms is a very powerful tool in chemical analysis. It allows for the separation of individual members of groups of closely related compounds. Among the substances capable of being separated in such a way are the carbohydrates. Simple procedures for the separation and identification of sugars in urine by paper and thin-layer chromatography follow. Only those considerations of direct practical importance to the methods employed will be discussed. For other theoretical considerations the reader is referred to one of the standard textbooks on chromatography.

In all chromatographic procedures the following items must be considered:

1. The sample.
2. Method.
3. Support medium.
4. Stationary phase.
5. Mobile phase.
6. Setting-up procedure.
7. Time of run.
8. Location and identification.

Paper chromatography of urine sugars

1. Sample

A fresh sample taken after a meal is preferable; however, random or 24-hour collections may be used.

2. Method

One-way ascending (i.e. the solvent is allowed to run *up* the paper).

3. Support medium

Paper: Whatman No. 4 or No. 1 (No. 4 gives quicker separation).

4. Stationary phase

Chromatography depends partly upon the continuous partitioning of the substances being separated between the stationary and the mobile phase. In this method the stationary phase is the water contained within the paper (about 15% of the weight of the paper).

5. Mobile phase

Many solvents (mobile phase) have been described. Probably the most convenient and one of the least unpleasant solvent systems to use for sugars is:

Propan-2-ol   160 ml
Water   40 ml

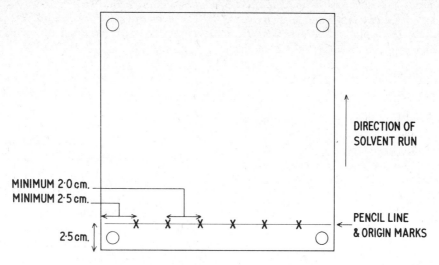

DIRECTION OF
SOLVENT RUN

MINIMUM 2·0 cm.
MINIMUM 2·5 cm.

2·5 cm.

PENCIL LINE
& ORIGIN MARKS

Fig. 40.2.   Paper chromatography; layout of sheet for one-way ascending chromatography.

6. *Setting-up procedure* (Using a standard 10-in. square paper)

Fig. 40.2 shows the layout of a sheet of paper for one-way ascending chromatography. Note the distance from the edge of the outside sample spots and the distance between them. The line, origin marks and any other inscriptions should be made faintly in *pencil*, ink will produce its own chromatogram with disastrous effect.

The diameter of the sample spots should be kept as small as possible. They can be applied by using a wire loop as used in bacteriology or, better still, by capillary pipette or microsyringe. If a pipette or syringe is used it is a good idea to put a little on at a time and dry by using a hair dryer after each application.

The optimum amount of sample will depend upon the concentration of the sugars present. Between $5\,\mu$l and $50\,\mu$l is usual; a rough guide can be obtained from the result of a Clinitest estimation. In addition to the test samples, spots of $5\,\mu$l and $10\,\mu$l of a standard made as follows should be run at the same time.

Glucose   0·5%
Galactose   0·5%
Fructose   0·5% } in 10% propan-2-ol- in water.
Xylose   0·5%
Lactose   0·7%

The above standard is satisfactory for general use, other sugars being added if required.

When all the spots are dry the paper is placed in the frame with any others to be run at the same time. The solvent is poured into the tray (Fig. 40.3) and the frame of papers lowered into the solvent. Care must be taken to ensure that the surface of the solvent is *below* the origin line on the paper. The lid is put in place and the solvent allowed to run.

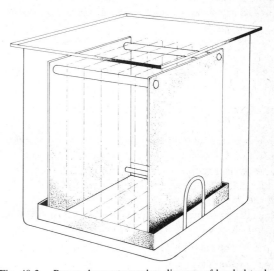

Fig. 40.3.   Paper chromatography; diagram of loaded tank.

7. *Time of run*

Usually overnight at room temperature. The solvent front will go to the top of the paper and solvent will then evaporate so that the flow is maintained; however, the speed of flow at this point will be increased if a pad of folded filter paper is fixed to the top of the chromatogram.

8. Location and identification

After being taken from the solvent the paper must be dried and again a hair dryer will be found to be satisfactory. Once dry, the chromatogram is ready for the locating reagent. Again many of these have been described but probably the most useful is aniline-diphenylamine.

Reagent

Aniline	1 ml
Diphenylamine	1 g
Acetone	100 ml
85% Phosphoric acid	10 ml

The chromatogram is sprayed (in a fume cupboard) using a glass spray bottle. These bottles are rather like scent sprays and can be obtained from any laboratory supplier. The spray should be held a few centimetres away from the paper and the reagent distributed evenly over the surface.

Heat for a few minutes at 95–100°C and observe for coloured spots, which will vary from grey-brown (pentoses, e.g. xylose) through greenish blue (e.g. glucose and galactose) to blue (e.g. lactose). The identification is helped by these differences in colour but more positive identification is necessary.

Chromatography employs as its basic measurement the so-called R_f value.

$$R_f = \frac{\text{distance substance travels from origin}}{\text{distance solvent front travels from origin}}$$

However, we have seen that in the separation of sugars we allow the solvent front to go, effectively, beyond the edge of the paper so that the denominator in the above ratio cannot be measured. This is done because many of the sugars have small and similar R_f values so that longer runs are necessary to allow sufficient separation. As an alternative to R_f we then use the R_g.

$$R_g = \frac{\text{distance substance travels from origin}}{\text{distance glucose travels from origin}}$$

These fractions (R_f and R_g) are physical constants of the substances concerned in a given solvent system and should be reproducible. However, in practice they can only serve as a guide since their reproducibility is not as a rule sufficiently good. It is for this reason that standards should always be run with the tests.

The approximate R_g values in the solvent system given for the suggested standards are as follows:

Xylose	1·30
Fructose	1·05
Glucose	1·00
Galactose	0·80
Lactose	0·32

Thin-layer chromatography (TLC) for urine sugars

TLC is much quicker and more sensitive than paper chromatography. Many of the factors governing paper chromatography also apply to TLC. In this case the separation is effected by, among other things, either absorption on to an inert medium or by partition of the substances of interest from a moving solvent.

1. Sample

As for paper chromatography.

2. Method

Thin-layer one-way chromatography.

3. Support medium

In this case the support medium is the substance to which is attached the thin layer of absorbent material. Glass is the most usual but plastic and metal foil can also be used.

4. Stationary phase

Silica gel G is recommended.

5. Mobile phase

n-butanol	75 ml
Glacial acetic acid	25 ml
Water	6 ml

6. Setting-up procedure

(a) Plates

The silica gel should be $250\,\mu\text{m}$ thick. Suitable plates can be obtained commercially, which is advisable if only small numbers of investigations are required. If the work load is sufficient the plates may be prepared as follows.

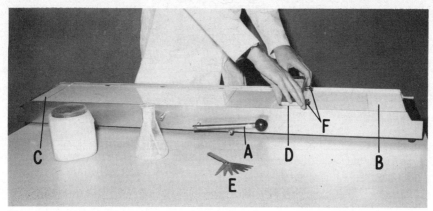

Fig. 40.4.   Thin-layer chromatography; making plates.

Glass plates 20×20 cm should be soaked in acid, washed and dried. It is essential that the surface of the glass is completely free of dirt or grease and is uniformly wettable.

A suitable plate-making apparatus is necessary, and Fig. 40.4 shows one type available from Shandon.*

The cleaned plates are placed in position and clamped with the handle *(A)*. At each end should be placed a half plate *(B* and *C)*. The front one *(B)* is used to rest the spreader *(D)* whilst the slurry is being added, the rear one *(C)* is where the spreader comes to rest at the end of the spreading action. The clearance between the plates and the front edge of the spreader is measured using the feeler gauge *(E)* and adjusted by use of the adjusting screws *(F)* on the spreader. (For this method we are using 250μm.) The edge of the spreader must be completely clean and free of dried slurry.

The spreader should now be placed on the leading half plate *(B)* and drawn slowly and gently back towards the operative finishing on half plate *(C)*. This dry run is done to ensure that the plates are level and that no obstruction to a smooth movement of the spreader is present. The best way of producing the smooth, steady motion will depend upon the person concerned. Probably the best way is to keep the arms straight, the spreader against one edge of the plate clamp, and to pull the spreader by stepping back. Do not exert any downward pressure on the spreader.

When the plates are ready and the spreader is adjusted and has been tested for free running, place it on *(B)*. The slurry can now be made. Mix 30 g of silica gel G with 60 ml distilled water and shake vigorously for 90 sec (this time is critical). Pour the slurry into the spreader and spread.

* Shandon Southern Instruments Ltd. Camberley, Surrey.

The technique of plate making requires some practice before reasonable results are obtainable. Allow the plates to dry for a few minutes, remove and dry for 10 min at 110°C in the horizontal position in a suitable rack. Activate for approximately a further 25 min at 110°C in a vertical position. The plates are now ready for use or can be stored in a desiccator.

(b) Application of samples

About 2μl of sample should be used, a little being put on at a time and dried. The origin should be about 2 cm from the bottom edge of the plate and the samples about 1 cm apart. Standards should again be run simultaneously. When the spots are dry the plates are placed in the tank and the solvent carefully run in. Again be sure that the solvent surface is below the origin line.

7.   *Time of run*

Allow the solvent to run about 15 cm which usually takes about 2 hr.

8.   *Location and identification*

Remove from solvent, dry and spray as for paper. Since the solvent front is still apparent, use may be made of the R_f values which for this solvent are approximately as follows.

Lactose	0·14
Galactose	0·35
Fructose	0·39
Glucose	0·42
Pentoses	0·5–0·9

KETONE BODIES

Ketosis

When there is insufficient utilisation of glucose due, for example, either to the inability of the body to metabolise it efficiently (as in diabetes mellitus) or to lack of intake (starvation), the body obtains the energy required by increasing the utilisation of fat. Normally fats are oxidised to CO_2 and water; however, under conditions of increased fat metabolism the oxidation is incomplete and there is a build-up of intermediate products. These are known as *ketone bodies* and are mainly acetoacetic acid, acetone and β-hydroxybutyric acid. This build-up of ketone bodies is termed *ketosis*. Testing urine for these substances is an important part of the routine investigation of diabetic patients.

Detection of ketone bodies in urine

There is no simple test for β-hydroxybutyric acid, which is not a ketone, but its presence has the same significance as acetone and acetoacetic acid.

1. Acetoacetic acid and acetone

Rothera's test

Take 5 ml of fresh urine. Saturate with ammonium sulphate. Add 0·5 ml of 2% aqueous sodium nitroprusside. Mix and add 0·5 ml of concentrated ammonia.

Result: The presence of acetone and/or acetoacetic acid is indicated by a purple colour which is most intense after about 15 min.

As alternatives to Rothera's test, Ames & Co. have produced two products, namely, Acetest and Ketostix. Acetest is in tablet form and ketostix is a test strip, and both give purple colours in the presence of ketones (see Chapter 45).

Rothera's, Acetest and Ketostix can all give false results in the presence of certain indicator substances used in diagnosis (e.g. bromsulphthalein). The colours are close enough to be mistaken for a true positive. If the presence of these substances is suspected the addition of alkali to the urine will reveal their presence by the change of colour in alkaline pH.

2. Acetoacetic acid (and salicylates)

Gerhardt's test

10% aqueous ferric chloride is added drop by drop to a few ml of fresh urine. Acetoacetic acid and salicylates give a purple colour. To differentiate between the two, thoroughly boil a sample of the urine and repeat the test. If the original result was due to acetoacetic acid this will be converted to acetone on boiling and the repeated test will be negative. On the other hand, salicylates are unaffected and the result will remain positive after boiling.

41. Electrolytes

An electrolyte is a compound which when dissolved in water, or melted, will conduct electricity. Solutions of electrolytes normally carry the same number of positive and negative charges, and this is true of plasma (*see* Fig. 41.1).

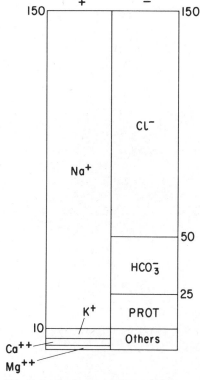

Fig. 41.1. Ionic composition of plasma.

As may be seen, sodium, potassium, chloride and bicarbonate account for most of the charged particles in solution in plasma water and in clinical chemistry these are collectively known as 'electrolytes'. This convention will be adopted here.

Sodium is the predominant extracellular (and therefore plasma—*see* Fig. 41.2) cation, and potassium is the predominant intracellular cation. The maintenance of correct water distribution between the body fluid compartments is essential for health, and is accomplished

by the regulation of intra- and extracellular electrolyte concentration as water will 'follow' the passage of electrolyte across cell membranes. The interpretation of electrolyte values is a difficult clinical matter.

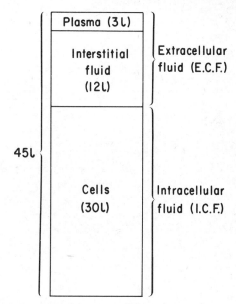

Fig. 41.2. Normal relative volumes of body fluid compartments.

Notes on units

This book has been written using as far as possible SI units. This being so, the values for Na$^+$, K$^+$, Ca^{++} and Cl$^-$ are given in the following methods in terms of mmol/litre. However, a measure of the weight per volume of an electrolyte gives no information about its activity. It is for this reason that some years ago the reporting of plasma electrolytes was changed from milligrams per 100 millilitres to milliequivalents per litre (mEq/litre). Now that SI units have been introduced we are reverting in effect to a weight per volume unit. However, for most of the substances referred to in this chapter a millimole is the same as a milli-equivalent since Na$^+$, K$^+$, Cl$^-$ and HCO$_3^-$ are all monovalent. It is only when we include such divalent ions as Ca^{++} or

Mg^{++} that difficulty arises when trying to add up a balance. Since these ions form only a small fraction of the electrolytes the difficulty does not arise in practice, and 'millimol/litre' is used for all analytes.

SODIUM AND POTASSIUM

Sodium and potassium are most commonly estimated by the technique of flame photometry. There are two types of flame photometry: emission and atomic absorption. Emission flame photometry is preferred for sodium and potassium estimation.

Principle

When energy in the form of heat from a flame is taken up by an atom, an outer electron is driven to an orbit with a higher energy state. There is a universal tendency for any system to revert to the state of least energy content (a battery running down is an example) and so the energised electron reverts to the original ground state. In doing so it must release energy, some of which is in the form of light. The wavelength of light depends upon its energy content, and as the electron conformations of no two elements are the same, the wavelength

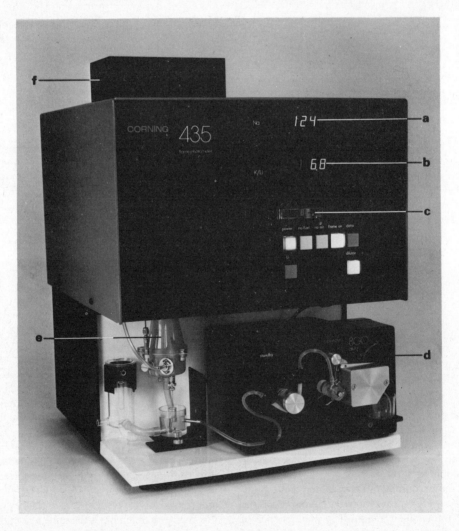

Fig. 41.3.   An emission flame photometer (Corning Ltd.) *(a)* Sodium display; *(b)* potassium display; *(c)* lithium indicator; *(d)* diluter; *(e)* nebuliser; *(e)* chimney.

of the emitted light is characteristic of each metallic element.

Instrumentation

A flame emission photometer has the following parts.

(1) A means of mixing the specimen with air as a finely divided spray—the nebuliser.
(2) A means of reducing the metal to the atomic state, and of exciting the atoms—the burner.
(3) A means of separating the wavelength of the emission to be measured from the background colour of the flame—the monochromator (*see* Chapter 5).
(4) A means of detecting and recording the intensity of the light emitted—a photosensitive element (*see* Chapter 5) and a read-out device.

There are several models of flame photometer available. A typical system is shown in Fig. 41.3.

The sample, and the standard, are diluted by hand, or more usually by a peristaltic pump which is a part of the instrument. The diluent contains lithium. The diluted sample is presented to a capillary tube (*a*) (*see* Fig. 41.4). The sample is drawn through the tube by a stream of air (*b*) provided by a compressor. The air stream causes the sample to be split into a cloud of tiny droplets—nebulised. Large droplets fall to the bottom of the nebulising chamber (*c*) and go to waste. The remaining cloud of small even-sized droplets is mixed with propane (*d*), the mixture passes through a baffle plate (*e*) and the fuel–air stream is ignited and burns, converting the metals present to their atomic form (*f*).

Light from the flame is measured at appropriate wavelengths by the photodetectors. The signals from sodium and potassium are compared with that from lithium, the concentration of which is constant. Any alterations in the signal which are due to fluctuations in the flame are compensated by a similar change in the lithium channel.

The results are presented simultaneously on a digital display panel, and are also printed, by some instruments, to provide a permanent record.

Automated methods

The automated estimation of sodium and potassium is, of course, possible. An example of the technique is the Technicon AutoAnalyzer (*see* Chapter 47) which uses a flame photometer capable of measuring both sodium and potassium simultaneously and incorporating the use of lithium as an internal reference.

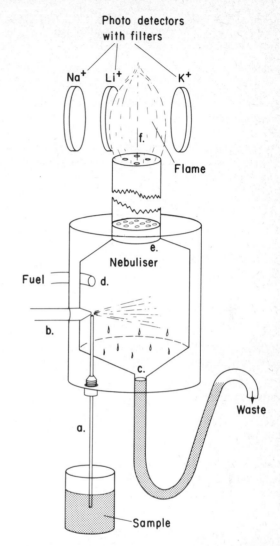

Fig. 41.4. The nebuliser and flame assembly of a flame emision photometer, (for explanation *see* text).

Most instruments now available incorporate a sample dilution device, and some have integral dialysers.

Standardisation

Modern instruments give a linear response to sodium and potassium over physiological ranges. It is usual to measure plasma against a standard with 140 mmol/litre sodium, and 5 mmol/litre potassium. Urines may be analysed using a standard with 100 mmol/litre of each. The linearity of response should be confirmed at least once a month using standards with 120/2 and 160/8 mmol/litre sodium and potassium respectively.

Standards

(a) Stock sodium standard 1·0 M. 58·44 g sodium chloride (dried to constant weight) dissolved in distilled water and made up to 1 litre.

(b) Stock potassium standard 1·0 M. 74·55 g potassium chloride (dried to constant weight) dissolved in distilled water and made up to 1 litre.

Dilutions of stock standards

Sodium/Potassium (mmol/litre)	Sodium stock (ml)	Potassium stock (ml)
120/2	120	2
140/5	140	5
160/8	160	8
100/100	100	100

These volumes are made up to 1 litre, with distilled water, for each standard.

Note: These standards are treated in the same way as patient samples.

Method

The method employed in flame photometry will depend on the particular instrument in use, but some points have general importance and will be discussed here.

Flame

The flame must be steady, the ratio of the gases (which determines the temperature of the flame) must be constant, and the rate of gas flow must be that recommended by the manufacturer.

Nebuliser

The rate of sampling must be kept constant. The chamber and capillary tube should always be clean, and adequate washing after use is essential.

Standards

A small aliquot of standard for use each day should be taken, and solution must never be replaced into a storage bottle. It is also better not to introduce a suction probe directly into a storage bottle, as to do so may contaminate the standard. For the most accurate work, standards which have the same viscosity as plasma are used with instruments which have a diluter.

Internal reference

Standards and samples are diluted in a solution containing 15 mmol/litre of lithium nitrate (1·85 g/litre), where an internal reference is used.

Note

Instruments using ion-selective electrodes are becoming more widely available.

Reference range—plasma

Sodium 135–146 mmol/litre.
Potassium 3·5–5·2 mmol/litre.

Estimation of sodium and potassium in urine

The same technique can be used as for plasma. The most suitable dilution of each urine has to be found because of the wide variations in concentration found. It is well to remember that the concentration of potassium in urine is normally much higher than in plasma.

CALCIUM

Calcium forms part of the structural mineral in bone, and is the most abundant cation in the body. It is also required at an optimum concentration for nerve conduction, especially in the heart.

Several methods have been used to measure plasma or serum calcium. Atomic absorption flame photometry and titration with EDTA have been most widely used, along with methods depending on the precipitation of an insoluble calcium salt. Dye-binding techniques have recently found much more favour, cresolphthalein complexone (metalphthalein) being used on automatic analysers. A dye-binding method incorporating methyl thymol blue is presented.

Estimation of serum calcium[1]

Principle

Calcium ions form a deep blue complex with methylthymol blue. Interference from magnesium is reduced by the addition of 8-hydroxyquinoline, with which it preferentially combines.

Reagents

(a) *Dye solution*

Methylthymol blue, sodium salt	0·18 g
Polyvinyl pyrrolidone	6·0 g
8-hydroxyquinoline	7·2 g
Hydrochloric acid, concentrated	10 ml
Distilled water	to 1 litre.

(b) *Diluent*

Sodium sulphite	24 g
Ethanolamine	220 ml
Distilled water	to 1 litre.

(c) *Working reagent*

Mix equal volumes of reagents (a) and (b).

Standards

(a) *10 mmol/litre*. Place 1·00 g dry calcium carbonate in a 1 litre volumetric flask, add 7·3 ml of concentrated hydrochloric acid, and make up to volume with distilled water.

(b) *2·5 mmol/litre*. Dilute 25 ml of the 10 mmol/litre standard to 100 ml.

Method

(a) 3·0 ml of working reagent is added to 50 μl of 2·5 mmol/litre standard, and to 50 μl of the test.

(b) Read the absorbances against the working reagent as blank at 612 nm.

Calculation

The concentration of calcium is given by:

$$\frac{\text{Abs. test}}{\text{Abs. standard}} \times 2·5 \ (\text{mmol/litre}).$$

Reference range

2·3–2·7 mmol/litre.

Note

Do not use plasma from blood which has been anti-coagulated with EDTA. Use serum or plasma from heparinised blood (*not* calcium heparin!).

CHLORIDE

Estimation of plasma chloride

There have been many methods developed for the estimation of plasma chloride. Those that follow are each based on a different principle; only the first will be given in detail.

Method of Schales and Schales[2]

This method employs an adsorption indicator, diphenyl-carbazone, and the chloride is titrated against mercuric nitrate.

Reagents

(a) *Mercuric nitrate*. About 3·0 g $Hg(NO_3)_2$ is dissolved in about 500 ml of water. Add 20 ml of 2 M HNO_3 and make up to 1 litre with distilled water.

(b) *Standard chloride*. 0·585 g NaCl (dried to constant weight) is dissolved and made up to 1 litre with water. This gives a solution of 10 mmol/litre.

(c) *Indicator*. 0·5 g diphenylcarbazone is dissolved in 50 ml of 95% ethanol. Store in the dark at 4°C.

Method

(a) *Standardisation of mercuric nitrate*. Take 2 ml of standard NaCl, add two drops of indicator and titrate with mercuric nitrate using a 2 ml burette. Repeat until results agree.

(b) *Estimation of plasma chloride*. Add 0·2 ml of plasma to 1·8 ml of water. Add two drops of indicator and titrate with mercuric chloride. When titrating plasma the solution will change from salmon pink to deep purple on the addition of the mercuric nitrate, this will soon disappear on further addition of titrant and the end-point is given by a sudden change from pale yellow to pale violet.

Calculation

$$\text{mmol/litre of chloride} = \frac{\text{Titration of test}}{\text{Titration of standard}} \times 100.$$

Note

The above titration can be carried out on a protein-free filtrate of plasma, when the end-point is somewhat easier to detect. With a little practice, however, the end-point in the method described is quite satisfactory and therefore the time taken in processing the samples is saved.

Mercuric thiocyanate/ferric nitrate method

This method is the one used by Technicon for the estimation of chloride on the AutoAnalyzer. The principle is that mercury reacts with chloride ion to form a non-ionised but soluble compound. Thus if chloride ion is reacted with mercuric thiocyanate, thiocyanate ions are released and the reaction can be written as follows:

$$Hg(SCN)_2 + 2Cl^- \longrightarrow HgCl_2 + 2(SCN)^-$$

If the thiocyanate is now reacted with a ferric compound red $Fe(SCN)_3$ is formed:

$$3(SCN) + Fe^{+++} \longrightarrow Fe(SCN)_3$$

The colour formed is read at 480 nm.

Note

A small amount of mercuric nitrate can be added to the system to adjust the sensitivity since this will react with the chloride before the mercuric thiocyanate. This has the property of reducing the sensitivity which is necessary for plasma chloride estimation on the Auto-Analyzer I; it is not necessary on the AutoAnalyzer II.

Reference range

95–105 mmol/litre.

Chloride can also be estimated with a chloride meter (*see* p. 351).

BICARBONATE

Bicarbonate (hydrogen carbonate) is the second most abundant cation in the plasma. It exists in equilibrium with carbonic acid and with dissolved carbon dioxide:

$$H^+ + HCO_3^- \rightleftharpoons H_2CO_3 \rightleftharpoons H_2O + CO_2$$

Because these equilibria are constantly maintained, any attempt to measure bicarbonate chemically results in a shift to the left so that all forms of carbon dioxide are measured. TCO_2 (total carbon dioxide) is the total amount of carbon dioxide released from the plasma by the action of a strong acid, which shifts the equilibria almost completely to the right, so that bicarbonate, carbonic acid, and dissolved carbon dioxide are measured. The carbon dioxide may be measured volumetrically or manometrically, as in the classical Van Slyke methods, or by dissolving in a weak buffer and measuring the resultant fall in pH with an indicator. A method has been described which uses the enzymatic incorporation of bicarbonate into phosphoenol pyruvate to form oxaloacetate which is measured by complexing with fast violet B.* Bicarbonate may be calculated from measurements of pH and P_{CO_2} by a blood gas analyser.

Reference range

23–30 mmol/litre.

REFERENCES

1. Gindler, E.M. and King, J.D. (1972). *Am. J. Clin. Path.*, **58**, 376.
2. Schales, O. and Schales, S.S. (1941). *J. Biol. Chem.*, **140**, 879.

   * Vickers Medical, Millbank Tower, London.

42. Kidney function tests

The major function of the kidneys is to help to regulate the composition of the body fluids (see Fig. 42.1). This function is carried out by:

acids. The efficiency of reabsorption, which mainly occurs in the proximal tubules, will affect the urine levels of these constituents.

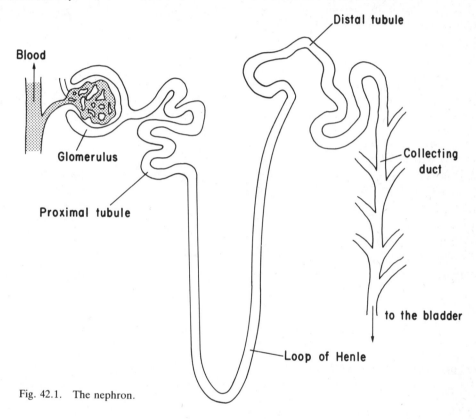

Fig. 42.1. The nephron.

Filtering the blood so that the constituents of plasma, except proteins which are comparatively large, pass into the urine. This process is carried out by the glomerulus and is called ultrafiltration. The glomerular filtration rate (GFR) measures the efficiency of this filtration and is measured by creatinine or urea clearance tests. Plasma urea and creatinine are also raised when the glomerulus fails to filter them. Urine protein is increased when the glomerulus is damaged.

Re-absorbing the desirable constituents from the filtrate. They include water, sodium, glucose, and amino

Excreting further unwanted substances such as potassium, hydrogen ion and ammonia from the cells which line the nephron. Urine acidification tests and acid–base studies are used to investigate this function.

Concentrating the urine by reabsorption of water in the distal tubules and collecting ducts. Specific gravity and osmolality are used to measure urine concentration without measuring any specific substance. The loop of Henle is also involved in the process of concentration.

315

UREA

Urea is the main end-product of protein metabolism; it is formed in the liver and excreted by the kidney. A raised plasma urea is therefore usually due to impaired renal function, but that impairment may not be due to renal disease. Gross dehydration will lower the GFR and will cause a rise in blood urea, as will any obstruction of the urinary tract which causes a back pressure of urine to the kidney. A pathological (disease-produced) decrease in plasma urea is rare, occurring in severe liver disease. In pregnancy, in growing children, and with a very low protein diet, plasma levels are lower than normal.

Estimation of plasma urea

The most common method of measuring urea in the UK is that based on the yellow colour formed when diacetyl monoxime is heated with urea. This method is confined to automated equipment almost exclusively, and will not be considered in detail.

Almost all other techniques depend initially on the action of urease, which is very specific:

$$NH_2.CO.NH_2 + 2H_2O \xrightarrow{\text{Urease}} 2NH^+_4 + CO_3$$
$$\text{(urea)}$$

The reaction may be followed kinetically by measuring the rate of increase of conductivity (*see* Chapter 47) or by measuring the amount of ammonia produced at equilibrium. A semi-quantitative method is employed by Urastrat* which indicates the volume of ammonia produced. The most usual manual technique is the colorimetric method using the Berthelot reaction.

Estimation of plasma urea by the Berthelot reaction

1. Principle

The ammonia formed by the action of urease on urea is determined by measuring the blue colour formed with phenol and hypochlorite, using sodium nitroprusside as a catalyst. EDTA is used to buffer the urease and to complex inhibiting metal ions.

2. Reagents

(a) *Buffered urease reagent.* 150 mg urease Type II[†] and 1·0 g ethylenediaminetetraacetic acid (EDTA) are

* From Wm. R. Warner, Ltd., Eastleigh, Hampshire.
† From Sigma London Chemical Co. Ltd., Fancy Road, Poole, Dorest.

shaken with distilled water. The pH is adjusted to 6·5, and the reagent is made up to 100 ml. Store at 4°C. Stable for 1 month.

(b) *Phenol colour reagent.* 50 g analytical grade phenol and 250 mg sodium nitroprusside are dissolved in distilled water and the volume is made up to 1 litre. Store cool and away from light.

(c) *Alkali–hypochlorite reagent.* 25 g sodium hydroxide and 2·1 g sodium hypochlorite are dissolved in distilled water and made up to 1 litre. Store cool and away from light.

3. Standard (10 mmol/litre)

Place 600 mg urea in a 1 litre volumetric flask. Add distilled water to dissolve and make to the mark. Add a few drops of chloroform as a preservative. Store at 4°C.

4. Method

(a) Set up test tubes as follows:

	Blank	Test	Standard
Buffered urease reagent	200 μl	200 μl	200 μl
Test plasma	—	20 μl	—
Standard	—	—	20 μl

(b) Incubate at 37°C for 15 min.

(c) Add 1·0 ml phenol colour reagent to each tube. Mix.

(d) Add 1·0 ml hypochlorite reagent to each tube. Mix.

(e) Incubate at 37°C for 20 min.

(f) Add 5·0 ml distilled water to each tube.

(g) Read absorbances of the test and standard against the blank at 630 nm.

5. Calculation

The plasma urea concentration is given by:

$$\frac{\text{Abs. test}}{\text{Abs. standard}} \times 10 \text{ (mmol/litre)}.$$

6. Notes

(a) Urine urea may be measured by this method, but a blank must be set up without urease to measure the preformed ammonia.

(b) If the absorbance of the standard does not lie

between 0·4 and 0·8 adjust the amount of added water until it does so.

(c) Urea is equally concentrated in plasma and cell water, and whole blood was formerly used. There is a small discrepancy, however, and plasma is now the sample of choice.

7. Reference range

(Adults) 2·5–6·5 mmol/litre.

URINE EXAMINATION

Much valuable information may be obtained by simple visual inspection of the urine, a fact that is often forgotten in these days of advanced technology. Table 42.1 shows some of the possible abnormal appearances

Table 42.1

Appearance of urine	Possible cause
Cloudy	(1) Blood (*see* p. 55)
	(2) Leucocytes (*see* p. 55)
	(3) Bacteria (*see* p. 55)
	(4) Fat*
	(5) Crystals, e.g. phosphate, urate, oxalate*
Red	(1) Oxyhaemoglobin
	(2) Porphyrins*
	(3) Beetroot*
Orange	(1) Some aperients (rhubarb, senna)*
	(2) High concentration of urates*
Brown	(1) Bilirubin (*see* p. 323)
	(2) Phenolic compounds*
Brown-black	(1) Melanin* } This darkening may occur on standing
	(2) Homogentisic acid }
	(3) Methaemoglobin*
Green or blue	(1) Dyestuffs (methylene blue, indigo carmine)*
	(2) Carbolic acid*

Notes (a) Each of the colours is typical, other shades occur.
  (b) This is not intended to be a comprehensive list.

of urine and their causes. The sections marked with an asterisk in the table are not discussed further in this book but are included to ensure that they are not ignored, but reported so that they may be investigated.

DETECTION AND MEASUREMENT OF PROTEIN IN URINE

Protein excretion in urine is normally less than 70 mg per day. This small amount is not detected by the qualitative tests given below.

Boiling test

The classical method of urine protein detection is the boiling test, and so long as this is carefully done it is still a simple and useful test. On heating, proteins are denatured and coagulate as, for example, boiling an egg will show.

1. Method

(a) A few ml of urine are centrifuged and the supernatant transferred to a clean test tube.

(b) Boil the upper part of the column of urine by gently agitating in a flame. Take care to point the tube away from yourself and anybody else, keep the tube moving and heat only the upper part of the urine as heating the lower part will increase the chances of boiling over.

(c) Compare the upper boiled region with the lower against a dark background. A cloudy precipitate will be due to the presence of protein or phosphates.

(d) Add a couple of drops of strong acetic acid and boil again. Precipitates due to protein will remain and those due to phosphates will disappear.

2. Notes

(a) Occasionally the precipitate only appears after the addition of acetic acid and reboiling; consequently this step must be carried out even if no precipitate is present after the first boiling.

(b) This method gives only a qualitative estimate of the protein present, so results are reported as: Trace, +, ++, etc., according to the degree of turbidity and the custom of the laboratory.

Quantitative method

1. Principle
Protein is precipitated from urine, redissolved, and measured using the biuret reagent of Weichselbaum. The test is done on a 24 hr urine collection.

2. Reagents

(a) 0·9% sodium chloride solution ⎱ As for serum
                                   ⎰ protein

(b) Working biuret reagent   ⎰ (see p. 325).

(c) 20% trichloroacetic acid (TCA) solution.

(d) 1 M sodium hydroxide solution.

3. Standard

A serum of known value (P) is diluted 1 in 10.

4. Method

(a) To 1 ml of urine or dilute protein standard in a test tube add 1 ml of TCA solution. Mix and stand at room temperature for 10 min.

(b) Centrifuge the test tubes.

(c) Decant the supernatant fluid and discard it. Allow the protein deposit to drain dry.

(d) Dissolve the protein in 0·5 ml of the sodium hydroxide solution.

(e) Add 2·5 ml of the sodium chloride solution. Mix.

(f) Add 2·5 ml of the biuret reagent. Mix. Incubate at 37°C for 5 min, or at room temperature for 30 min.

(g) Read the absorbance against a blank using 0·5 ml of NaOH at (d) at 540 nm.

5. Calculation

$$\frac{\text{Abs. test}}{\text{Abs. standard}} \times \frac{\text{Value of standard (P)}}{10}$$

$$= \text{urine protein in g/litre}$$

6. Note

If turbidity occurs, which is not deposited on the bottom of the tube during centrifugation—report as trace.

Salicylsulphonic acid test

Method

A few drops of 25% salicylsulphonic (sulphosalicylic) acid are added to a few millilitres of clear urine. A precipitate is formed if protein is present. False positives can occur after the use of certain radio-opaque substances for pyelograms. Whilst being a simple and quick test, it cannot be recommended in place of the other tests mentioned here. A very rapid and convenient method for the detection of urine protein is the use of the commercial test strips described in Chapter 45.

Bence-Jones protein

Bence-Jones protein is a group of small-molecule (mol. wt. c. 22,500) proteins that are excreted in the urine from some cases of a malignant bone disease known as multiple myeloma.

An important property of Bence-Jones protein is that a precipitate occurs on heating to between 40° and 60°C which is lower than with the other proteins that occur in urine. This property forms the basis of the test that follows. This is a relatively insensitive test. If a negative result is obtained in spite of a suspicion that the patient has the disease, then further specialised testing is required. A positive test is found in 6 out of 10 patients with Bence-Jones proteinuria.

Method

Filter the urine, make just acid to litmus and place about 5 ml in each of three tubes. Add 1 drop of 33% acetic acid to one tube, 2 drops to a second tube and nothing to the third. Place the tubes in a beaker of cold water with a thermometer. The thermometer is best placed in one of the tubes of urine for more accurate control. Heat the beaker; if Bence-Jones protein is present a precipitate will form between 40° and 60°C which will redissolve on boiling. Turbidities starting at 60°C or higher will be caused by albumin and other proteins.

Frequently other proteins are present with Bence-Jones in which case it will not be possible to observe the disappearance of the precipitate on boiling. In order to do so, filter the urine whilst hot and retest the filtrate.

URINARY ACIDIFICATION TEST

An oral dose of ammonium chloride normally causes the production of an acid urine. The ammonium ion is converted to urea by the liver, while the chloride is excreted by the kidney in association with hydrogen ions.

After the dose, timed urine samples are collected and the pH, which normally falls below 5·3, measured with a pH meter (see Chapter 4).

SPECIFIC GRAVITY OF URINE

The measurement of the specific gravity of urine can be of importance in detecting any abnormalities of the concentrating abilities of the kidneys. This test is frequently performed in the ward, but is sometimes done in the laboratory.

The simplest method, assuming an adequate volume of urine, is the use of a urinometer, which is a hydrometer calibrated over the range of expected values for urine.

1. Method

The urinometer is allowed to float in the urine. The calibration figure level with the surface of the urine is noted. This figure has then to be corrected. This is done as follows: 0·001 is added for each 3°C above the calibration temperature marked on the instrument or 0·001 subtracted for each 3°C below.

For example:

Urinometer reading	1·020
Urine temperature	19°C
Calibration temperature	15°C
Correction	+0·001 (nearest 3°C above calibration temperature)
SG of urine	1·021.

2. Notes

(a) Sufficient volume of urine is required for the urinometer to float freely without coming in contact with the vessel containing the urine.

(b) The decimal point is often omitted from specific gravity readings, i.e. 1·010 becomes 1010. There is no reason for this except tradition.

(c) The presence of large quantities of albumin or glucose will also affect the specific gravity. 0·003 should be subtracted from the observed value for each gram per 100 ml.

(d) Normally a 24-hour urine would have a specific gravity of around 1·020; random specimens may vary between 1·001 and 1·040 depending upon such factors as the amount of fluid intake, perspiration and the content of the urine.

(e) Specific gravity tests are sometimes carried out as part of concentration or dilution tests in the investigation of renal disease.

3. Alternative methods

The above method requires a relatively large volume of urine. This, of course, is not always available. Smaller quantities of urine can be weighed, using either a specific gravity bottle or by pipetting a known quantity and comparing the weight with an equal volume of water under the same conditions.

Osmolality

Urinometers are convenient to use but not particularly accurate. The specific gravity of urine depends upon the weight of substances dissolved whereas the kidney's ability to concentrate urine is related to the concentration of osmotically active particles (see Chapter 47).

43. Tests of liver function

The liver is the largest organ in the body and weighs about 1·5 kg in an adult. It has many functions of which only two are considered here; they are the excretion of bile and protein metabolism.

EXCRETION OF BILE

A knowledge of the metabolism of bile is necessary to understand the forms of jaundice that occur and the reason why certain tests are requested. Bile is secreted by the liver, stored and concentrated in the gall bladder and released into the duodenum, where it helps to emulsify dietary fat. One of the constituents of bile is bilirubin, and the detection and measurement of bilirubin and its breakdown products is described in this chapter. Figure 43.1 is a simplified diagram of bile pigment metabolism.

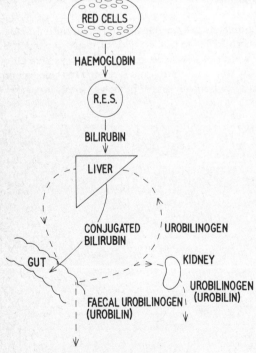

Fig. 43.1. Bile pigment metabolism.

Bilirubin

The bilirubin present in normal blood is largely derived from the breakdown of haemoglobin in the reticulo-endothelial system (RES) which is a system of cells in the spleen, liver, lymphoid tissue and bone marrow. It passes from the RES to the liver where it is conjugated with glucuronic acid and passes into the bile. Bilirubin is insoluble in water, it is carried in the blood attached to albumin and so it cannot be excreted by the kidney. This bilirubin will not react with aqueous reagents in the absence of a solubilising agent or accelerator, and is termed *indirect reacting bilirubin*. When bilirubin has been conjugated with (joined to) glucuronic acid in the liver, it is made water-soluble, is excreted from the liver into the gall bladder, and is termed *direct reacting* as it reacts with aqueous reagents.

Jaundice

Jaundice is the name given to the conditions in which the patient has a yellow coloration of the skin and eyes, due to the presence of a raised serum bilirubin. Jaundice may be divided into three types.

1. Pre-hepatic. The bilirubin load is too much for the liver to conjugate, usually because haemoglobin is being broken down quickly—such as in haemolytic disease. The bilirubin is mostly direct.

2. Hepatic. Liver cell damage, for example in infective hepatitis, prevents conjugation. In the early stages the bilirubin is indirect, but as the cell damage affects the structure of the liver, conjugated bilirubin may be increased.

3. Post-hepatic. When bilirubin which has been conjugated cannot be excreted because there is some obstruction, the conjugated bilirubin 'spills over' into the blood. This bilirubin, remember, is water-soluble and may be excreted by the kidney.

TESTS OF BILE PIGMENT METABOLISM

Serum bilirubin[1,2]

Total bilirubin is determined by diazotisation in the presence of caffeine which is an accelerator of the diazo reaction with unconjugated bilirubin. Direct-reacting (conjugated) bilirubin is measured without caffeine at an acidic pH at which unconjugated bilirubin does not react. The sensitivity of the method is increased by converting the red azo-dye into the blue form by alkalinisation. Ascorbic acid is used to stop the reaction and to eliminate interference by haemoglobin.

1. Reagents

(a) *Sulphanilic acid reagent*

Sulphanilic acid	5·0 g
Hydrochloric acid, concentrated	15 ml
Distilled water	to 1 litre

(b) *Sodium nitrite solution*

Sodium nitrite	0·50 g
Distilled water	to 100 ml

Note: This reagent must be made fresh each week, and be kept at 4°C.

(c) *Diazo reagent*

Sodium nitrite acid solution (b)	0·25 ml
Sulphanilic acid solution (a)	10 ml

Note: Make fresh for each batch of analysis, the reagent is stable for about 3 hr only.

(d) *Caffeine reagent*

Sodium benzoate	75 g
Caffeine	50 g
Sodium acetate, anhydrous	75 g
Ethylene diamine tetra-acetic acid, disodium salt (EDTA, disodium salt)	1 g
Distilled water	to 1 litre

(e) *Alkaline tartrate reagent*

Sodium hydroxide	100 g
Sodium potassium tartrate	350 g
Distilled water	to 1 litre

(f) *Ascorbic acid solution*

Ascorbic acid	0·20 g
Distilled water	5 ml

Note: Make fresh every day.

2. Standards

The standardisation of bilirubin methods is full of problems as pure bilirubin is insoluble in aqueous media. A good, but time-consuming and technically complex standard has been proposed by Billing *et al.*[3] Use aliquots of a freeze-dried material such as Versatol Paediatric,* which has a known value.

3. Method

Set up test tubes as follows, thoroughly mixing after each addition.

	TOTAL		DIRECT	
	Blank (ml)	Test (ml)	Blank (ml)	Test (ml)
Serum (or standard)	0·2	0·2	0·2	0·2
Water	0·8	0·8	0·8	0·8
Caffeine reagent	—	2·0	—	—
Ascorbic acid solution	0·1	—	0·1	—
Diazo reagent	0·5	0·5	0·5	0·5

Keep all tubes in the dark for 10 min then add:

	TOTAL		DIRECT	
	Blank (ml)	Test (ml)	Blank (ml)	Test (ml)
Ascorbic acid	—	0·1	—	0·1
Caffeine reagent	2·0	—	2·0	2·0
Alkaline tartrate	1·5	1·5	1·5	1·5

Read the absorbance of each 'Test' tube against the relevant blank in 1 cm cuvettes at 600 nm. The colour is stable for up to 30 min.

4. Calculation

$$\frac{\text{Abs. 'serum'}}{\text{Abs. 'standard'}} \times \text{conc. 'standard' } (\mu\text{mol/litre})$$
$$= \text{conc. 'serum' } (\mu\text{mol/litre}).$$

5. Notes

(*a*) Bilirubin is unstable. Direct sunlight can cause a loss of half of the value in 1 hr. Keep specimens and tests in dim light for the whole procedure.

* From Wm. R. Warner, Eastleigh, Hampshire.

(b) On rare occasions the direct-reading bilirubin value may be higher than that of the total bilirubin. This phenomenon is probably due to mild inhibition of diazotisation by caffeine.

6. Reference range

Up to $17\,\mu$mol/litre.

Urine urobilinogen

Bilirubin that enters the gut in bile is reduced by bacterial action into a group of substances known collectively as urobilinogen. Most of this is excreted in the faeces but some is reabsorbed into the blood, from which it is taken up by the liver, to be re-excreted in bile, and by the kidney; so it appears in the urine. It is absent from the gut, and from the urine in obstructive jaundice, because no bilirubin is secreted. On exposure to atmospheric oxygen, urobilinogen is oxidised to urobilin. A fresh specimen of urine is therefore essential.

1. Reagent (Ehrlich's)

p-dimethylaminobenzaldehyde	2 g
Concentrated HCl	20 ml
Distilled water	to 100 ml

2. Method

Add 1 ml of reagent to 10 ml of urine
Stand for 5 min.

3. Result

An increased concentration of urobilinogen will yield a red coloration. It should be noted that normally a fresh urine will contain some urobilinogen so that a slight coloration should be ignored.

4. Notes

(a) If bilirubin is present it should first be removed in the following manner. To 10 ml urine add 2 ml 10% calcium chloride, mix and filter. Perform test on filtrate.

(b) A normal fresh urine should be treated at the same time as the test to assist in assessing the significance of any colour change.

(c) In certain types of a rare condition known as porphyria a substance called porphobilinogen is excreted in the urine. This will also give a positive reaction to Ehrlich's reagent. To differentiate, the test urine should first be saturated with sodium acetate. A few millilitres of chloroform or amyl alcohol should then be added and the mixture shaken. The colour produced by urobilinogen is extracted into the chloroform whereas that due to porphobilinogen remains in the aqueous phase. It may be necessary to repeat the chloroform extraction to remove all the coloured complex due to urobilinogen.

(d) Commercial tests are available (see Chapter 45).

Urine urobilin (Schlesinger's test)

1. Reagents

(a) Tincture of iodine (tincture = alcoholic solution)
(b) Ethanol
(c) Zinc acetate.

2. Method

(a) To 5 ml of urine add 2 or 3 drops of tincture of iodine.

(b) In a second test tube put about 1 g zinc acetate and 5 ml of ethanol and shake.

(c) Mix the contents of both tubes by repeatedly pouring backwards and forwards between the tubes.

(d) Filter.

3. Result

Zinc urobilin gives a greenish yellow fluorescence.

4. Notes

(a) The iodine is added to oxidise any urobilinogen present to urobilin.

(b) Bilirubin, if present, should be removed in the same way as described under 'Urobilinogen'.

(c) Normal urine will contain a little urobilin so that a faint fluorescence is ignored. If it is found difficult to decide whether there is or is not an increased fluorescence then the test can usually be said to be negative.

(d) Positive results can be confirmed by spectroscopic analysis where a dark band due to zinc urobilin can be seen in the green part of the spectrum at the junction between green and blue.

Urine bilirubin

A large number of tests for bilirubin in urine have been described. Those given below will be found to be most satisfactory.

Fouchet's test

1. Reagents

(a) 10% barium chloride
(b) Fouchet's reagent:
25g trichloroacetic acid are dissolved in water, 10 ml of 10% ferric chloride is added and the mixture is made up to 100 ml with water.

2. Method

(a) Add 5 ml of 10% barium chloride to 10 ml of urine, mix and filter.
(b) Allow filter paper to drain for a few minutes after filtration is complete.
(c) Spread filter paper on to a second dry, clean paper.
(d) Add 1 or 2 drops of Fouchet's reagent to the edge of the precipitate.

3. Result

The presence of bilirubin is indicated by a greenish blue colour.

4. Notes

(a) The barium chloride is added to produce a precipitate of insoluble barium sulphate to which the bilirubin is adsorbed. If only a small amount of precipitate is formed this can be increased by the addition of a few drops of dilute sulphuric acid.
(d) Colours other than the greenish blue referred to above are not due to bilirubin but to some other substance in the urine, either contaminant or drug metabolite.

Ictotest and Ictostix

These tests, obtainable from Ames & Co., are based on the diazo reaction (see p. 321). They are both suitable for the detection of bilirubin in urine. The manufacturers' instructions must, of course, be adhered to.

Significance of bilirubin and urobilinogen tests

The following table must be taken only as a rough guide, particularly as more than one of the groups referred to on p. 320 can exist concurrently.

Disease group	Serum bilirubin Direct	Indirect	Urine bilirubin	Urine urobilinogen
Pre-hepatic	Normal	Raised	Negative	Raised
Hepatic	Raised	Normal	Positive	Raised
Post-hepatic	Raised	Normal	Positive	Normal (or low)

THE PLASMA PROTEINS

Another important aspect of liver function is protein metabolism. Many proteins are synthesised in the liver from amino acids derived from dietary proteins. The estimation of proteins in plasma or serum is of considerable value not only in diseases affecting the liver but also in a wide variety of other conditions.

If the amount of protein circulating in the plasma is reduced (hypoproteinaemia) a disturbance of water balance results, and this is one of the causes of oedema. Oedema is an excess of fluid in the cells, tissue spaces and serous cavities of the body. Hypoproteinaemia may occur as the result of, for example:

(a) Starvation, where insufficient dietary protein is available for proper metabolism.
(b) Liver disease leading to disturbed protein metabolism.
(c) Gross loss of protein, particularly albumin, via the urine as, for example, in nephrotic syndrome.
(d) Loss of protein in extensive burns or crush injuries.

The estimation of total protein concentration alone does not provide a great deal of information. The proteins in plasma can be divided into three groups: albumin, globulins, and fibrinogen. Protein estimations are usually performed on serum which, of course, does not contain fibrinogen. A method giving an indication of the amount of fibrinogen present in plasma can be found on p. 243. The globulins can be divided into three main groups, α, β, and γ which themselves can be further subdivided into numerous fractions. Studies of increases or decreases in these fractions are of great importance, as is the detection of various abnormal proteins that may occur.

Methods of estimating total serum proteins

A very large number of methods for the estimation of total serum proteins have been described. These include:

1. Kjeldahl methods

The proteins are digested by boiling in the presence of sulphuric acid and a catalyst (e.g. selenium dioxide). The amount of protein present is calculated by estimating the nitrogen released either by the use of Nessler's reagent or by titration (as ammonia) with standard acid. The nitrogen content of protein is usually taken as 16%, so that the result for nitrogen is multiplied by 6·25 to give the protein concentration. This factor has been used for many years and despite many arguments as to its validity, looks likely to remain in use. Kjeldahl methods are too time-consuming to be of value for routine use but have been used extensively as reference methods.

2. Biuret methods

These methods depend upon the production of purple colours by the action of alkaline copper sulphate solutions on substances containing either two or more peptide linkages, or two $-CONH_2$, $-CH_2NH_2$ or some similar groups joined directly or through single carbon or nitrogen atoms. Proteins therefore give this reaction which takes its name from biuret ($CO.NH_2-NH-CO.NH_2$) which is the simplest substance having the necessary structure. One of the many 'biuret' methods described is given below. These methods can be recommended for routine use and can be easily automated for total protein estimation.

3. Other colorimetric methods

These include those which estimate specific amino acids by a suitable reagent and extrapolate to give the total protein. These methods are not recommended, as different proteins vary considerably in their amino acid make-up. Albumin is capable of binding certain dyes, for example, Bromocresol green (BCG); this has formed the basis of a number of methods and is particularly useful in automated procedures where the fractionation of proteins is not convenient.

4. Physical methods

These include the estimation of refractive index, specific gravity (by flotation in copper sulphate solutions) and ultra-violet spectrophotometry.

Methods of fractionating proteins

1. 'Salting-out' techniques

Globulins (and fibrinogen if present) can be precipitated by high concentrations of various salts, for example, ammonium sulphate, sodium sulphate or sodium sulphite. Various strengths have been used, and one example can be seen in the method below. All the globulins may be precipitated, or by varying the concentration of salt γ- or β- + γ-globulins can be precipitated thus further fractionating the proteins.

Methanol and ethanol have also been used to precipitate globulins.

2. Electrophoresis

Electrophoresis is the migration of charged particles through a liquid medium under the influence of an applied e.m.f. The technique has been applied to the separation of serum proteins and has proved to be of great value. The serum is applied as a narrow band to a suitable supporting medium (e.g., cellulose acetate membrane). At pH 8·6 on cellulose acetate the α-globulins split into two fractions so that the serum separates into albumin, α_1-, α_2, β- and γ-globulin with albumin nearest the positive pole. The fractions can then be located using a suitable stain, e.g. Ponceau S. By using other supporting media, such as starch gel, many more fractions can be obtained.

The technique of electrophoresis can also be used to separate other closely related charged compounds, an example being the separation of abnormal haemoglobins.

3. Other methods of protein fractionation

Protein fractions can also be identified by gel diffusion techniques (sometimes in conjunction with electrophoresis) using specific immune sera. It should be remembered that all the serum protein fractions referred to above are mixtures of many individual proteins.

Estimation of total protein in serum

1. Principle

Copper in alkaline solution reacts with peptide bonds to give a violet colour; the simplest compound to give this colour is biuret, from which the reaction takes its name.

2. Reagents

(a) Sodium chloride solution (0·9%). 9 g sodium chloride are dissolved in distilled water and made up to 1 litre.

(b) Stock biuret reagent. 45 g potassium sodium tartrate are dissolved in 400 ml 0·2 M sodium hydroxide. 15 g copper sulphate ($CuSO_4 . 5H_2O$) are added and dissolved. 5 g potassium iodide are added and the volume made up to 1 litre with 0·2 M sodium hydroxide.

(c) Stock biuret blank reagent. As for *(b)* but without the copper sulphate.

(d) Biuret diluent. 0·2 M sodium hydroxide containing 5 g potassium iodide per litre.

(e) Working biuret reagent. 50 ml of *(b)* are added to 250 ml of *(d)*.

(f) Working biuret blank. 50 ml of *(c)* are added to 250 ml of *(d)*.

3. Standard

Use a serum whose protein content has been determined by the Kjeldahl method, or a commercial standard of known protein content. Store as freeze-dried solid or as deep-frozen small aliquots.

4. Method

(a) Set up test tubes as follows:

	Reagent blank	Serum blank*	Serum test	Standard
Sodium chloride	6·0	5·0	5·0	5·9
Standard	—	—	—	0·1
Test serum	—	0–1	0·1	—
Biuret reagent	6·0	—	6·0	6·0
Biuret blank	—	6·0	—	—

* This tube is only required if the test serum is turbid or icteric.

(b) Mix the tubes and incubate at 37°C for 10 min. Cool to room temperature.

(c) Read the standard and test against the reagent blank at 540 nm. If a serum blank has been set up, read the test against it.

5. Calculation

The protein concentration is given by:

$$\frac{\text{Abs. test}}{\text{Abs. standard}} \times \text{Standard value (g/litre)}.$$

6. Reference range

62–80 g/litre.

7. Note

Haemolysed sera should not be analysed, as the haemoglobin will be measured.

Estimation of serum albumin

1. Principle

Globulins are precipitated by sodium sulphite and the subnatant used to measure the concentration of albumin by the biuret method. The use of Span 20 in ether allows the floating precipitate to form a compact button which may easily be by-passed to allow an aliquot of the subnatant to be taken for analysis.

2. Reagents

As for total protein with the following additions.

(g) Sodium sulphite solution (28%). 140 g sodium sulphite are dissolved in warm distilled water and made up to 500 ml. Store at 37°C.

(h) Ether–Span 20 reagent. 1 ml Span 20 (Sorbitan monolaurate) is shaken with 90 ml of diethyl ether. After mixing the solution is stored at 4°C.

3. Standard

As for total protein.

4. Method

(a) Add 0·2 ml serum to 5·8 ml sodium sulphite solution in a glass-stoppered test tube.

(b) Add 1 ml ether–Span reagent. Stopper the tube and mix by gently inverting 20 times. Vigorous mixing will destroy some of the protein.

(c) Remove the stopper (to prevent sticking). Centrifuge. The globulins separate as a button at the ether–water interface.

(d) Gently tilt the tube to disengage the button from the side. Insert a volumetric (bulb) pipette and remove 3 ml of the lower layer.

(e) Set up the following tubes:

	Reagent blank	Serum blank*	Test	Standard
Sodium chloride solution	—	—	—	5·9
Sodium sulphite	3·0	—	—	—
Standard	—	—	—	0·1
Subnatant layer	—	1·5	3·0	—
Biuret reagent	3·0	—	3·0	6·0
Biuret blank	—	1·5	—	—

* This tube is only required for turbid or icteric sera.

(f) Mix the tubes and incubate for 10 min at 37°C. Cool to room temperature.

(g) Read the standard and test against the reagent blank at 540 nm. If a serum blank has been set up, read the test serum against it.

5. *Calculation*

The albumin concentration is given by:

$$\frac{\text{Abs. test}}{\text{Abs. standard}} \times \tfrac{1}{2} \times \text{Standard total protein value (g/litre)}.$$

6. *Note*

Globulins may be calculated by subtracting the albumin from the total protein.

7. *Reference range*

30–53 g/litre.

REFERENCES

1. Jendrassik, L. and Grof, P. (1938). *Biochem. Z.*, **297**, 81.
2. Michaelsson, M. *et al.* (1965). *Paediatrics*, **35**, 925.
3. Billing, B. *et al.* (1971). *Ann. Clin. Biochem.*, **8**, 21.

44. Chemical tests for diseases of the alimentary tract

In this chapter we will deal with some of the tests that are used in the laboratory investigation of diseases of the alimentary tract, particularly those of the stomach and duodenum. Before going into these tests let us consider briefly the common conditions that occur in this region and some of the associated terminology (Fig. 44.1).

value both in diagnosis and, in the case of vagotomy, the assessment of effectiveness of the treatment of peptic ulceration.

Cancer

In some parts of the world (e.g. Japan) the stomach is

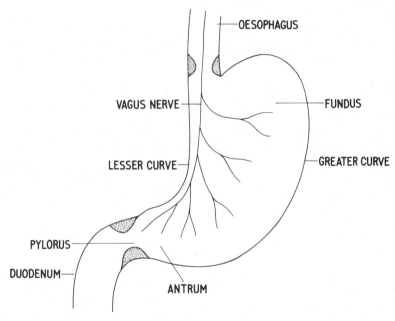

Fig. 44.1. Diagram of the stomach

Peptic ulcers

Ulcers of the stomach (gastric) and duodenum are very common. The cause of such ulceration is still subject to doubt; however, it is usual to find increased acid secretion particularly in cases of duodenal ulcer which is 4 or 5 times more common than gastric ulcer. The treatment is mostly directed at lowering the acid content of the gastric juice. This can be done by chemical neutralisation (antacids) or surgically, by removing part of the stomach (partial gastrectomy) or cutting gastric branches of the vagus nerve (vagotomy) which is part of the control system for gastric acid secretion. Thus measurement of the acidity of gastric juice can be of

the most common site of malignant tumour; in Britain it is second only to the bronchus. The measurement of gastric acidity is in general less useful in conditions of the stomach than in those of the duodenum; however, an ulcer seen on X-ray examination associated with a high acidity, is less likely to be malignant than one associated with a low acidity.

Achlorhydria

Achlorhydria is the complete absence of acid in gastric juice, it is one of the constant findings in pernicious anaemia.

327

Free and total acidity

In the past, gastric juice was first titrated to about pH 4 to give the so-called 'free' acid and then to pH 7 to get the 'Total acid'. This is no longer recommended as being a useful exercise and is therefore not discussed further.

MEASUREMENT OF GASTRIC ACIDITY

The collection of gastric juice through a naso-gastric tube is a ward procedure, so details will not be given here. There have been in the past a number of 'test meals' devised, ranging from gruel to alcohol. Histamine has also been used to stimulate gastric activity, but it can have unpleasant side effects and is not specific in its action. All these tests are open to a number of criticisms and they are now being superseded by the 'Pentagastrin test'. Pentagastrin is a synthetic drug which resembles the active part of the gastric hormone gastrin and mimics its action. The following comments are based, therefore, on the Pentagastrin test but, of course, the technique of titrating the acidity of the gastric juice samples is equally applicable to those obtained during the performance of a 'test meal' type of investigation.

Pentagastrin test

The patient is fasted overnight and a naso-gastric (Ryles) tube is passed. The stomach is emptied and this specimen is known as the *resting juice*. The gastric juice is then collected for 1 hour and this sample is labelled *basal juice*. The patient is given an intramuscular injection of Pentagastrin ($6\,\mu$g/kg body weight) and the juice is then collected for 4 consecutive 15-minute periods. All this is, of course, done on the ward. The laboratory should receive the following samples:

Resting Juice
Basal Juice
Post-Pentagastrin Samples 1, 2, 3, 4

The volume of each specimen should be measured and recorded. The presence of blood or bile should also be noted. For this, visual inspection is usually adequate. Blood will usually be brown owing to the change of haemoglobin to acid haematin. Bile, from regurgitated duodenal juice, will colour the gastric aspirate green. If only a few flecks of blood are present, particularly in the resting juice, they are of little significance.

The pH of the juice should then be ascertained. This is conveniently done using indicator papers, and any with a pH of greater than 7 will, of course, not require titration.

The acid concentration should now be measured, either by manual or automatic titration, in the basal and post-pentagastrin samples.

Manual titration

1. Reagents

(a) Standard Alkali: 0·01 M NaOH made fresh daily by dilution of 1·0 M NaOH.

(b) Indicator: Neutral Red, 0·1% in 70% alcohol.

2. Method

The juice should be spun down hard in a centrifuge particularly if much mucus is present. 1 ml of juice is pipetted into a small flask (or large diameter test tube) and 2–3 drops of indicator are added. Titrate, using the standard alkali. The end-point is denoted by a change in the indicator from yellow to red.

3. Notes

The flask should be agitated continuously during the titration. The first *permanent* red colour is taken as the end-point.

4. Calculation

Titration in ml of 0·01 M NaOH × 10 = mmol HCl/litre. For Pentagastrin tests 'mmol HCl/Total volume of specimen' is required:

$$\frac{\text{Titration in ml} \times 10 \times \text{volume of specimen in ml}}{1000}$$
$$= \text{mmol/TV}$$

5. Reference ranges

	Mean	Males Upper limit	Mean	Females Upper limit
Basal	1·3	4·3	1·1	4·6 mmol/hr
Total post-pentagastrin	17·1	40·9	9·4	23·8 mmol
Peak ½ hour	10·8	24·6	6·1	14·9 mmol
(i.e. highest sum of two consecutive ½-hour samples)				

Automatic titration

Automatic titration assemblies are available. In these, the burette is mechanically filled and emptied and is controlled by a specially designed pH meter. The sample is kept mechanically stirred and titrant is added until the required pH is obtained. This apparatus is suitable for use in titrating gastric juice and is set for an end-point of pH 7 for this purpose.

Insulin 'test meal'

This is a test carried out to test the efficiency of a vagotomy. The patient is given insulin to lower the blood sugar; normally this would cause the vagus nerve to stimulate the secretion of gastric acid. If the vagus has been effectively cut this stimulation will not occur.

The samples of gastric juice are titrated in the same way as described above. Samples of blood for glucose are taken during the test and are analysed in the usual way (*see* p. 302). This is to see if the blood glucose falls far enough to stimulate the vagus nerve.

BLOOD IN FAECES

Blood in faeces can occur as a result of many conditions of the alimentary tract. Usually this blood is not apparent to the naked eye and is termed 'occult'. If large amounts of such blood are present the stools will take on a black tar-like appearance. Fresh blood on the surface of a stool may be seen as a result of rectal or vaginal bleeding. This blood should *not* be reported as a positive 'occult blood' as this will be misleading. (It will, of course, give a positive reaction to 'occult blood' methods which are therefore without value if fresh blood is visible.) Most tests are based on the detection of the peroxidase-like activity of haemoglobin and some of its derivatives. Unfortunately the most satisfactory of these tests were formally carried out using such reagents as benzidine and *o*-toluidine which have since been shown to be carcinogenic so that their use can no longer be justified. The method that follows has the advantage of using non-carcinogenic agents.

Occult blood in faeces[1]

1. Reagents

(a) Hydrogen peroxide (Analar): Dilute to 10 vols* strength for use.

* The term 'vol.' (volume) represents the strength of a solution of hydrogen peroxide. For example, '10 vols' means that 1 volume of the H_2O_2 will yield 10 volumes of oxygen at NTP on complete degradation. H_2O_2 is obtainable commercially at various strengths, it should be stored at 4°C in plastic bottles and diluted as required.

(b) Acetic acid (Analar): 50% solution.

(c) Bicine (N, N–bis–(2-hydroxyethyl) glycine): as powder.

(d) Diphenylamine (Analar): 1% in glacial acetic acid.

2. Method

(a) Add 10 ml of 50% acetic acid to a pea-sized specimen of faeces in a test tube and place in a boiling water-bath for 10 min.

(b) Place a knife-point (about 100 mg) of Bicine into a clean test tube.

(c) Add to the Bicine 0·2 ml of cooled faecal suspension.

(d) Add 0·5 ml of 1% diphenylamine.

(e) Add 0·1 ml of 10 vols H_2O_2, mix well and start stopwatch.

3. Result

Positive: green colour within 90 sec. Weak positive: green colour between 90 and 120 sec. Any colour developing after 2 min is ignored. A weak positive control consisting of a 1/4000 dilution of blood (Hb > 12 g/100 ml) in water should be included with each batch of analysis.

4. Notes

(a) Samples from at least 3 different days should be examined.

(b) The faeces are boiled to destroy any enzyme peroxidase present that would give false positive results. The haemoglobin derivatives are more heat-resistant.

(c) The Bicine is included to prevent false positives from patients undergoing oral iron therapy.

(d) If bile is present, a green suspension will be produced. The test should be carried out as stated, and at the end of 2 min about 2 ml of diethyl ether is added. Colour due to bile is unaltered, that due to blood will become purple.

(e) The sensitivity of the test is such that it is unnecessary to put the patients on to any special diet so long as certain blood-rich foods, for example liver, are avoided for a few days prior to testing.

(f) No attempt should be made to use any of the test strips available for urine testing for blood, for example Ames' Hemastix, as they are far too sensitive for use with faeces where there is normally a small blood loss each day.

MALABSORPTION

This condition is investigated in two parts.

1. Is malabsorption present?

The best answer to this question is provided by the estimation of faecal fat. A long (3–5-day) collection of faeces is homogenised. The fatty acids present are released from the compounds in which they occur by treatment of an aliquot of the homogenate with 5% alcoholic potassium hydroxide. This process is saponi-fication and the fatty acids are in the form of potassium salts. The salts are converted to acids by the addition of hydrochloric acid. The fatty acids thus formed are extracted into an immiscible solvent (petroleum ether) and titrated against a standardised alkali such as tetra methyl ammonium hydroxide (TMAH), a strong alkali soluble in organic solvents. The titration figure gives the amount of fatty acids present.

2. What is the cause?

A dose of the pentose xylose is normally absorbed from the gut, enters the blood stream and is excreted by the kidney. If the gut wall is diseased or abnormal this will not happen, and no xylose will be detected in the blood or urine. Xylose is measured by its reaction with thio-urea in acetic acid to form a furfurol, which forms a coloured complex with p-bromo aniline.

If malabsorption is present but there is no reduction of xylose absorption there is a strong possibility that the condition is due to pancreatic insufficiency. A tube is passed into the duodenum and the contents are aspi-rated, often after hormonal stimulation of the pan-creas. Tests for enzyme activity are performed on the aspirate to confirm the reduced levels of digestive enzymes.

REFERENCE

1. Woodman, D.D. (1970). *Clin. Chem. Acta*, **29,** 249.

45. Miscellaneous tests

COMMERCIAL URINE TESTS

Commercial systems are available for testing urine for several substances. The principles of analysis will be presented here. It is important to remember that the manufacturer's instructions must be read carefully and followed closely to ensure good results. It is all too common to blame a test strip for giving an incorrect result when the real cause of error is the manner in which the strip was used or stored.

Bilirubin

The reaction is that of bilirubin with a solid diazonium salt in an acid medium to give a purple or blue colour.

Ames* Ictotest and Bililabstix use *p*-nitrobenzene-diazonium *p*-toluene sulphonate.

BCL† Bilur-Test uses 2,6-dichlorophenyldiazonium fluoborate.

Blood

Nascent (newly formed, reactive) oxygen is evolved by the peroxidase-like activity of haemoglobin on a peroxide. The oxygen is accepted by an indicator which changes colour when in the oxidised form (a redox indicator).

Ames Hemastix uses *o*-toluidine as the indicator and gives a blue colour when positive.

BCL Sangur-Test uses 2,5-dimethylhexane 2,5-di-(hydroperoxide) as the peroxide.

Ketone bodies

Aceto acetic acid and acetone give a purple colour when reacted with sodium nitroprusside and glycine in an alkaline medium.

Ames Ketostix and BCL Ketur-Test both use this principle.

* Ames Ltd., Stoke Poges, Bucks.
† BCL, Lewes, Sussex.

Notes

(1) Phenyl ketones give an atypical colour with this test, which may be misinterpreted as a positive result. Such colours should be further investigated (*see* phenylketones).

(2) Ames Acetest uses the same reagents. It may be used for detecting ketone bodies in whole blood as well as urine and plasma or serum.

(3) 3-hydroxybutyric acid is also a ketone body but it is not detected by this reaction.

Glucose

Glucose oxidase catalyses the formation of gluconic acid and hydrogen peroxide from glucose. The hydrogen peroxide is degraded by peroxidase to give oxygen which is taken up by an oxygen acceptor to give a colour change.

Ames Clinistix uses the blue colour of oxidised orthotoluidine to indicate the amount of glucose.

Ames Diastix uses the brown colour of iodine which is released from potassium iodide on oxidation. The colour is blended with that of a blue background dye to give good differentiation of glucose levels.

BCL Diabur-Test uses 3-amino,6-chloro,9-(3-dimethylaminopropyl)carbazole which gives a brown colour.

Reducing sugars

A reagent tablet is used, Ames Clinitest, which contains copper sulphate, sodium hydroxide, sodium carbonate and citric acid. Sodium carbonate and citric acid form an effervescent couple which encourages the other reagent to dissolve. Some heat is also generated by the couple, and by the dissolution and partial neutralisation of sodium hydroxide. In the resultant alkaline medium copper sulphate is reduced by sugar to reddish insoluble cuprous oxide. Carbon dioxide from the sodium carbonate displaces air from the reaction mixture and prevents re-oxidation of the cuprous oxide by atmospheric oxygen. The resultant colour of the mixture indicates the amount of sugar in the original urine.

Note

This test is much less specific than strips which use glucose oxidase, as any reducing substance may give a positive result.

pH

A double indicator is used to give a broad range of colours covering the entire urinary pH range. Colours range from orange through yellow and green to blue. Ames (various) and BCL Nephur-Test use a mixture of methyl red and bromothymol blue.

Phenylketones

Phenylketonuria is an inborn error of amino-acid metabolism. The patient is unable to convert phenylalanine to tyrosine. If untreated, severe mental retardation may result, so early diagnosis is essential.

Ames Phenistix uses the reaction between phenyl-pyruvic acid and ferric ammonium sulphate to give a grey-green colour in an acid medium provided by cyclohexyl-sulphamic acid. Magnesium ions are present to reduce possible interference by phosphate.

Note

This test is routinely done on babies at about 4 weeks.

Protein

A buffered indicator will give the wrong pH value in the presence of protein. This is referred to as the protein error of indicators. The error is proportional to the concentration of protein in solution.

Ames Albustix uses tetrabromophenol blue.

BCL Albym-Test uses tetrachlorophenol tetra-bromosulphonphthalein.

Urobilinogen

Ames Urobilistix uses Ehrlich's reaction. *p*-dimethyl-aminobenzaldehyde and urobilinogen react to give a reddish colour in an acid medium. Porphobilinogen will give a false-positive reaction which should be investigated further.

BCL Ugen-Test uses the reaction between urobili-nogen and *p*-methoxyphenyldiazonium fluoborate to give a red azo-dye. This reaction is more specific than the classical Ehrlich's reaction.

CEREBROSPINAL FLUID (CSF)

The estimation of glucose and protein in CSF are frequently requested. Since it is not usually possible to remove a large volume from the patient, care must be taken to ensure the best use of what is available. The clinician should be instructed to use two sterile containers, the first part of the collection for chemical analysis, the second for microbiology. If very little fluid is obtained, it is better to take the specimen for chemical analysis into a fluoride-oxalate tube than to split the sample or use a plain container only, as protein may be measured on a specimen from a tube with preservative, but glucose quickly disappears from a plain tube.

Estimation of glucose in CSF

Any of the methods used for blood glucose are suitable. (*See* Chapter 40).

Reference range

3·0–4·5 mmol/litre.

Estimation of protein in CSF

1. Principle

Proteins are measured by the turbidity of a fine suspension after precipitation with trichloroacetic acid. The turbidity is affected only slightly by the relative concentrations of the different protein fractions, which is not so with sulphosalicylic acid.

2. Reagent

3% w/v trichloroacetic acid.

3. Standard

A clear serum of known protein concentration is diluted 1 in 100. Make fresh each week.

4. Method

(*a*) Pipette 0·5 ml of unknown, standard, and isotonic saline into three tubes.

(b) Add 3·0 ml 3% TCA into each tube, mixing on a vortex mixer immediately.

(c) Stand at room temperature for 10 min.

(d) Read the absorbances of the test and standard against the saline blank at 450 nm.

5. Calculation

The CSF protein is given by:

$$\frac{\text{Abs. test}}{\text{Abs. standard}} \times \text{Value of original standard serum} \times \frac{1}{100} \text{ g/litre.}$$

6. Reference range

0·15–0·45 g/litre (for lumbar fluid).

7. Note

If the value of the test is higher than that of the standard, the test is repeated on a diluted fluid. If there is insufficient fluid to repeat, the test may be diluted with 3% TCA.

The appearance of CSF is important and should be reported.

46. Enzymes

Enzymes are proteins that act as organic catalysts. The estimation of enzyme activities in body fluids and tissue extracts has become an extremely useful tool both in diagnosis and in following the course of a wide variety of pathological conditions.

This chapter will serve as an introduction to enzyme analysis. We will restrict ourselves to a brief discussion of the major factors affecting the analysis of enzymes in clinical chemistry and to giving methods for the estimation of a few commonly used enzymes. No attempt will be made to discuss the setting up of new methods or modifying those already in use. However, the following list of factors will call attention to their importance and enable us to make a sensible guess at the cause of any error that becomes apparent.

FACTORS AFFECTING ENZYME ANALYSIS

The following factors are all important in the management of enzyme activity, and changes in any of them may result in a wrong answer.

Temperature

The effect of temperature is complex and is illustrated in Fig. 46.1. As the temperature rises the activity increases, in common with many biological functions, and very roughly doubles for every 10°C rise. At higher temperatures, however, more and more active sites become denatured, until the enzyme is inactivated completely.

Practical measures

Include the choice of a suitable temperature. Workers are presently divided into three camps: those who think that room temperature (25°C) is best; those who prefer normal body temperature (37°C); and those who suggest a compromise of 30°C. A device is required which ensures an even temperature, kept within ±0·5°C from day to day. Changes in the room temperature should be kept to a minimum. It may be noted that water baths which employ only heating elements will not be satisfactory to maintain a temperature which is close to the ambient temperature.

Substrates should be briefly pre-heated so that the reaction starts at the correct temperature.

Time

As enzymic reactions are catalytic they proceed fairly rapidly. This means that if one of a group of tests is allowed to react for longer than the others, then it will give a higher result, and that if the time varies from day to day, so will the results.

Practical measures

Each enzyme test, rather than each batch, should be carefully timed. This may be achieved by the staggered addition of substrate, and of the reagent used to stop the reaction.

pH

For an enzyme to work the configuration of the active site must be in the correct ionic form. This ionic configuration is affected by the pH, so that the activity

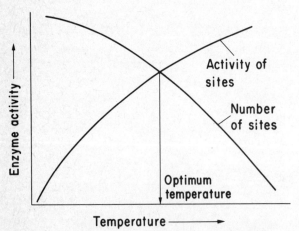

Fig. 46.1.   The effect of temperature on enzyme activity.

of an enzyme decreases if the optimum pH is not maintained.

Practical measures

Buffer systems are used to obtain and maintain the desired pH, which may otherwise be altered by the catalysed reaction. It should be mentioned here that the chemical nature of the buffer is important. A 'transphosphorylating' buffer such as diethanol amine will increase the activity of alkaline phosphatase by entering into the reaction itself. Different buffers may also change the optimum pH.

Co-factors

These include all the non-protein components of an enzyme system including co-enzymes and activators. Co-factors may be simple inorganic ions or complex organic substances. They may be essential to the activity of an enzyme or merely enhance its activity.

Practical measures

It is essential to ensure that the presence and concentration of co-factors is precisely controlled, to avoid changes in activity from day to day.

Inhibitors

Many substances inhibit enzyme activity, by occupying or altering the active site. They include heavy metals, fluoride, cyanide and some drugs. Other substances may inhibit an enzyme reaction by reacting with a co-factor, and so removing it from the enzyme. Sometimes the product of an enzyme reaction is itself an inhibitor, or even the substrate at high concentrations.

Practical measures

The maintenance of a clean environment and the use of high-quality distilled water and reagents go some way to ensure that inhibitors are kept to a minimum.

Substrates

The speed of an enzyme reaction depends upon the concentration of substrate, until a certain substrate concentration is reached. In Fig. 46.2 this is shown, and

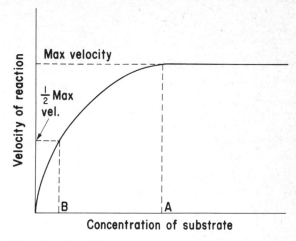

Fig. 46.2. The effect of substrate concentration of the velocity of an enzyme-catalysed reaction.

the substrate concentration must be higher than that at point A, so that the speed of reaction is not dependent on the substrate concentration. The molar concentration of the substrate, which results in a speed of reaction which is half the maximum speed, is a constant for a given enzyme system of measurement (point B). The constant is known as the Michaelis constant.

The substrate used may affect the speed of reaction; for example, different triglycerides are cleaved at different rates by lipase.

Practical measures

The substrate concentration given in a method will have been defined with these factors in mind. It must be adhered to.

METHODS OF MEASUREMENT

(a) Kinetic

If the course of a catalysed reaction is closely followed, it will be seen that the early part of the reaction is linear, but that the speed slows down as time proceeds because the equilibrium point is being approached. If the rate of product formation (or substrate utilisation) is measured during the early linear part of the reaction a true comparison of enzyme activities may be gained (see Fig. 46.3). Instruments are available which measure this rate of change and they are known as kinetic enzyme analysers. The method is a kinetic method. Some analysers take a measurement of the activity at

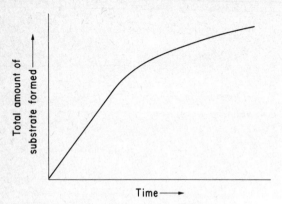

Fig. 46.3. The course of an enzyme reaction.

zero time and at two or three times later, but these are not true kinetic analysers.

(b) End-point

Kinetic analysers were not available to early workers, who allowed the reaction to carry on for a given time and then stopped it by drastically changing one of the factors given above, or by inactivating the enzyme. Continuous-flow analysers stop enzyme reactions by dialysing away the product and substrate from the enzyme protein.

UNITS OF ENZYME ACTIVITY

In recent years attempts have been made to standardise the units of enzyme activity, so that the results obtained in one hospital or country may be comparable to those from another laboratory. The unit which is used most in this country is the International Unit (IU), which is defined as follows: one unit of any enzyme is that amount which will catalyse the transformation of 1 micromole (μmol) of the substrate per minute under standard conditions.

Such a definition is useful only when there is widespread international agreement about the standard conditions. Various bodies have produced proposals for a few enzymes which have been adopted locally, but general acceptance has not so far been gained. All the factors already discussed affect enzyme analyses, and until these are defined the IU will have limited practical use. Each laboratory should publish reference ranges for all the enzymes which it measures. The most usual unit in clinical laboratories is the International Unit per litre (IU/litre).

SERUM ALKALINE PHOSPHATASE

Alkaline phosphatase is one of a number of enzymes occurring in serum that are capable of hydrolysing phosphate monoesters. It is most active between pH 8 and 10 (hence its name) and is relatively non-specific, being able to degrade a variety of phospho-monoesters. Alkaline phosphatase is found in bone and is also present in liver, kidney, intestine and placenta. Increases in serum alkaline phosphatase occur in various conditions affecting bone, and in liver disease. The method that follows is an example of a colorimetric method of enzyme analysis.

Estimation of serum alkaline phosphatase[1]

1. Principle

The enzyme acts on a substrate of disodium phenyl phosphate to release phenol. The phenol is estimated by reaction with 4-aminophenazone in the presence of alkaline potassium ferricyanide and measurement of the resulting red colour.

2. Reagents

(a) Buffered substrate
  (i) Disodium phenyl phosphate (0·01 M).
  Dissolve 1·09 g disodium phenyl phosphate in distilled water and make up to 500 ml. Bring quickly to the boil and then cool. The cooled solution should be preserved by the addition of a few drops of chloroform and storage in a refrigerator.
  (ii) Buffer
  3·18 g sodium carbonate (anhydrous)
  1·68 g sodium bicarbonate
  Dissolve and make up to 500 ml with distilled water.
  (iii) Working buffered substrate (pH 10)
  Make equal volumes of (i) and (ii).

(b) Sodium hydroxide. 0·5 M.

(c) Sodium bicarbonate. 0·5 M.

(d) 4-aminophenazone. 3·0 g dissolved in water and made up to 500 ml.

(e) Potassium ferricyanide. 12·0 g dissolved and made up to 500 ml with distilled water.

3. Standards

(i) Stock. Dissolve 1·0 g pure crystalline phenol in 0·1 M HCl and make up to 1 litre using the acid (1 mg/ml).

Standardise as follows:

Add 50 ml of 0·1 M NaOH to 25 ml of stock standard. Warm to 65°C add 25 ml 0·05 M I_2. Stopper and stand at room temperature for about 30 min. Add 5 ml concentrated HCl. Titrate excess iodine with 0·1 M sodium thiosulphate ($Na_2S_2O_3 . 5H_2O$) using starch as indicator (1 ml of 0·05 M I = 1·57 mg phenol).

(ii) Working standard (0·01 mg/ml). Dilute stock standard 1 in 100 with 0·1 M HCl.

(iii) Working standard (0·03 mg/ml). Dilute stock standard 3 in 100 with 0·1 M HCl.

4. Method

Two tubes are used for each estimation, one being serum blank, the other the test.

(a) Add 2·0 ml buffer substrate to each of two tubes, place in 37°C water bath for a few minutes to warm to incubation temperature.

(b) To one tube add 0·1 ml serum (test).

(c) Incubate for exactly 15 min at 37°C.

(d) Remove from bath and immediately add 0·8 ml of 0·5 M NaOH to both tubes, mix.

(e) Add 1·2 ml 0·5 M $NaHCO_3$ to each tube, mix.

(f) Add 0·1 ml of serum to blank tube.

(g) Standards. To each of three tubes add 1·1 ml buffer. To one add 1·0 ml water (standard blank); to the next 1·0 ml of working standard (0·01 mg/ml); to the last 1·0 ml of working standard (0·03 mg/ml). Add 0·8 ml 0·5 M NaOH and 1·2 ml of 0·5 M $NaHCO_3$ to all three tubes.

(h) Add 1·0 ml of 4-aminophenazone solution to all tubes; mix.

(i) Add 1·0 ml of potassium ferricyanide solution to all tubes; mix.

(j) Read to 520 nm.

5. Calculation

$$\frac{\text{Abs. of test (T)} - \text{Abs. of serum blank (B)}}{\text{Abs. of std (S)} - \text{Abs of std. blank (SB)}}$$

$$\times \text{ conc. of std.} \times \frac{100}{0·1}$$

= King Armstrong (KA) units/100 ml

i.e. $\dfrac{T - B}{S - SB} \times 0·01 \text{ (or } 0·03) \times \dfrac{100}{0·1} = $ KA units/100 ml.

6. Notes

(a) The order of adding reagents is important and the contents of the tube should be well mixed after each addition.

(b) Specimens giving a result of more than 40 KA units should be diluted 1/10 with isotonic saline and repeated as the method is not linear above this level.

(c) Units: 1 KA unit = amount of enzyme in 100 ml serum which will liberate 1 mg phenol in 15 min at 37°C at pH 10. To convert KA units to the international system, 1 KA unit = 7·1 IU/litre.

7. Reference range

3–13 KA units/100 ml, equivalent to 21–92 IU/litre.

ESTIMATION OF TRYPSIN IN DUODENAL CONTENTS

Method A[2]

The estimation of trypsin in duodenal juice after a standard test meal is occasionally done to assist in the diagnosis of pancreatic disease.

1. Principle

Trypsin acts on the specific substrate N-benzoyl-L-arginine ethyl ester (BAEE) to release H^+, and the rate of this reaction is measured by timing the neutralisation of a known amount of alkali. The range of pH used is narrow so that change in enzyme activity due to pH is minimal.

2. Reagents

(a) 0·05 Molar acetate buffer, pH 5·8

(i) 6·805 g of Analar sodium acetate (CH_3COONa) are dissolved in CO_2-free distilled water and diluted to 1 litre.

(ii) Dilute 29 ml of Analar glacial acetic acid (CH_3COOH) to 1 litre with CO_2-free distilled water. Titrate against 0·5 M NaOH, dilute to exactly 0·5 M then further dilute 1 in 10.

(iii) Working buffer: mix 94·0 ml of solution (i) with 6·0 ml of solution (ii) and add 0·05 g calcium chloride ($CaCl_2$).

(b) Substrate. Dissolve 0·5 g BAEE in 10 ml of 0·1% sodium barbiturate. Adjust to pH 9. Check pH prior to use.

(c) 0·04 M NaOH.

3. Method

The reaction is carried out in a small beaker on a magnetic stirrer and the pH is read using a suitable pH meter with small electrodes in the beaker. The reaction vessel should be placed in a large beaker and surrounded with water kept at 25°C. The solutions should all be at 25°C before use.

(a) Mix 1·0 ml of duodenal content with 9·0 ml of buffer.

(b) Mix 1·0 ml of diluted duodenal content with 5·0 ml of substrate in the reaction vessel.

(c) Place reaction vessel on to stirrer, insert electrodes. The pH will be about 8·5 and falling.

(d) When pH reaches 8·0 add 0·1 ml of 0·04 M NaOH and start a stopwatch.

(e) The pH will rise, then fall back to 8·0; when this figure is reached stop the timer.

4. Calculation

The elapsed time corresponds to the release of 4 μmol of H^+

$$\frac{4}{\text{Time in min}} \times \text{dilution of duodenal contents (10)}$$

$= \mu\text{mol } H^+/\text{min/ml} = \text{mIU/litre}.$

5. Notes

(a) This method gives results directly in international units.

(b) If the time exceeds 10 min repeat using 1 in 5 dilution: if time still exceeds 10 min report as <2 mIU/litre.

6. Reference range

Up to 40 mIU/litre.

Method B[3] (modified)

This method is particularly suitable as a screening test for the estimation of trypsin in duodenal contents from children suspected of having fibrinocystic disease of the pancreas. It can also be used for faeces.

1. Principle

The enzyme utilises as substrate the gelatin coating of unused X-ray film.

2. Reagent

1% sodium carbonate.

3. Method

A series of dilutions of duodenal contents in 1% sodium carbonate is made at 1:10, 1:100, 1:1000.

A small piece of unused X-ray film is marked out in labelled squares. One drop of neat duodenal content and of each of the dilutions plus a drop of sodium carbonate solution as a control are placed, using Pasteur pipettes, in the relevant squares of the X-ray film. Care should be taken that the area of each drop is roughly constant. The film is then placed on damp filter paper in a Petri dish, covered and placed in a 37°C incubator for 30 min. On removal from the incubator place in the freezing compartment of a refrigerator for 15 min. Wash under running cold tap water.

4. Results

Tryptic activity is shown by clear areas of film. The control should only show slight roughening of the surface but no digestion of the gelatin. Report as highest dilution giving clear area.

5. Notes

(a) Care must be taken at all stages to prevent the drops running into each other.

(b) Normal duodenal juice should give a completely clear area 1:10 or above.

(c) Other dilutions can be made if an end-point is desired.

(d) Faecal tryptic activity can be estimated by making a suspension of faeces in 1% sodium carbonate and treating as described above.

AMYLASE

It is difficult to produce consistent results for amylase, because the substrate starch is a variable mixture of two different compounds, amylose and amylopectin. This difficulty is reflected in the reliance of 9 out of 10 laboratories taking part in the Wellcome quality control programme on commercially produced starch preparations. Such substrates should be used according to the manufacturers' recommendations.

Amylase catalyses the reaction

$$\text{Amylose} \xrightarrow{\text{Amylase}} \text{Maltose}.$$

Methods divide into those which monitor the disappearance of starch (amyloclastic) and those which determine the maltose or glucose produced (saccharogenic). There are theoretical and practical difficulties with both methods.

Amylase in urine

The method described is included as an example of a urinary enzyme determination and is a useful practical exercise. Urine amylase is raised in pancreatitis, and may remain raised after the serum level has returned to normal. The method is a classic among enzyme techniques, having been originally described by Wohlgemuth in 1908, and modified by Harrison.

1. Principle

The amylase present in urine splits starch progressively into smaller compounds and ultimately to maltose. Whereas starch gives a blue colour with iodine, when it has been broken down to a molecule containing in the region of 10 glucose units, a red colour is produced and on further degradation to below about 5 glucose units, no colour is given.

2. Reagents

(a) Starch solution
  (i) Stock.
  2 g of soluble starch are made into a paste with a few ml of distilled water and washed into about 60 ml of boiling water. Add 10 g sodium chloride, dissolve, cool, transfer to a 100 ml volumetric flask and make up to volume with distilled water.
  (ii) Working starch solution.
  Dilute (i) 1:20 with water.

(b) Iodine solution
  (i) Stock iodine (approx. 0·05 M).
  Weigh 6·4 g into a 500 ml flask add 10–12 g KI (Analar, free from KIO_3) and 20 ml water.
  Stopper flask, shake until dissolved. Make up to mark with distilled water.
  (ii) Working iodine solution (approx. 0·01 M).
  Dilute (i) 1:5 with water.

3. Method

(a) Adjust pH of urine to be just less than 7 using concentrated acid or alkali as required.
(b) Put up a series of tubes as follows:

Tube number	1	2	3	4	5
Urine (ml)	1·0	0·5	0·3	0·2	0·14
Water (ml)	0·0	0·5	0·7	0·8	0·86
Working starch solution (ml)	2·0	2·0	2·0	2·0	2·0

Tube number	6	7	8	9	10	11	12	13
Urine diluted 1 in 10 (ml)	1·0	0·7	0·5	0·4	0·3	0·2	0·15	0·12
Water (ml)	0·0	0·3	0·5	0·6	0·7	0·8	0·85	0·88
Working starch solution (ml)	2·0	2·0	2·0	2·0	2·0	2·0	2·0	2·0

(c) Incubate at 37°C for 30 min.
(d) Cool immediately in cold water.
(e) Add working iodine solution drop by drop to each tube, watching carefully for the appearance of a blue colour.
(f) Note the smallest volume of urine not giving a blue colour.

4. Calculation

Diastatic index = ml of 0·1% starch digested by 1 ml of urine at 37°C in 30 min.

$$= \frac{2}{\text{smallest volume of urine not giving a blue colour}}.$$

Example. On completion of test a blue colour was first seen in tube 7.
∴Smallest volume not giving blue colour (in tube 6) is 1·0 ml of urine diluted 1 in 10 (i.e. 0·1 ml).
∴Diastatic index = (2/0·1) = 20 units.

5. Notes

(a) The term 'diastatic index' (DI) comes from the alternative (obsolete) name for amylase—diastase.
(b) DI units cannot be directly converted to international units because of the varying molecular sizes of starches.
(c) As amylase (being of course a protein) may be degraded by bacteria, care must be taken not to leave the urine at room temperature for long periods.
(d) The working starch and iodine solutions should be made freshly each day.

(e) If no end-point is reached, further tubes may be set up using urine diluted 1 in 100.

6. Reference range

24 hour urine   5–20 units.
Random urine   <50 units.

ULTRAVIOLET SPECTROPHOTOMETRIC METHODS OF ENZYME ANALYSIS

An important group of methods for the estimation of enzyme activity is based on the difference in absorption at 340 nm between oxidised and reduced pyridine nucleotides. In general they are superior to colorimetric methods.

One such method is that for serum lactate dehydrogenase (LDH), the technical details for which are given below. LDH catalyses the reaction:

$$CH_3CHOH . COO + NAD \rightleftharpoons$$
$$\underset{Lactate}{}$$
$$CH_3 . CO . COO + NADH_2$$
$$\underset{Pyruvate}{}$$

NAD (nicotinamide-adenine dinucleotide) does not absorb at 340 nm whereas reduced nicotinamide-adenine dinucleotide ($NADH_2$) absorbs strongly at this wavelength.

Coupled enzyme methods

Other enzyme reactions that do not directly involve NAD can be measured by 'coupling' the reaction to another that can involve NAD. An example of this is the estimation of aspartate aminotransferase, an enzyme of importance in the diagnosis of myocardial infarction. Aspartate aminotransferase catalyses the reaction:

L-aspartate + α-oxoglutate $\rightleftharpoons$
$$+ \alpha\text{-oxaloacetate} + \text{L-glutamate}$$

The oxaloacetate so formed can react with $NADH_2$ in the presence of malate dehydrogenase (MDH) in the following reaction:

$$\text{Oxaloacetate} + NADH_2 \overset{MDH}{\rightleftharpoons} \text{malate} + NAD.$$

thus producing the necessary change in absorption at 340 nm.

Other enzymes coupled in this way include alanine aminotransferase and creatine kinase.

LACTATE DEHYDROGENASE

Serum LDH increases a few hours after a myocardial infarction and remains raised for between 1 and 2 weeks. It can also increase, although less markedly, in other conditions, including hepatitis and some malignancies. Since LDH is very widely distributed throughout the body an increase is not a specific indication of myocardial infarct or of any other condition. The usefulness of LDH in diagnosis is enhanced by studying the isoenzymes (see note below).

Estimation of serum LDH[4]

1. Principle

See above. The reaction from pyruvate to lactate is utilised.

2. Reagents

(a) Phosphate buffer (pH 7·4)
Potassium dihydrogen phosphate (K_2PO_4)   2·69 g
Dipotassium hydrogen phosphate (K_2HPO_4)   13·97 g
Distilled water   to 1 litre

(b) $NADH_2$ solution
2·5 mg $NADH_2$/ml of phosphate buffer.
Prepare fresh daily.

(c) Sodium pyruvate solution
2.5 mg sodium pyruvate per ml of phosphate buffer.
Store deep-frozen.

3. Method

(a) Add 2·7 ml buffer, 0·1 ml serum and 0·1 ml $NADH_2$ to a 1 cm cuvette (silica or quartz) and mix.
(b) Stand at room temperature for 20 min.
(c) Add 0·1 ml sodium pyruvate solution, and start a stopwatch.
(d) Read absorbance at 340 nm at 1 min intervals for 5 min.

4. Calculation

One unit of LDH activity produces a decrease in absorbance of 0·001 per min at 340 nm.

$\therefore$ units per ml of serum

$$= \frac{\text{Average decrease in absorbance (A) per min}}{0 \cdot 001} \times \frac{1}{0 \cdot 1}$$

= Average decrease in (A) per min × 10,000

(for international units per litre multiply the above results by 0·482).

5. Notes

(a) The mixture is allowed to stand for 20 min in step 3(b) above to allow any keto acids present in the serum to be reduced. Some workers prefer to check that no further change in optical density is taking place before the addition of pyruvate.

(b) If an ultraviolet spectrophotometer is not available then the test may be read at 366 nm and the result multiplied by 1·89.

(c) Results should be read at 25°C; the reaction rate increases 7% for each 1°C increase in temperature. The temperature within the cuvette holder of the spectrophotometer may be several degrees above room temperature. Instruments with cuvette holders capable of being thermostatically controlled are therefore preferable, otherwise the temperature should be measured and the result adjusted accordingly.

(d) High levels of activity may produce non-linear results over the 5 min reading period in which case the serum should be diluted 1 in 10 in physiological saline and the test repeated.

(e) Non-haemolysed serum should be used for the test. Haemolysis increases the activity since the LDH activity in red cells is more than 100 times greater than in serum. Heparin is said not to interfere but most other anticoagulants lower the enzyme activity; it is preferable, as with other enzyme estimations, to use serum.

6. Reference range

200–650 units per ml (95–300 IU/litre).

ISOENZYMES

Many enzymes have been found to be groups of proteins showing similar catalytic activity, but being separable by physical and chemical means, these proteins are isoenzymes.

The most commonly measured isoenzymes are shown in Table 46.1.

Some separation methods for isoenzymes

(1) *Electrophoresis*, on cellulose acetate or polyacrylamide gel. Enzymes separated in this way include creatine kinase and alkaline phosphatase.

Table 46.1.   Commonly measured isoenzymes

Enzyme	Isoenzymes	Most important organs of origin
Creatine kinase	BB	Brain
	MB	Heart muscle
	MM	Skeletal muscle
Alkaline phosphatase	'B'	Bone
	'L'	Liver
	'I'	Intestine
	'P'	Placenta
Lactate dehydrogenase	LD_1	Heart (hydroxy
	LD_2	butyrate
	LD_3	dehydrogenase)
	LD_4	
	LD_5	Liver

(2) *Chromatography on DEAE-cellulose*. This technique is sometimes used for creatine kinase.

(3) *Heat stability* has been used to distinguish alkaline phosphatase which is stable (from the placenta) from that which is labile (liver and bone) when heated at 56°C for 30 min.

(4) *Inhibition*. Intestinal and placental alkaline phosphatase is inhibited by L-phenylalanine, other isoenzymes are not so affected. Urea has also been used to inhibit the liver component.

(5) *Immunological techniques* depend on antibodies to the enzymes which prevent catalytic activity. Thus an antibody to CK isoenzyme will prevent a reaction due to the isoenzyme, and the loss of activity may be measured.

(6) *Substrate specificity*. LD_1 will catalyse the reaction:

oxobutyrate + $NADH_2 \rightleftharpoons \alpha$-hydroxybutyrate + NAD

to a much greater extent than LD_{2-5}. Thus the use of α-oxobutyrate as a substrate will separate LD_1 from the other isoenzymes. LD_1 is broadly equivalent to hydroxybutyrate dehydrogenase (HBD).

ENZYMES AS REAGENTS

It has already been seen (Chapter 40) that the enzyme glucose oxidase is used as a reagent in the measurement of glucose. You will have seen that the enzyme malate dehydrogenase is used in the coupled enzyme method for aspartate aminotransferase (AsAT). These two are just part of the large and growing number of enzyme reagents. Some of the advantages and disadvantages of using enzymes are set out below.

Advantages

(1) Enzymes employ mild reaction conditions; they require pH's which are not extreme. An example of this is the replacement of alkaline saponification of triglycerides by the action of lipase.

(2) Enzymes are specific. Of all the substances present in blood, glucose is the only one which is a substrate for glucose oxidase. In some previous methods, which depended upon the reducing properties of glucose, other metabolites interfered with the colour reaction.

(3) Because enzyme methods do not employ extremes of heat, acidity or alkalinity, they are inherently safer than some reactions which they replace. Enzymatic cholesterol methods are much less dangerous than the colorimetric methods employing concentrated acids.

(4) The features mentioned above mean that enzyme-dependent methods are usually simpler than the methods which they replace, and often one- or two-step methods are possible. These simpler methods are usually less prone to operator error.

(5) Enzymes are re-usable so that the incorporation of an enzyme into a solid matrix from which the reaction mixture can be moved means that the same reagent may be used for many tests.

Disadvantages

(1) Enzymes are expensive. They are produced by biological systems; sometimes they are harvested from an animal source. The price of an enzyme, however, usually decreases as the demand increases. Higher demand prompts large-scale manufacture, which is cheaper per unit of enzyme.

(2) The biological nature of enzyme reactions means that an equilibrium is reached. In an inorganic reaction an almost instantaneous result occurs, with no further chemical change. Some means of stopping the reaction, or of timing all tests, is therefore required.

(3) Earlier in this chapter we saw the different factors affecting enzyme reactions. The same scrupulous attention to detail is required when enzymes are being used as reagents.

(4) As enzymes are proteins, the proteins in serum are present in the reaction. The presence of proteins may make the design of a method using enzyme reagents difficult.

The advantages of enzyme reagents may be brought to many biological compounds not immediately obvious as substrates for enzymic measurement. Cholesterol, triglyceride and creatinine may be measured, as well as glucose and other monosaccharides, urate, lactate and pyruvate. Almost any metabolite is capable of being altered catalytically, and the range of substances measured with enzyme reagents will continue to grow.

REFERENCES

1. Kind, P.R.N. and King, E.J. (1954). *J. Clin. Path.*, **7**, 322.
2. Wiggins, H.S. (1967). *Gut*, **8**, 415.
3. Gordon, I., Levin, B. and Whitehead, T.P. (1952). *Br. Med. J.*, **1**, 463.
4. Wroblewski, F. and LaDue, J.S. (1955). *Proc. Soc. Exp. Biol. Med. N.Y.*, **90**, 210.

47. Automation in clinical chemistry

All the quantitative methods described in this section require instruments. Automation may be applied to most of these methods, which means that a proportion of pipetting, timing and manipulation of analytical processes is done by machine. The proportion may be very large, as in multi-channel analysers, or quite small as in automatic diluters and dispensers.

For the purposes of this chapter automation will be taken to mean the performance by instruments of most of the processes concerned with the production of a result from a specimen. Automatic processes mimic at least the effect of manual ones. Fluid handling is carried out by automatic pipettes or by metering pumps; timing and incubation are done within the instrument; readings are gained in the same reaction vessel as the chemical reaction or after transfer into the light path of a spectrometer by automatic means.

Automatic chemical analysers can be subdivided as in Table 47.1. No single analyser will be considered in detail, but some principles and examples are given.

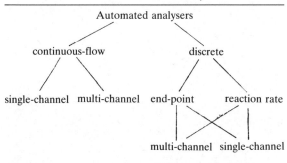

Table 47.1. Automatic analysers

slowed down by friction (*see* Fig. 47.1). The introduction of bubbles of air, which are large enough to scrub the sides of the tube, ensures a minimum of mixing from sample to sample because each air bubble maintains the integrity of the plug of liquid in front of it and produces a turbulent flow in that plug which is a very efficient mixing agent.

A continuous-flow analyser may be thought of in five parts: sampler; pump; manifold; photometer; recorder.

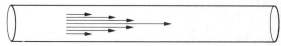

a. Laminar flow

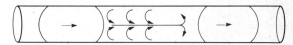

b. Turbulent flow

Fig. 47.1. The effect of bubbles on hydraulic system.

CONTINUOUS-FLOW SYSTEMS

Continuous-flow systems employ, as their name implies, one single hydraulic line in which all the reactions and incubations take place in solution. The major practical problem with this means of handling fluid is that of laminar flow where the fluid travels faster in the centre of the tube than it does at the sides where it is

Sampler

A Technicon* sampler is shown in Fig. 47.2. The probe dips in turn into each sample on a turntable and continuous suction which is applied to a line attached to the probe allows aspiration. A suitable wash solution is aspirated from a continuously replenished container. Standards and control sera are placed into cups and are aspirated in the same way as the samples. The rate of aspiration is controlled either by an electric timer or by a mechanical cam.

Pump

The pump is the heart of any continuous-flow system. It drives the fluids around and it is also responsible for the metering or pipetting of each of the fluid components. A Technicon sampler is seen in Fig. 47.3. The rollers

* Technicon Instrument Corporation.

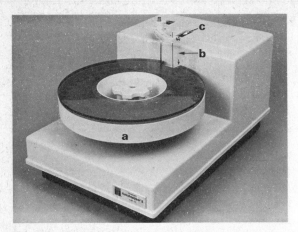

Fig. 47.2. Sampler module (Technicon Instruments Corp.). *(a)* Turntable; *(b)* probe; *(c)* wash receptacle.

drive fluid along the pump tubes by pressing against a platen (not shown) and rolling forward. The pump lines are colour-coded so that their value in ml/min can be seen at a glance. The air bar is a device to ensure the correct size and timing of the air bubbles.

Manifold

The manifold contains most of the hydraulic tubing between the pump and the spectrometer. It may contain elements which mix, incubate, and mimic protein precipitation and time delay which is necessary for organic reactions to come to completion or to achieve a steady state. Mixing is achieved as has been described before; incubation occurs when a section of the manifold tube has its temperature raised above that of room temperature, a simple heating bath achieves this. The heating medium may not be aqueous, especially for high temperatures when mineral oil is used. Protein precipitation is not achieved in continuous-flow analysers. Proteins are removed from the chemical reaction by moving the reactants which are generally of small molecular size across a semi-permeable membrane (*see* Fig. 47.4). This membrane allows small molecules to pass but prevents large protein molecules from crossing. Protein molecules are undesirable in chemical reactions involving serum or plasma because they contain carbohydrate, lipid and inorganic parts of the molecule which may themselves enter into a reaction. Proteins may also be precipitated by adverse reaction

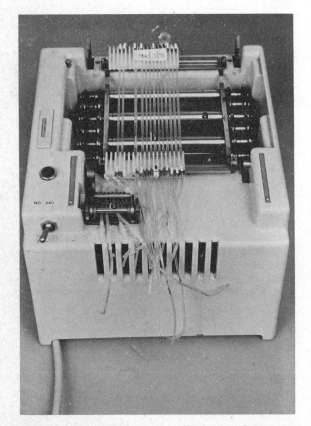

Fig. 47.3. Proportioning pump (Technicon Instruments Corp.).
(a) Rollers; *(b)* pump tubes; *(c)* air bar.

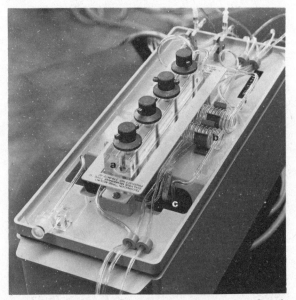

Fig. 47.4. The manifold (Technicon Instruments Corp.). *(a)* dialyser; *(b)* mixing coil; *(c)* heating bath (inlet and outlet only are shown)

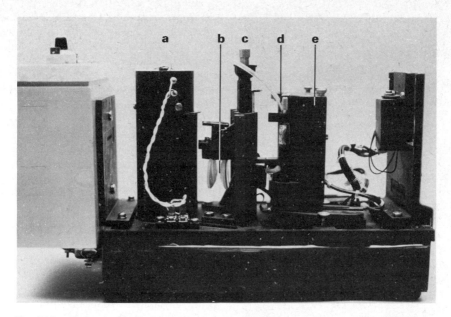

Fig. 47.5. Photometer/side view (with outer casing removed) (Technicon Instrument Corp.).
(a) Lamp housing; *(b)* collimator; *(c)* slit and filter; *(d)* flow cell; *(e)* photo-
detector.

conditions like high acidity. Time delay is achieved by sending the reaction mixture through one or more delay coils, which means that time delay is really incubation at room temperature.

Photometer

The photometer continuously measures the absorbance, at a given wavelength, of the solution which is going through the flow cell, as can be seen in Fig. 47.5. The photometer contains all the elements which are found in a normal spectrophotometer (*see* Chapter 5). The lamp housing contains a tungsten bulb and a fan which maintains a constant cool temperature in the spectrophotometer. The collimator consists of two lenses which together make the light converge through a slit the width of which controls the sensitivity of the spectrophotometer. The light then passes through an interference filter and thence to the flow cell and onto a photoemissive tube. When the substance to be analysed is itself coloured at the wavelength of measurement then a blank channel is run so that the colour of the analyte may be electrically subtracted from the colour of the solution. A blank channel may also be used to compensate for turbid, haemolysed, or jaundiced samples (*see* Fig. 47.6).

The streams are 'de-bubbled' just before entering the flow cell, so that bubbles do not affect the absorbance measurement. In some newer instruments the bubbles are left in the stream and a microprocessor removes the effect electrically.

Recorder

The light which the photodetector in the photometer detects causes a voltage change in the photodetector. This voltage is constantly measured and monitored by the recorder (*see* Fig. 47.7), the pen travelling to indicate the voltage at the photodetector. The pen builds up a trace which can be read by a bench-worker, or the voltage which it indicates can be accepted by a microcomputer and analysed so that the microcomputer will give the value of all the results sequentially and without transcription errors.

Figure 47.8 shows a complete system. Samples are loaded onto the sampler on the extreme right, are pulled through the pump together with reagents. The manifold contains those elements in which the chemical reaction takes place and in which proteins are eliminated by dialysis. The resultant coloured solution is read in the colorimeter, together with the blank channel if necessary, and the results are presented on the recorder. These may be further analysed by a microcomputer or calculator and the results presented in numerical

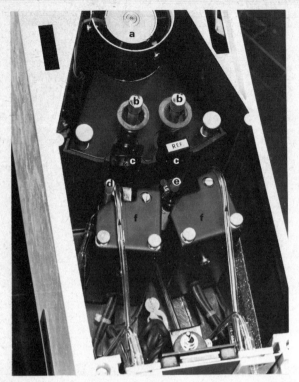

Fig. 47.6. Photometer—top view (Technicon Instruments Corp.).
(a) Lamp housing; (b) slit; (c) filter holder; (d) flow cell; (e) blank flow cell; (f) photo-detector housing.

electrodes. As can be seen from the figure, the chemical analysis occupies only part of the equipment. A computer is necessary for constant monitoring of the chemical reactions, a task which would be too time-consuming for the operator, and to calibrate the machine with reference sera at set intervals. The computer also performs statistical analyses on each of the channels and diagnoses faults both in itself and in the analyser. Information concerning the patient, his diagnosis, his address and his supervising clinician may also be entered so that a report, which is produced by the printer, may be addressed correctly. The specification of the computer is beyond the scope of this book.

SMALL DEDICATED ANALYSERS

Small dedicated analysers are becoming more widely used both in the laboratory and close to the patient. There is a potential danger in the use of any instrument by inadequately trained operators. A deterioration in performance of the analyser, resulting in spurious answers, may go undetected. This problem is made worse by the fact that the operation of the machine will be designed to be simple and it may be possible for answers to be obtained when the technique is inadequate. Some modern analysers overcome this by monitoring their own performance constantly. The laboratory can minimise poor use by offering a quality control scheme for these machines and a training scheme for the operators.

Small analysers may be considered by the method of detection of the end-point of measurement.

A. Photometric analysers

1. Reflectometry

Test strips are used which are impregnated with the dry chemicals necessary to produce a colour, when a drop of blood is applied, which depends upon the concentration of the substance being measured. When the blood is washed off, after a given time, the test strip is ready to be used. It is inserted into the reflectance meter which measures the light reflected from the surface of the test strip. As the colour becomes darker less light is reflected and a higher result is indicated. These meters are calibrated directly in concentration units. They are more reproducible and accurate than reading such test strips by eye, and they have the advantage of being usable by the patient who can follow his own blood glucose on a regular basis without having to report to a laboratory.

form. Such analysers have been in use for over 20 years and have remained a central part of the analytical instrumentation in most laboratories. In some instances, however, their advantages are not as great as those of discrete analysers which will be considered later in this chapter.

Multi-channel analysers

It is often convenient for substances which are frequently requested together to be analysed together in the laboratory. As a result of this instrument companies have produced large-scale machines which analyse twenty or more channels at the same time. Such an analyser is the SMAC (Sequential Multiple Analyser with Computer, which is produced by Technicon, see Fig. 47.9). The principles of analysis are the same as those for single channels, with the exception that sodium and potassium are measured by ion-selective

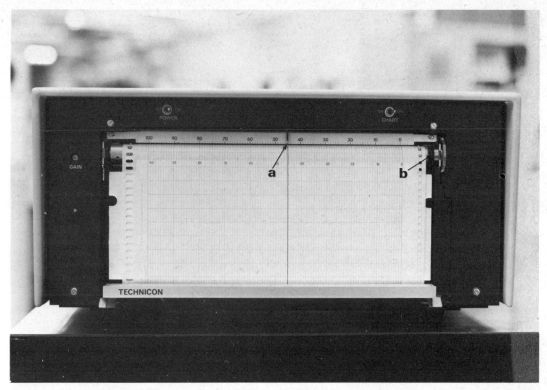

Fig. 47.7.   A recorder (Technicon Instruments Corp.). *(a)* Pen; *(b)* paper drive.

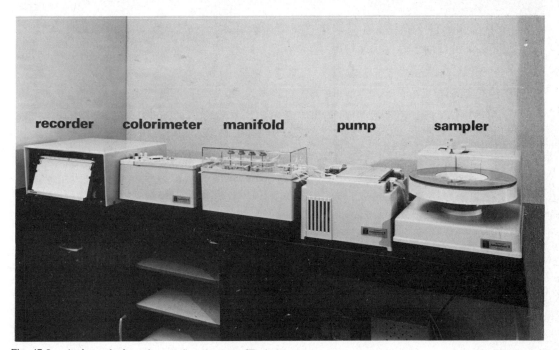

Fig. 47.8.   A channel of continuous-flow analysis (Technicon Instrument Corp.).

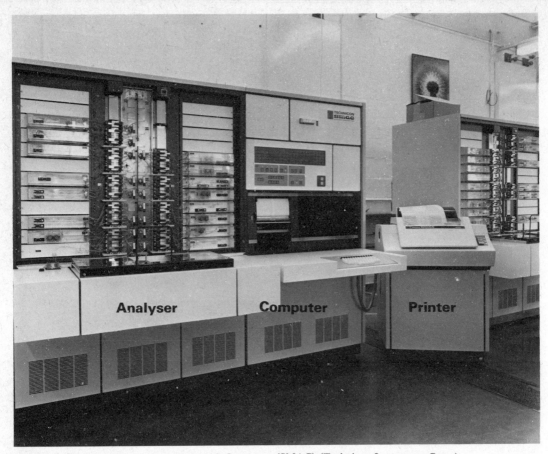

Fig. 47.9.   Sequential Multiple Analyser with Computer (SMAC) (Technicon Instrument Corp.).

2. Fluorimetry

Fluorescence photometry differs from normal photometry in that the detector is at right-angles to the original beam of light (see Fig. 47.10). Photometry measures the amount of light taken up by a sample (Chapter 5) and fluorescence measures the light given out by a sample which has been excited by an incident beam. To avoid interference from the incident light, the emitted light is measured at an angle, usually 90°.

An example is the Corning* calcium analyser (see Fig. 47.11) which uses a tungsten halogen lamp and a blue filter to provide the primary wavelength to the cuvette (see Fig. 47.12). When a sample containing calcium is added to the buffered indicator in the cuvette, the level of the resulting fluorescence is proportional to the amount of calcium. The current gener-

---

* Corning Ltd., Halstead, Essex.

---

ated by the photodetector is converted into a pulse signal which controls an automatic burette dispensing EDTA titrant into the cuvette. The amount of titrant required to reduce the fluorescence to a pre-set level is measured, and is proportional to the calcium concentration in the sample. The amount of titrant is compared with that required for a standard solution and the result is displayed directly as mmol/litre.

3. Nephelometry

Nephelometry is the measurement of scattered light at the same wavelength as the incident light. The scattering is caused by reflectance from particles in suspension, and the measurement is usually at 90°C from the incident light. For some instruments where the incident light is from a laser source the measurement is at a more acute angle.

Small dedicated analysers have used this principle to

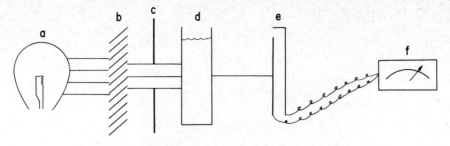

Absorbance photometry

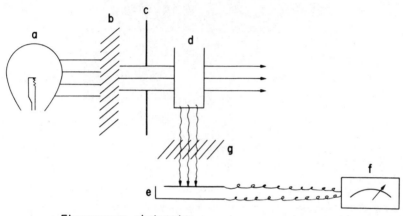

Fluorescence photometry

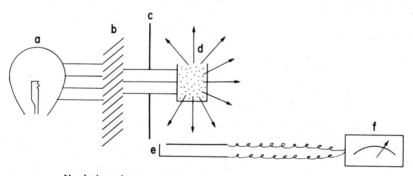

Nephelometry

Fig. 47.10. Photometric measurement (a) Lamp; (b) filter; (c) collimator; (d) cuvette; (e) photo-detector; (f) meter/recorder; (g) secondary filter.

monitor the breakdown of a particulate substrate by an enzyme, for example starch being degraded by amylase, or a lipid emulsion by lipase.

B. Electrometric analysers

Spectrophotometers measure the voltage produced by a photo-detector and are therefore electrometers. The term is used here, however, to signify measuring devices other than photo-detectors.

1. Amperometry

There are several analysers available which have an electrode sensitive to the level of oxygen. The electrode consists of a wire which is kept at a constant voltage.

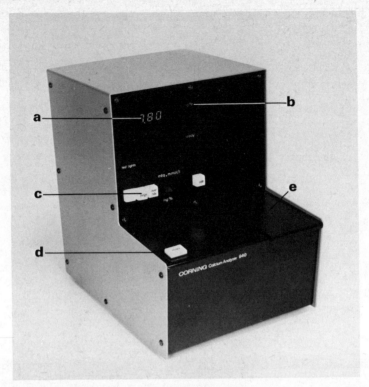

Fig. 47.11. Fluorescence calcium analyser (Corning Ltd.).
(a) Result display; *(b)* units; *(c)* controls; *(d)* titrate start; *(e)* analytical compartment.

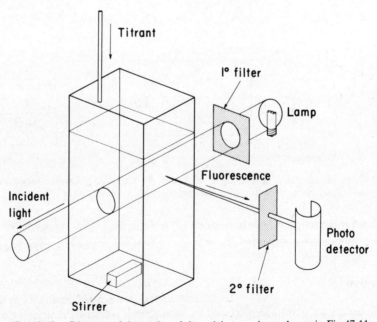

Fig. 47.12.   Diagram of the optics of the calcium analyser shown in Fig 47.11.

Oxygen is reduced at the end of the wire, and thus uses up electrons and in doing so reduces the charge in the wire. The current needed to replace the electrons and maintain the voltage is dependent on the concentration of oxygen. The instruments in use all depend upon enzyme reagents to produce a change in oxygen concentration and have been used to measure glucose, urate and cholesterol as in the equations below. Some analysers are designed to be used for any or all of the reactions. Others are designed to measure only one of them.

$$\text{Glucose} + \text{oxygen} \xrightarrow{\text{glucose oxidase}} \text{Gluconic acid} + \text{hydrogen peroxide.}$$

$$\text{Uric acid} + \text{oxygen} \xrightarrow{\text{uricase}} \text{Allantoin} + \text{carbon dioxide.}$$

$$\text{Cholesterol} + \text{oxygen} \xrightarrow{\substack{\text{cholesterol} \\ \text{oxidase}}} \text{Cholesterone} + \text{hydrogen peroxide.}$$

(Hydrogen peroxide is degraded chemically to avoid the reappearance of oxygen.)

2. Conductometry

(a) When a chemical reaction results in a change of conductivity that change may be used to indicate the end of a titration. This is the principle of a chloride meter* (see Fig. 47.13). The first pair of electrodes release silver ions into the reaction cup at a steady rate. The silver chloride formed is precipitated until no further chloride is available, when the excess silver ions produce a sudden increase in conductivity which is detected by the second pair of electrodes and the current is stopped.

The time taken for this process to occur is measured and compared with that taken for a standard chloride solution. Thus conductivity is used as an indicator for the end of the reaction.

$$\underset{\substack{\text{silver} \\ \text{from} \\ \text{electrode}}}{\text{Ag}^+} + \underset{\substack{\text{from} \\ \text{serum}}}{\text{Cl}^-} \longrightarrow \underset{\text{precipitate}}{\text{AgCl}}$$

---

* Corning Ltd., Halstead, Essex.

(b) The rate of change in conductivity may itself be measured as in a urea analyser where the reaction

$$(\text{NH}_2)_2\text{CO} + 2\text{H}_2\text{O} \xrightarrow{\text{urease}} 2(\text{NH}_4)^+ + \text{CO}_3^{--}$$

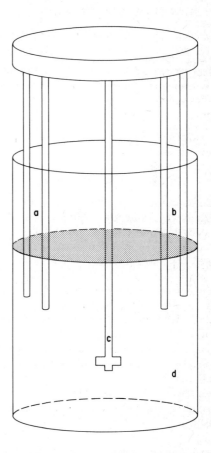

Fig. 47.13.   The electrodes of a chloride meter (a) Silver ion generating electrode pair; (b) conductivity sensing electrode; (c) stirrer; (d) sample in solution.

takes place. The maximum rate of increase in conductivity is proportional to the level of urea. Serum or plasma samples are compared with a standard solution, and the results indicated directly in concentration units.

3. Coulometry

This is the measurement of a quantity of electricity and is used in an iron analyser. Here the amount of electricity, at a specified voltage, is measured which is required to convert the iron in serum, which is all in the ferric form (Fe^{+++}) to the ferrous form (Fe^{++}). The voltage is specific for every metal which can be present in two forms in solution so that several metals could (in theory) be measured in a single sample.

4. Thermometry

Osmolality is one of a group of related properties of solution known as 'colligative properties'. Colligative properties depend only upon the concentration of the substances in solution and include:

    osmotic pressure increase;
    freezing temperature decrease;
    boiling temperature increase;
    saturated vapour pressure decrease.

In clinical chemistry osmolality (mol/kg solvent) rather than osmolarity (mol/litre solution) is used. Instruments in common use either measure freezing temperature decrease or indirectly measure saturated vapour pressure.

Freezing point measurement. Cryoscopic methods employ a process where a super-cooled but still liquid solution is suddenly frozen by vigorous stirring. The heat given out during the process of freezing is enough to melt some of the frozen solution. The liquid/frozen solution mixture is at the freezing point of that solution (by definition!), and is measured very accurately. The freezing temperature is compared with that of a standard solution and becomes lower as the osmolality increases.

Saturated vapour pressure measurement. The second method measures the amount of heat needed to keep a thermistor probe which is above a solution at a given temperature. The amount of heat depends upon the vapour pressure of the solution which in turn depends upon the number of dissolved particles.

5. Voltametry

Electrodes which are sensitive to the concentration of hydrogen ions in solution have already been considered in Chapter 4. Electrodes are now available, however, which are sensitive to one of several ions, and elec-

trodes which have found use within clinical chemistry include those which are sensitive to sodium, potassium and calcium. They have been called ion-specific electrodes, but 'ion-selective electrode' is a better term, as none is completely specific.

CENTRIFUGAL ANALYSERS

Samples in sequence, and reagents, are automatically distributed radially in wells in a specially designed centrifuge rotor (*see* Fig. 47.14, which shows a detail of the Centrifichem* system). Centrifugal force drives the samples and reagents together, and changes in the centrifugal speed effect efficient mixing. The resultant reaction mixture is driven into a series of associated cuvettes and measurement occurs of the absorbance. A computer takes measurements over a period of time, analyses them, compares them with those of standards and converts them into direct concentration units. Centrifugal analysers may be used for end-point or reaction-rate methods, which makes them versatile. They are particularly useful for the analysis of a relatively few samples (less than 50) for each of several tests. They have also been used as back-up equipment for large multiple analysers, and for fast analysis of emergency specimens.

REACTION RATE ANALYSERS

In these machines a sample is automatically taken from a specimen container, diluted in buffer, pipetted into a reaction vessel, brought to the measuring temperature and the reaction started by adding a substrate. The rate of reaction is measured by following the decrease of substrate or a co-factor, or the increase in product or a co-factor. Often NADH is measured at 340 nm.

MULTIPLE DISCRETE ANALYSERS

These are the largest of the discrete analysers and may be capable of doing up to 20 different analyses on one sample. They most commonly use photometric methods, often using well-established chemical principles using a sample blank instead of protein precipitation. Sodium and potassium are most usually measured using flame-emission photometry. For most other ana-

---

* Union Carbide (UK) Ltd. Amersham, Buckinghamshire.

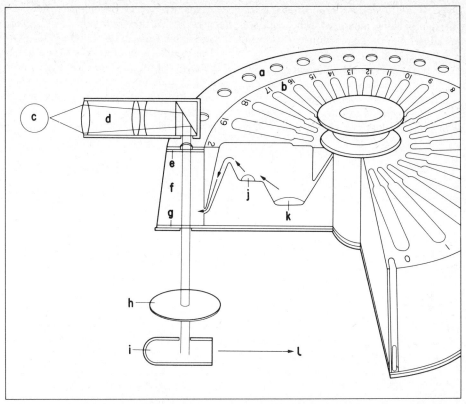

Fig. 47.14. Diagram of a centrifugal analyser (Union Carbide (UK) Ltd.)
(a) Rotor; (b) transfer disc; (c) light source; (d) collimator; (e) quartz ring; (f) reaction mixture; (g) quartz disc; (h) filter; (i) photomultiplier; (j) sampler and diluent; (k) reagent; (l) signal.

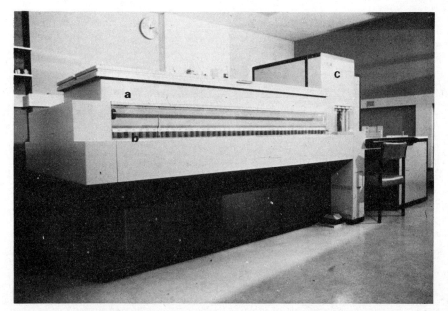

Fig. 47.15. The Greiner Selective Analyser, GSAII (Greiner Electronics Ltd.)
(a) Refrigerated reagent store; (b) analytical console; (c) computer console.

lytes a colour is produced which is proportional to the amount of substance being measured. The measurement may be end-point or of the reaction-rate type and may be done at more than one wavelength.

The most significant operational difference between multi-channel discrete analysers and multi-channel continuous-flow analysers is that the discrete can usually be programmed by the operator to do less than the full complement of tests available on that machine. This means that the clinicians are not bombarded with answers that they have not requested and do not want. Such a machine is the Greiner GSA II (*see* Fig. 47.15). The sample is placed on a turntable and the request pattern is programmed into a computer. The sample is then pipetted into the correct number of reaction cups for the pattern. Reagents are added and the reaction vessels are incubated according to the computer program.

Index

ABO blood groups, 267
  sub-groups, 269
Absolute values, 239
Absorbance, 32
Absorption spectrum of haemoglobins, 253
Accuracy of methods, 298
Acetest, 308, 331
Acetic ethanol fixative, 211
Acetoacetic acid in urine, 308
Acetone in urine, 308
Achlorhydria, 327
Acid alcohol fast organisms in sections, 202
Acid decalcifying fluids, 179
Acid elution test, 279
Acid formaldehyde haematin, 176
  removal of, 194
Acid mucopolysaccharides, alcian blue method for, 199
Act, Health & Safety at Work, 4
Adhesives for sections, 193
Aerobes, 44
Aerosols, 5
Aesculin hydrolysis test, 72
Agar
  in culture media, 118, 122–131
    see also 'Culture media'
  nutrient, 125
Agglutination reactions, in microbiology, 139, 140
Agglutinins, 139
Aggregometers, 250
Albumin, serum, estimation of, 325
Albustix, 332
Albym-Test, 332
Alcaligenes faecalis, 90
Alcaligenes species, 89
Alcian blue method for mucins, 199
Alcian blue/PAS stain, 199
Alkalescens-dispar group, 97
Alkaline phosphatase
  in neutrophils, 237
  in serum, 336

isoenzymes of, 341
Allele, 266
Allelomorph, 266
Alpha-haemolysis, 69
Alum haematoxylin
  celestine blue and, 196
  Cole's, 195
  eosin and, 195
  Harris's, 208, 211
Ammoniacal silver for sections, preparation of, 198
Amoebae in meningitis, 53
Amperometry, 349
Amylase, 338
Anaemia
  screening test for, 283
  sickle-cell, 252
Anaerobes
  culture of, 46
  facultative, 44
Anaerobic cocci, 74
Analysers
  centrifugal, 352
  continuous flow, 343–346
  dedicated, 346–352
  discrete, 352–354
  electrometric, 349–352
  photometric, 346–349
  reaction rate, 352
Anaphase, 266
Ancylostoma duodenale, 116
Animals
  cages for, 166
  euthanasia of, 166
  feeding, 165
  hygiene, 165
  laboratory, 165 et seq
  marking for identification, 166
  post-mortem examination of, 167
Anisocytosis, 233
Ante-natal screening, 279
Anti-activators, 242
Anti-D, 271
  prophylactic treatment with, 280

Anti-human globulin, 265
  preparation of reagent, 276
Anti-nuclear factor, 257
Anti-plasmins, 242
Anti-roll plate in cryostat, 206
Antibiotic
  assay techniques, 150–152
  combinations, 153
  sensitivity, testing for, 146
Antibodies 139
  anti-human species, 277
  blood group, 263–264
  immune, 265
  incomplete, 265
  production of, 264
Anticoagulant therapy, 244
Anticoagulants
  for transfusion blood, 284
  in haematology, 217
Antigen-antibody reactions, demonstrations of, 264–265
Antigens
  bacterial, 139
  blood group, 263–264
Antisera, 141
API 20A, 103
API 20E, 91
Aplastic marrow, 236
Aqueous mountant for sections, 207
Artifact pigments
  chrome fixation and, 177
  formalin, 176
  mercury, 176
  removal of, 194
Artifacts in tissue sections, 173
Ascaris lumbricoides, 115
Ascoli test, 78
Aspergillus species, 108, 112
Aspirates, bronchial, culture of, 58
Auramine stain in bacteriology, 64
Autoclaves, 157–159
  bottled-fluid, 159
  downward-displacement, 158
  pressure-cooker, 157

Autolysis in tissues, 175
Automatic tissue processing, 185
Automation
  in blood group serology, 280
  in clinical chemistry, 343–354
  in haematology, 246–250
Autosome, 266
Avidity of grouping sera, 271
Azoeosin stain, 201
Azure A stain, 200

B antigen, bacterial, 139
B-lymphocytes, 232
Bacillus
  anthracis, 77
  cereus, 77
  species, 77
  subtilis, 77
Bacitracin sensitivity test, 70
Bacteria
  cultivation of, 43–48
  in sections, 202
Bacterial count in urine, 55
Bacteriophages, 69
Bacteroides fragilis, 103
  in blood culture, 52
Balance, analytical, 25
Balance, top-pan, 26
Band forms, 231
Barr body, stain for, 213
Base sledge microtome, 187
Basophilia, 235
Basophilic stippling, 234
Basophils, 231
Beer-Lambert Laws, 32
Behaviour, code of, 3
Benedict's test, 304
Benzene as clearing agent, 182
Benzyl penicillin, *Str. pyogenes*
  sensitive to, 70
Berthelot reaction, 316
Beta-haemolysis, 69
Beta lactamase, 73
Bicarbonate in plasma, 314
Bile, excretion of, 320
Bile pigments metabolism, tests of,
  321–323
Bile-solubility test, 72
Bililabstix, 331
Bilirubin, 320
  commercial tests for, 331
  in urine, 323

serum, estimation of, 321
serum, reference range, 322
Bilur-Test, 331
Biochemical tests in microbiology,
  132–137
Biopsy specimens, culture of, 59
Biuret, 324
Blast cells, 217
Blastomycetes species, 108
Bleeding time methods, 243
Blood
  collection of, 218–219
  commercial tests for, 331
  count, 223–227
  film, 228
  films, staining methods, 228–230
  for clinical chemistry, 295
  in culture media, 119
  in faeces, 329
  leucocyte-poor, for transfusion, 285
  nature of, 217
  occult, in faeces, 329
  platelet-free, for transfusion, 285
  rapidly frozen, for transfusion, 285
  storage of, for clinical chemistry, 297
  storage of, for transfusion, 284
  transfusion, history of, 263
Blood bank documentation, 290
Blood culture, 51
  media for, 124
Blood donors, 283
Blood film staining methods,
  supplementary, 236
Blood group serology, automation in,
  280
Blood grouping
  ABO methods, 267–270
  Rh. methods, 272–273
  Rh., albumin displacement method,
    272
  Rh., enzyme techniques, 272, 275
  Rh., saline method, 272
  Rh., Stratton sandwich method, 272
  selection and preparation of
    ABO sera, 270
  selection and preparation of
    Rhesus grouping sera, 273
  tile method, 268
  tube method, 268
Blood groups
  ABO system, 267
  inheritance of, 265

Rhesus system, 271–273
systems other than ABO and Rh.,
  273
Blood transfusion compatibility tests,
  275–276
Body fluids, culture of, for
  mycobacteria, 87
Bohr effect, 223
Bone decalcification, 179–180
Bone marrow
  as site of haemopoiesis, 217
  biopsy, 236
  buffered formalin as fixative for, 176
  culture of, 52
Bordet-Gengou medium, 130
Bordetella
  parapertussis, 101
  pertussis, 101
  pertussis, features of, 99
  pertussis, in per-nasal swabs, 50
Borrelia
  species, 104
  vincentii, 103, 104
Botulism, 85
Bouin's fixative, 177
Branhamella catarrhalis, 75
Breed count, 142
Broth
  glucose, 121
  liver digest, 121
  nutrient, 120
  selenite F, 121
  serum, 120
  tetrathionate, 121
  Todd-Hewitt, meat infusion, 121
  tryptone soya, 122
Brown's opacity tubes, 145
Browne's
  TST, 159
  tubes, sterilisation indicators, 156,
    159
Brucella
  abortus, 100
  abortus, in Widal reaction, 94
  in blood culture, 51
  melitensis, 100
  melitensis, in Widal reaction, 94
  milk ring test, 101
  species, 100
  species, features of, 99
  suis, 100
Buffer solutions, 19

Burr cell, 234

Cabinets, safety, biological, 7
Cages, animal, 166
Calcium
  as coagulation factor, 240
  in serum, estimation of, 312
  reference range, in serum, 313
  salts in sections, removal of, 179–180
  Von Kossa method for, 202
Calgon Ringer solution, 138
Cambridge rocking microtome, 187
Campylobacter
  jejuni, 107
  jejuni, in faeces, 57
  species, 107
Candida
  albicans 108, 109
  albicans, in faeces, 57
  albicans, in vaginal swabs, 116
  species, Feinberg's medium for, 123
  species, in nasal swabs, 58
Capsule, bacterial, 140
  demonstration of, 65
Carbol fuchsin, 202
Carbon dioxide, bacterial cultivation
  in, 47
Carbowax fixative, 210
Carboxyhaemoglobin, 253
Carboxyphiles, 44
Carnoy's fixative, 177
  in cytology, 211
Carriers of typhoid fever, 93
Castaneda's medium, 124
Castaneda's method of blood culture,
  51
Casts in urine, 55
Catalase test, 132
Cedar wood oil as clearing agent, 182
Celestine blue, preparation of, 196
  with haematoxylin, 196
Cell barrier layer, 35
Cell counts
  differential, 231
  electrical resistance method, 246–248
  electro-optical method, 248–249
  visual methods, 225
Celloidin
  embedding, 185–186
  section preparation, 193
  section staining, 203
Centrifugal force, relative, 238

Centrifuges, 27–28
Centromere, 266
Cerebrospinal fluid, 332–333
  culture of, 52
  for clinical chemistry, 296
Cervical swabs, culture of, 59
Chelating agents for decalcification,
  179
Chemotaxis, 231
Chemotrophs, 43
Chloride in plasma, estimation of, 313
Chloride reference range, in plasma,
  314
Chlorides in distilled water, test for, 18
Chloroform as clearing agent, 182
Chromaffinoma, fixation of, 178
Chromatids, 266
Chromatin, 231
Chromatography, 304–307
Chrome fixative deposit, 177
Chromic acid for cleaning microscope
  slides, 61
Chromosomes, 265
Citrate dextrose (ACD) anticoagulant
  for transfusion blood, 284
Citrate-phosphate dextrose solution,
  anticoagulant for transfusion
  blood, 284
Clearing agents for histology, 181–182
Clinistix, 331
Clinitest, 331
Clostridia
  in blood culture, 52
  species, 82–85
Clostridium
  tetani, 84
  welchii, 82
  welchii, in faeces, 57
Clothing, protective, 6
Clotting time
  Kaolin-cephalin, 243
  whole-blood, 243
Co-factors, 335
Coagulase test, 74
Coagulation factors, 240
Coagulometers, 249–250
Cocci, Gram-positive, 69–75
Coccidioides immitis, 108
Codes of practice
  ionising radiations, protection from,
  23
  prevention of infection, 4

Coefficient of variation, 298
Cold agglutinins, 270
Cole's haematoxylin, 195
Collimator, 33
Colonies, shapes of, 68
Colorimetry, sources of error in, 37
Compatibility tests
  albumin technique, 276
  enzyme techniques, 275
  in blood transfusion, 275–276
  indirect antiglobulin technique, 276
Conductometry, 351
Connective tissue, stain for, 196
Containers
  for culture media, 119
  specimen, 49
Continuous flow methods of analysis,
  343–346
Control sample, 298
Controls for sensitivity testing, 148
Coombs' technique, 276
  automated, 282
Cord blood, 281
Corpuscular defects, 255
Corynebacterium
  diphtheriae, 78
  diphtheriae, granule stain for, 62
  diphtheriae, in nasal swabs, 57
  species, 78–81
  species, appearance on Albert
    stained films, 79
Cough plates, culture of, 58
Coulometry, 352
Count
  Breed, 142
  dilution, 143
  membrane filter, 144
  Miles and Misra, 144
  pour plate, 143
  presumptive coliform, 143
  surface colony, 144
  total, bacterial, 142
  viable, bacterial, 142
Counter-current immuno-
    electrophoresis, 139
Counting chamber
  Helber, 142
  Neubauer, 225
Coverslips, mounting sections with, 195
Craigie's tube, 96
Creatine kinase, isoenzymes of, 341
Creatinine in urine, 303

Crenated cells, 234
Cresyl fast violet stain, 213
Cross match
    emergency, 278
    protocol for, 277
    saline technique, 277
Cryoprecipitate, 287
Cryostat, 205
    rapid H & E method, 208
Cryptococcus neoformans, 108
Culture in meningitis, 53
    anaerobic, 45
    requirements for, 66
Culture media
    Bacto fluid thioglycolate, 124
    blood agar, 125
    Bordet-Gengou, 130
    brain-heart infusion, 124
    Brewer's thioglycolate, 122
    Castaneda's, 124
    chocolate agar, 126
    crystal-violet blood agar, 126
    cystine serum tellurite, 127
    deoxycholate citrate, 128
    DNase agar, 127
    egg-yolk neomycin agar, 130
    Elek's, 130
    Feinberg's, 123
    for blood, 124
    glucose broth, 121
    glucose phosphate, 135
    Hoyle's, 127
    identification of, 120
    kanamycin blood agar, 126
    liver digest broth, 121
    liver infusion agar, 128
    Loeffler's, 131
    Lowenstein-Jensen, 131
    lysed blood agar, 126
    MacConkey's agar, 128
    MacConkey-aesculin, 128
    nutrient agar, 125
    nutrient broth, 120
    ONPG, 136
    oxidation-fermentation, 135
    peptone water, 123
    phenolphthalein phosphate agar, 127
    potassium cyanide, 137
    Robertson's cooked meat, 122
    Sabouraud agar, 131
    salt mannitol agar, 127
    selenite F broth, 121

    sensitivity test agar, 128
    serum agar carbohydrate, 134
    serum broth, 120
    serum water carbohydrate, 134
    Skirrow's, 126
    sterilisation of, 120
    tetrathionate broth, 121
    Thayer-Martin, 126
    thioglycolate, fluid, 123
    thiosulphate-citrate-bile-salt sucrose, 129
    Todd-Hewitt meat infusion broth, 121
    transport, Stuart's, 123
    tryptone soya broth, 122
    urea agar slopes, 134
    vancomycin chocolate agar, 126
    xylose lysine deoxycholate agar, 129
Cultures
    disposal of, 9
    stock, 47
Cupboards
    fume, 7
    storage, 22
Cusum, 300
Cuvette, 34
Cyanmethaemoglobin method for haemoglobin, 223
Cylinders
    gas, 30
    graduated, 13
Cytofix, 210
Cytology
    cresyl fast violet stain for, 213
    fixatives for, 210–211
    May-Grunwald Giemsa stain for, 212
    of effusions, 209
    Papanicolaou stain for, 211
    specimens, 209

D antigen, 271
Dacie's fluid, 225
Daily means, 299
Decalcification, 179–180
    electrolytic, 180
    surface, 180
    test for, 180
Defibrination, 218
    syndrome, 242
Dehydration of tissues, celloidin and LVN, 186
    paraffin wax, 181

Dermatophytes, 109
Desiccants, 15
Desiccators, 15
Detectors, photosensitive, 35
Dextran, 289
Diabur-Test, 331
Diastix, 331
Didymium filters, 297
Differential counts, 231
    automatic, 249
Dilutions, 21
Diphtheria toxin, 80
Diphtheroid bacilli, 81
Direct antiglobulin test, 281
Discs, gelatin charcoal, 131
Disinfectants, properties of, 162–163
Disinfection, 155 *et seq*
Dispensers, 13
Distilled water
    production of, 18
    pyrogen free, 284
Documentation in haematology, 220
Drabkin's solution, 224
Drift control, 298
Duke's method for bleeding time, 243

Ear swabs, culture of, 56
Ectothrix, 110
EDTA
    as anticoagulant, 217
    decalcifying fluid, 179
Effusions, cytology of, 209
Ehrlich's reagent, 133
El Tor vibrio in faeces, 57
Elastic tissue
    orcein stain for, 197
    resorcin fuchsin stain for, 197
Electrodes
    calomel, 29
    pH measuring, 29
Electrolytes, 309
Electrophoresis of plasma proteins, 324
Elek's medium, 130
Elliptocytosis, 233
Embedding
    gelatin, 205
    media, 181
    moulds, 182–183
Endothrix, 110
Enterobacter, 92
Enterobacteria, 90–98
    in blood culture, 51

Enterobacteria – *contd*
  in meningitis, 53
Enterobius vermicularis, 115, 116
Enzyme analysis, factors affecting,
  334–335
Enzymes, 334–342
  as reagents, 341–342
  methods of measurement, 335
  units of activity, 336
Eosin, haematoxylin and,
  for frozen sections, 208
  for paraffin sections, 195
Eosinophilia, 231, 235
Eosinophils, 231
  in sections, 201
  stain for, 201
Epidermophyton
  floccosum, 111
  genus, 108, 109
Epstein-Barr virus, 258
Errors
  random, 298
  systematic, 298
Erysipelothrix
  culture for, 58
  rhusiopathiae, 81
Erythrocyte sedimentation rate, 257
  Westergren method, 258
Erythrocyte transketolase, 295
Erythrocytes, 230
  for clinical chemistry, 295
  life span of, 230
  morphology of, 233–234
Erythropoietin, 230
Escherichia
  coli, 91
  coli, enteropathogenic, 91
  coli, enteropathogenic, in faeces, 57
  coli, in blood culture, 51
Ethanol 95% as fixative, 210
Eubacteria, 66
Eukitt mountant, 211
Euthanasia for laboratory animals, 166
Extinction, 32
Extinguishers, fire, 7
Extracorpuscular defects, 255
Extrinsic system of blood coagulation,
  241
Eye swabs, culture of, 56

Faeces
  blood in, 329
  culture of, 56
  examination for parasites, 114
  occult blood in, 329
  specimens for clinical chemistry, 296
Fat in sections, 207
Feinberg's medium, 123
Ferric iron, Perl's method for, 201
Fetal cells, detection of, 281
Fetal haemoglobin, 251
  in acid elution test, 281
Fibrin
  Gram's stain for, 202
  in sections, 200
  trichrome stain for, 196
Fibrin(ogen) degradation products, 242
Fibrinogen, 240
  for treatment of fibrinolytic disorders,
    288
  titre, 243
Fibrinolytic system, 241
Filde's extract, in culture media, 118
Filter
  flasks, 13
  funnels, 13
  pumps (Venturi), 15
Filters
  didymium, 297
  membrane, 160
  membrane, in cytology, 210–211
  sintered glass, 160
  wavelength selection, 33
Filtration in microbiology, 160–161
Fire, 7
First Aid, 9
Fixation, 175–178
  aims of, 175
  chromaffinoma for, 178
  cytology, 210–211
  general, 175
  ideal, 175
  of blood films, 229
  phaeochromocytoma for, 178
  rapid frozen sections for, 208
  rapid paraffin sections for, 177, 183
  secondary, 175–176
  smears in histology, 178
Fixatives
  absolute methanol, 210
  acetic ethanol, 211
  Bouin's, 177
  buffered formalin, 176
  Carbowax, 210

Carnoy's, 177
Carnoy's in cytology, 211
Cytofix, 210
'dry', 210
ethanol 95%, 210
formal-sublimate, 176
formalin, 176
Heidenhain (Susa), 177
Helly's, 177
ideal, 175
Orth's, 177
Schaudinn's, 177
Schaudinn's in cytology, 211
Susa, 177
Zenker's, 177
Flagella, 140
Flame photometry, 310–312
Flasks, 13
  volumetric, use of, 20
Fluorimetry, 348
Food-poisoning, clostridial, 84
Formal-sublimate 10%, as fixative,
  176
Formalin
  10%, as fixative, 176
  10% buffered, as fixative, 176
  pigment, 176
    removal of, 194
Formic acid decalcifying fluid, 179
Fouchet's test, 323
Francisella, 102
Freeze dried plasma, 288
Freezing microtome, 188
  cryostat, 205
  use of, 205
Fresh frozen plasma, 287
Frozen sections
  preparation of, 205
  stains on, 207–208
Fructose in urine, 303
FTA-ABS, 105
Fungi
  dimorphic, 108
  filamentous, 108
  in sections, 203
  in sections, Gram's stain for, 202
  in sections, PAS stain for, 198
  yeast-like, 108
Funnels
  filter, 13
  separating, 13
Fusiformis fusiformis, 103, 104

Galactose in urine, 303
Gamma-haemolysis, 69
Gastric acidity, measurement of, 328
Gastric lavage, culture of, 57
Gelatin embedding for frozen sections, 205
Genes, 265–267
Genotype, 267
Gentamicin assay, 151
Gerhardt's test, 308
Giardia lamblia, 116
Giemsa stain, 229
Glassware, 10–17
  borosilicate, 10
  cleaning of, 16
Globin, 223
Glomerular filtration rate, 315
Glucose
  blood, method for, 302
  commercial tests for, 331
  homeostasis, 302
  in CSF, 332
Glycogen, PAS method for, 198
Glycosuria, 303
Gomori hexamine silver stain, 203
Gram's stain
  for sections, 202
  in bacteriology, 62
Granulocytes, 231
Grating diffraction, 34
Guide plate cryostat, 206
Guinea-pigs, 168
Gum arabic for frozen sections, 207

H antigen, 140
Haem, 223
Haemalum, Mayer's, 237
Haematin acid formaldehyde, 176
  removal of, from sections, 194
Haematocrit
  micro method, 238
  Wintrobe method, 238
Haematoxylin
  celestine blue and, 196
  Cole's, 195
  eosin and, 195–208
  Harris's, 208, 211
  Van Gieson and, 196
  Weigert's iron, 204
Haemochromatosis, 236
Haemoglobin, 223–225
  by cyanmethaemoglobin method, 223

estimation of, 223–225
  in erythrocytes, 230
Haemoglobin A, 251
Haemoglobin C, 252
Haemoglobin F, 251
Haemoglobin M, 253
Haemoglobin S, 252
Haemoglobinopathies, 251
Haemolysis
  extravascular, 255
  intravascular, 255
Haemolytic disease of the newborn, 273, 279
  treatment of infants with, 280
Haemolytic disorders, 255–256
Haemophilus
  influenzae, 99
  influenzae, in meningitis, 53
  species, 98–100
  species, growth factors, 119
Haemopoiesis, 217
Haemosiderin, Perl's method for, 201
Haemostasis, 240–245
Harris's haematoxylin, 208, 211
Hazards
  chemical, 7
  electrical, 8
Heaf test, 89
  for staff, 3
Heat-resistance test for *Str. faecalis*, 72
Heidenhain's fixative, 177
Heinz bodies, 234
Helber counting chamber, 142
Helly's fixative, 177
Hemastix, 331
Henle, loop of, 315
Heparin
  as anticoagulant, 218
  in anticoagulant therapy, 245
Hepatitis B antigen
  safety precautions, 289
  testing blood donors for, 288, 289
Hess's test, 242
Hexamine silver stain, 203
Histoplasma species, 108
Holding time, 156
Honing of microtome knives, 189
Howell-Jolly bodies, 234
Hoyle's medium, 127
Hydrogen sources for bacterial
  cultivation, 47

Hydrogen sulphide test, in
  microbiology, 137
Hygiene, personal, 6
Hyperglycaemia, 302
Hyperplastic marrow, 236
Hypochromia, 233
Hypoglycaemia, 302
Hypoplastic marrow, 236
Hypoproteinaemia, 323

Ictostix, 323
Ictotest, 323, 331
Ideal fixative, 175
Immune antibodies, 265
Immunisation, protective, 4
Immunoglobulin A, 264
Immunoglobulin D, 264
Immunoglobulin E, 264
Immunoglobulin G, 264
Immunoglobulin M, 264
Incubation of cultures, 47
Indole reaction, 133
Infectious mononucleosis, 258
Inhibisol
  for clearing tissues, 181
  for mounting sections, 194
Inhibitors of enzymes, 335
Inoculation
  loops, 45
  of animals, material for, 167
  of culture media, 44–45
Insulin test meal, 329
Intrinsic system of blood coagulation, 241
Iodine
  in Gram's stain, 202
  removal of mercury pigment with, 194
Ion-exchange resins for decalcification, 180
Iron in haemoglobin, 223
Iron haematoxylin, 204
Iron pigment in sections, Perl's method for, 201
Irradiation, ultra-violet, 161
Isoenzymes, 341
Ivy's method for bleeding time, 243

Jaundice, 320

K antigen, 92, 139, 140
Kaolin-cephalin clotting time, 243

Ketone bodies, 308
  commercial tests for, 331
Ketosis, 308
Ketostix, 308, 331
Ketur-Test, 331
Kidney, functions of, 315
Kininogen (high molecular weight), 241
Kjeldahl method of estimating
        proteins, 324
Klebsiella, 92
  aerogenes, 92
  in sputum, 58
  pneumoniae, 92
Knives
  automatic machine sharpening, 190
  honing, 189
  microtome, 188–189
  stropping, 190
Kovac's reagent, 133

Laboratory records in haematology,
        222
Lactate dehydrogenase,
  isoenzymes of, 341
Lactobacilli, 82
Lactose in urine, 303
Laminar flow, 343
Lancefield grouping, 70, 139
Laryngeal swab, culture of, 57
LE cells, 257
Lectins, 271
Leishman's stain for blood films, 229
Lepromin, 89
Leptocytes, 234
Leptospira
  icterohaemorrhagiae, 104
  interrogans, 104
  species, 104
  in meningitis, 53
Leuckhart's embedding moulds, 182
Leucocytes, differential count, 234
Leucocytosis, 230
Leucopenia, 230
Leukaemia, 235
Lipids, method for, in sections, 207
Liquoid
  in blood culture media, 51
  in brain-heart infusion, 124
Listeria
  in meningitis, 53
  monocytogenes, 81

monocytogenes, motility of, 61
Liver digest, in culture media, 118
Locus, 267
Loeffler's serum medium, 131
Low viscosity nitro-cellulose (LVN)
  embedding, 186
  sections, 193
Low-ionic-strength saline, 278
Lowenstein-Jensen medium, 131
Lymphatic system, 217
Lymphocytes, 232
Lymphocytosis, 232, 235
Lymphopenia, 235
Lysine/cyanide reagent, 224
Lysogeny, 80

MacConkey's agar, 128
MacConkey-aesculin agar, 128
Macrocytosis, 233
Macrophages, 230
Malabsorption, 330
Malachite green, counterstain for
        Ziehl-Neelsen, 62
Malassezia furfur, 111
Mantoux test, 89
  for staff, 3
Marrow needle, 236
Martius scarlet blue stain, 200
Mast cells in sections, 200
May-Grunwald–Giemsa stain for blood
        films, 229
May-Grunwald stain, 229
Mayer's haemalum, 237
McFadyean's reaction, 62, 78
Mean cell haemoglobin, 239
Mean cell haemoglobin concentration,
        239
Mean cell volume, 239
Meat extract, in culture media, 118
Medium, Stuart's, transport, 50
Megakaryocytes, 233
Meiosis, 266
Meningitis, causative organisms, 53
Mercuric chloride-formalin fixative,
        176
Mercury pigment in sections, 176
  removal of, 194
Mesophiles, 44
Metabolism, bacterial, biochemical
        tests for, 68
Metaphase, 266
Methaemoglobin, 223, 252, 253

Methanol fixative, 210
Methyl green-pyronin stain, 200
Methyl-red test, 136
Methylene blue staining method, 62
Mice, 169
Michaelis constant, 335
Micro-aerophiles, 44
Micro-organisms, Classification
        (Howie), 5
Micrococci in nasal swabs, 58
Micrococcus species, 74
Microcytosis, 233
Microhaematocrit method, 238
Microprocessor in balances, 25
Microscope, 38–40
  lenses, 38
  setting up, 39
  slides, cleaning of, 61
Microsporum species, 108, 109, 111
Microtome knives, 188–189
  bevel of, 189
  sharpening, 189
  slant, 192
  tilt, 189, 192
  types, 188–189
Microtomes, 187–188
Microtomy
  celloidin and LVN sections, 193
  frozen sections, 205
  paraffin wax sections, 191
Miles and Misra colony count, 144
Minimal inhibitory concentration,
        152
Minimum bactericidal concentration,
        153
Monochromator, 33
Monocytes, 231
Monocytosis, 232, 235
Motility, 61
Moulds, 108
Mountants
  Eukitt, 211
  Styrolite, 211
Mounting media
  for sections, aqueous, 207
  for sections, resinous (histology), 195
        (cytology), 211
MSB stain, 200
Mucin in sections
  alcian blue method, 199
  PAS method, 198
  azure A method, 200

Mucor, 108
　species, 113
Mycobacteria, 85–89
　culture of, 86
　pathogenic, 88
Mycobacterium tuberculosis, 85
　in Category Bl, 5
　in meningitis, 53
Myeloid:erythroid ratio, 236
Myeloma, multiple, 318

Nagler reaction, 84
　medium for, 130
Nasal swab, culture of, 57
Nebuliser in flame photometry, 311
Necator americanus, 116
Neisseria
　gonorrhoeae, 76
　meningitidis, 75
　　in blood culture, 51
　　in meningitis, 53
　　in nasal swabs, 57
Nephelometer for bacterial counts, 145
Nephelometry, 348
Nephron, 315
Nephur-Test, 332
Neubauer counting chamber, 225
Neutropenia, 235
Neutrophil alkaline phosphatase,
　method for, in blood films, 237
Neutrophil leucocytosis, 235
Neutrophils, 231
Niacin test, 88
Nitric acid for decalcification, 179
Nitrocellulose, low viscosity (LVN)
　embedding, 185–186
　section cutting, 193
　staining, 203
Nomenclature, bacterial, 66
Novobiocin sensitivity test, 73–75

O antigen, 92
　bacterial, 140
Oil red O stain for lipids in sections, 207
Optical density, 32
Optochin test, 72
Orcein stain for elastic fibres, 197
Orth's fixative, 177
Osmosis, 255
Osmotic pressure, 255
Oxford Staphylococcus, 74
Oxidase test, 132

Packed-cell volume, 238
Papanicolaou stain, 211
Paraffin wax
　embedding, 182–183
　　processing schedules, 183–185
　sections
　　microtomy of, 191–193
　　staining of, 195–203
Pasteurella
　multocida, 102
　septica, 102
　species, 101–102
　　features of, 99
Pasteurisation, 156
Paul-Bunnell-Davidsohn test, 258
Penetration time, 156
Penicillin, destruction by beta
　lactamase, 73
Penicillium, 108, 112
Pentagastrin test, 328
Pentoses in urine, 303
Peptococcus, 75
Peptone
　in culture media, 118
　water, 123
　　sugars, 133
Peptostreptococcus, 75
Per-nasal swabs, culture of, 58
Periodic acid-Schiff
　method for sections, 198
　reaction, in blood films, 237
Perl's method for ferric iron, in
　sections, 201
Perl's Prussian blue reaction, 236
pH
　effect on enzyme analysis, 334
　commercial tests for, 332
　electrodes, 29
　for bacterial growth, 44
　measurement of, 30
　meters, 28–30
Phaeochromocytoma, fixation of, 178
Phage type, 73
Phagocytosis, 230, 231
Pharyngeal swabs, culture of, 58
Phenistix, 332
Phenyl-ketones, commercial test for,
　332
Phosphotungstic acid haematoxylin
　stain, 196
Photocell, 35
Photochromogens, 44

Photoemissive tube, 36
Photomultiplier, 36
Phototube, 36
Pigments
　artifact, 175
　formalin, 176
　haemosiderin, 201
　mercury, 176
　removal of, 194
Pipettes, 10–12
　cleaning of, 16
　Pasteur, 11
Plasma
　for clinical chemistry, 295
　freeze dried, 288
　fresh frozen, 287
　protein fraction, 288
　proteins, 323–326
　substitutes, 288
Plasma cells in sections, 200
Plasmapheresis, 284
Plasminogen, 242
Plastic embedding moulds, 183
Plasticiser in LVN embedding, 186
Plastics, 17
Plate diffusion test, 147
Platelet
　aggregation, 250
　concentrate, 287
　counts, visual method, 227
　　automatic, 247, 248
Platelets, 223
　function of, 240
　in blood film, 235
Pleural effusion fixation in histology,
　178
Pluripotential cells, 217
Poikilocytosis, 233
Polychromasia, 230, 233
Polymorphonuclear neutrophil, 231
Polyvinylpyrrolidone, 289
Post-mortem
　examination of animals, 167
　specimens, culture of, 58
Post-nasal swabs, culture of, 58
Potassium
　estimation of, 310–312
　in body fluids, 309
　in urine, 312
　reference range, in plasma, 312
Pre-kallikrein, 241
Precipitins, 139

Precision of methods, 298
Preparation of tissues for microtomy, 181–186
  celloidin and LVN, 185–186
  frozen, 205
  paraffin, 181–185
Prism, 33
Processing
  histology, celloidin, 185
    LVN, 185
    paraffin wax, 181
  machines, for histology, 183
  schedules for, 183–185
Proerythroblast, 230
Prophase, 266
Propionobacterium acnes, in blood culture, 51
Protein
  Bence-Jones, 318
  commercial tests for, 332
  in CSF, 332
  in urine, 317
Proteins
  methods of fractionation, 324
  plasma, 323–326
  serum, estimation of total, 324
  serum, reference range (total), 325
Proteinuria, 54
Proteus
  mirabilis, 98
  morgani, 98
  rettgeri, 98
  species, 97
  vulgaris, 98
Prothrombin, 240
Prothrombin time
  one-stage method, 244
  one-stage method, by coagulometer, 250
Protoporphyrin, 223
Prussian blue stain for iron, in sections, 201
Pseudomonas
  aeruginosa, 89
    in blood culture, 52
  pseudomallei, 89
  species, 89
    in meningitis, 53
Psychrophiles, 44
PTAH stain, 196
Pump filter, 15
Punctate basophilia, 234

Pus, culture of, 58
Pyocyanin, 89
Pyrogens, 284

Quality control
  charts, 299–300
  in blood group serology, 282
  in clinical chemistry, 295–301
  in haematology, 219
  in microbiology, 43
  of culture media, 138
  of gentamicin assay, 150
Quellung
  capsular swelling test, 99
  reaction, 92

R_f, 306
R_g, 306
Ralmount section mountant, 195
Rapid frozen sections, 208
Rapid paraffin wax schedule, 183
Rapid tissue fixation, Carnoy's fluid for, 177
RDC decalcifying fluid, 179
Rectal swabs, culture of, 56
Red cells, 230
  concentrated, for transfusion, 285
  in urine, 55
  osmotic fragility, 255
Red-cell count
  automatic, 246, 248
  visual method, 225
Reducing sugars, commercial tests for, 331
Reflectometry, 346
Refrigerators, 284
Reiter protein complement-fixation test, 105
Relative centrifugal force, 238
Renal threshold, 302
Resorcin fuchsin stain for elastic fibres, 197
Reticulin fibres in sections, method for, 198
Reticulocyte, 230, 234
  counts, 235
Rhizopus species, 113
Ribosomes, 230, 234
Ringer solution, 137
Roche Entero-tube, 91
Romanowsky stains, 228
Rotary microtome, 187

Rothera's test, 308
Rouleaux, 228, 234

Sabouraud agar, 131
Safety, 4–8
  cabinets, biological, 7
  officers, 4
Salicylates in urine, 303, 308
Salicylsulphonic acid test, 318
Saline, isotonic, physiological, 19, 137
Salmonella, 92–96
  food poisoning, 95
  paratyphi, 92
  serotypes, 95
  typhi, 92
    in faeces, 57
  typhimurium, 95
Sangur-Test, 331
Satellitism, 98
Schaudinn's fixative, 178
  in cytology, 211
Schick test, 79
Schiff's reagent, 198, 237
Schistocytes, 233
Schistosoma
  haematobium, 116, 117
  mansoni, 116
    examination for, 114
Schlesinger's test, 322
Secondary fixation, 175–176
Section cutting
  celloidin and LVN, 193
  frozen, 205
  paraffin, 191
Section mounting, 195
Selenite F broth, 121
Sensitivity
  of methods, 298
  tests, 147–150
    inoculation of plates for, 149
    on primary cultures, 149
Sequestrene as anticoagulant, 217
Serial sections, 192
Serology in microbiology, 69
Serratia marcescens, 98
Serum
  albumin, estimation of, 325
  alkaline phosphatase, 336
  bilirubin, estimation of, 321
  for clinical chemistry, 295
  lactate dehydrogenase, 340
  preservative, 141

Sex chromatin, stain for, 213
Shift to the left, 231
Shift to the right, 231
Shigella
    boydi, 96
    dysenteriae, 96
    flexneri, 96
    sonnei, 96
    species, 96–97
Sickle cells, 234
    demonstration of, 252
Sickle-cell anaemia, 252
Signs, warning
    biohazard, 5
    chemical hazard, 22
Silver impregnation for reticulin fibres
        in sections, 198
Skin, culture of, 58
Skirrow's medium, 126
Smears fixation, in histology, 178
Sodium
    estimation of, 310–312
    in body fluids, 309
    in urine, 312
    reference range, in plasma, 312
Solutions, 19–20
    buffer, 19
    preparation of, 20
Sörenson's buffer, 229
Specificity
    of grouping sera, 271
    of methods, 297
Specimen
    blood, for clinical chemistry, 295
    collection of in clinical chemistry, 295
    containers, 49
    disposal of, 9
    microbiological, 43
    plasma, for clinical chemistry, 295
    posting of, 8
    reception of, 8
        in histology, 173
    serum, for clinical chemistry, 295
    urine, for clinical chemistry, 295
Spectroscope, 253
Spherocytes, 255
Spherocytosis, 233
Spirilla, 107
Spirillum minus, 107
Spirochaetes, 103
Spore strips for autoclave testing, 159
Spores, recovery medium for, 122

Sporotrichum species, 108
Sputum
    culture of, 58
    cytology, 210
    fixation, in histology, 178
    smears, fixation in cytology, 210–211
    smears, fixation of in histology, 178
Staining methods
    Albert's, 65
    alcian blue, 199
    alcian blue/PAS, 199
    auramine, 64
    azoeosin-haematoxylin, 201
    azure A, 200
    capsule demonstration, 65
    connective tissue trichrome, 196
    cresyl fast violet, for cytology, 213
    Gomori hexamine silver, 203
    Gram's for sections, 202
    Gram's, in bacteriology, 62
    haematoxylin and eosin, 195
        rapid for frozen sections, 208
    haematoxylin and van Gieson, 196
    Martius scarlet blue, 200
    May-Grunwald–Giemsa, for cytology,
        212
    methyl green-pyronin, 200
    MSB, 200
    oil red O for neutral fats, 207
    orcein and methylene blue, 197
    Papanicolaou, for cytology, 211
    PAS for sections, 198
    Perl's, 201
    phosphotungstic acid haematoxylin,
        196
    PTAH, 196
    resorcin-fuchsin elastic stain, 197
    silver impregnation for reticulin
        fibres, 198
    trichrome, 196
    Van Gieson, 196
    Von Kossa's, 202
    Ziehl-Neelsen for sections, 202
    Ziehl-Neelsen, in bacteriology, 63
Staining sections
    celloidin and LVN, 203
    frozen, 207
    paraffin, 194
Staining techniques
    for cytology, 211–213
    for histology, 194–204, 207–208
    for microbiology, 62–65

Standard deviation, 298
Staphylococci
    in blood culture, 51
    in meningitis, 53
Staphylococcus
    albus, 73
    aureus, 72
        in faeces, 57
        in nasal swabs, 58
        satellitism, 98
    epidermidis, 73
        in nasal swabs, 58
    Oxford, 74
    pyogenes, 72
    saprophyticus, 74
Stem cells, 217, 231
Step sections, 192
Sterilisation, 155 *et seq*
    biological tests of, 164
    by chemical methods, 163
    by dry heat, 155
    by moist heat, 156
    by steam, 156
    by sub-atmospheric steam and
        formaldehyde, 159
Sterilisers, sub-atmospheric steam, 159
Sterilising time, 156
Stills, water, 18
Stock cultures, preservation of, 47
Storage of chemicals, 22–24
Streptococci in blood culture, 51
Streptococci in meningitis, 53
Streptococcus
    faecalis, 72
    pneumoniae, 69, 71
        in meningitis, 53
        in nasal swabs, 58
    pyogenes, 69
    viridans, 69, 71
Streptolysin O, 70
Strongyloides stercoralis, 116
Stuart's transport medium, 123
Styrolite mountant, 211
Substrates for enzymes, 335
Sulphaemoglobin, 224, 253
Sulphates in distilled water, test for, 18
Supravital stain, 235
Supravital staining, 230
Surface decalcification, 180
Susa fixative, 177
Swabs
    bacteriological, 49

Swabs – *contd*
 cervical, culture of, 59
 culture of, for mycobacteria, 87
 throat, culture of, 59
 urethral, culture of, 59
 vaginal, culture of, 59
 vaginal, parasites in, 116
 wound, culture of, 59
Syphilis, 105
 testing blood donors for, 289
Systemic lupus erythematosus, 257

T-lymphocytes, 232
Taenia
 saginata, 115
 solium, 115
Target cells, 233
Telophase, 266
Terpene mountant, 195
Tetrathionate broth, 121
Thalassaemia, 251
Thayer-Martin medium, 126
Thermometers, 13
Thermometry, 352
Thermophiles, 44
Throat swabs, culture of, 59
Thrombocytes, 233
Thrombocytopenia, 233, 287
Thrombocytosis, 233
Thromboplastin, 240
Thymus, 217
Tine test, 89
Tissue
 culture of, for mycobacteria, 87
 preparation of, for microtomy,
  181–186
 sections, frozen, preparation of,
  205–208
 specimens, culture of, 59
Titre, 140
Todd-Hewitt meat infusion broth, 121
Toluene as clearing agent, 182
Toxic granulation, 231
TPHA, 105
TPI, 105
Transfusion
 autologous, 285
 exchange, 281
 intrauterine, 281
 reaction, investigation of, 280
Transmittance, 32

Transport medium, Stuart's, 50
Treponema
 pallidum, 104–105
 species, 104
Trichomonas
 hominis, 116
 vaginalis, 116
  Feinberg's medium for, 123
Trichophyton
 genus, 108, 109
 mentagrophytes, 111
 rubrum, 111
Trichrome stain for sections, 196
Trichuris trichiura, 116
Triple vaccine, 101
Trisodium citrate as anticoagulant, 218
Trypsin in duodenal contents, 336–337
Tryptone soya broth, 122
Tube, photoemissive, 36
Tubercle bacilli, stain for, in sections,
  202
Tuberculin, 89
Turbulent flow, 343

Ugen-Test, 332
Ulcers, peptic, 327
Unna's van Gieson stain, 196
Urates in Von Kossa's method, 202
Urea, 316
 plasma, estimation of, 316
Urease, 316
Urethral swabs, culture of, 59
Uric acid in urine, 303
Urine
 acetoacetic acid in, 308
 acetone in, 308
 acidification test, 318
 amylase, 339
 bilirubin, 323
 blood cells in, 55
 casts in, 55
 culture of, for mycobacteria, 87
 cytology, 209
 examination of in clinical chemistry,
  317
 ketone bodies, detection of, 308
 microbiological investigation of,
  53–56
 osmolality, 319
 potassium, estimation of, 312
 preservation of, 296

protein, detection and measurement
  of, 317–318
 reducing substances in, 303
 sodium, estimation of, 312
 specific gravity of, 319
 specimens for clinical chemistry, 295
 specimens for cytology, 209
 sugars, paper chromatography of,
  304–306
 sugars, thin-layer chromatography
  of, 306–307
 tests, commercial, 331–332
 urobilin, 322
 urobilinogen, 322
Urinometer, 319
Urobilin, 322
Urobilinogen, 322
 commercial tests for, 332
Urobilistix, 332

V factor, 98
 culture medium, 137
Vaccine, triple, 101
Vacuum embedding, 182
Vaginal swabs, culture of, 59
Van Gieson method for sections, 196
Variation, coefficient of, 298
VDRL, 105
Veillonella species, 76
Venepuncture, 219
Venesection, 283
Vi antigen, 139
Vibrio cholerae, 106
 in faeces, 57
 cultivation in alkaline peptone
  water, 124
Vibrio
 El Tor, 106
  in faeces, 57
 para-haemolyticus, 106
  in faeces, 57
Vibrios, 105–107
Virulence, tests of, 69
Voges-Proskaur test, 136
Voltammetry, 352
Von Kossa's method for calcium in
  sections, 202
Von Willebrand's disease, 242

Wassermann reaction, 105

Water
  baths, 30
  CO$_2$ free, 19
  deionised, 18
  distilled, 18
  in culture media, 119
Wavelength
  checking, 37
  choice of, 37
Weigert's iron haematoxylin, 204
Wharton's jelly, 281
Whey agglutination test, 101
White cells, 230
  in urine, 55
White-cell counts
  automatic, 246, 248

differential, automatic, 249
  visual method, 226
Whole-blood clotting time, 243
Widal reaction, 93
Wintrobe haematocrit, 238
Worm
  hook, 116
  round, 115
  thread, 115
  whip, 116
Wound swabs, culture of, 59

X factor, 98
  culture medium, 137
X-ray for decalcification, 180

Xylene
  for clearing tissues, 182
  mounting sections from, 194

Yeast extract, in culture media, 118
Yeasts, 108
Yersinia
  pestis, 102
  pseudotuberculosis, 102
  species, 102
    features of, 99

Zenker's fixative, 177
Zeta potential, 265
Ziehl-Neelsen stain for sections, 202
  in bacteriology, 63